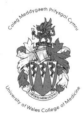

BREAST DISEASE
FOR CLINICIANS

BREAST DISEASE FOR CLINICIANS

EDITORS

Barbara Bourne Bennett, M.D.
Barbara G. Steinbach, M.D.
N. Sisson Hardt, M.D.
Linda S. Haigh, M.D., Ph.D.
University of Florida College of Medicine
Gainesville, Florida

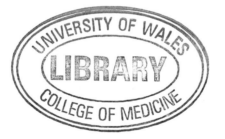

McGRAW-HILL
Medical Publishing Division

New York   Chicago   San Franciso   Lisbon   London   Madrid   Mexico City
Milan   New Delhi   San Juan   Seoul   Singapore   Sydney   Toronto

McGraw-Hill

A Division of The McGraw·Hill Companies

BREAST DISEASE FOR CLINICIANS

1 2 3 4 5 6 7 8 9 0 KGP KGP 0 9 8 7 6 5 4 3 2 1

ISBN 0-8385-0514-7

The book was set in Minion by Rainbow Graphics.
The editors were Andrea Seils, Susan R. Noujaim, and Lester A. Sheinis.
The production supervisor was Richard C. Ruzycka.
The text designer was Joan O'Connor.
The cover designer was Mary McKeon.
Cover art: "La Toilette" by Toulouse Lautrec.
The indexer was Alexandra Nickerson.
Quebecor World/Kingsport was printer and binder.

This book is printed on acid-free paper.

Library of Congress Cataloging-in-Publication Data

Bennett, Barbara B. (Barbara Bourne)
    Breast disease for clinicians/authors, Barbara B. Bennett, Barbara G. Steinbach,
  N. Sisson Hardt, Linda S. Haigh.
      p. ; cm.
    Includes bibliographical references and index.
    ISBN 0-8385-0514-7
    1. Breast—Diseases—Diagnosis. 2. Primary care (Medicine) 3. Breast—Cancer—Treatment.
I. Steinbach, Barbara G. II. Hardt, N. Sisson. III. Haigh, Linda S. IV. Title.
    [DNLM: 1. Breast Diseases—diagnosis. 2. Breast Diseases—therapy. 3. Physical Examination—
methods. 4. Primary Health Care—methods. WP 840 B471b 2001]
RG492.B46 2001
618.1'9—dc21
                                                     00-140210

In memory of Mr. William H. Bourne,
a consummate gentleman who was
a model of altruism, generosity,
dedication, and perseverance for
all who knew him.

CONTENTS

CHAPTER 14

CHAPTER 15

COLOR PLATES appear between pages 50 and 51.

PREFACE

Any clinician involved in the delivery of health care to women is likely, at some point in time, to be confronted with a breast-related question about which he or she knows relatively little. Medical schools devote insufficient time to didactic training about breast diseases. Residency programs, until recently, have perpetuated the problem by considering the breast to be in the domain of the general surgeon. Fortunately, with the current emphasis on primary care, the development of practical skills and understanding of breast complaints are being fostered in primary care specialties (e.g., obstetrics and gynecology, pediatrics, family practice, and internal medicine).

Patients may present with a wide variety of complaints, questions, and concerns. Symptoms of nipple discharge, breast pain, or the presence of a lump prompt many outpatient visits. Some patients simply seek an educated opinion and advice. A common topic for discussion is augmentation or reduction mammaplasty. Still other women present out of fear that they may have or be at high risk for development of breast cancer. A detailed history and thorough physical examination offers an ideal opportunity for discussing risk factors and screening recommendations.

Whether the clinician is a physician assistant, nurse practitioner, medical student, resident, or physician, this book is intended to serve as a succinct, easy-to-read reference. It is not expected to take the place of a timely surgical consultation, when indicated. However, this text supplies basic background information on anatomy and physiology, and discusses diagnostic and management strategies for both benign and malignant breast disease. We have addressed issues related to pregnancy and the puerperium, as well as cosmetic surgery to the breast. Numerous figures and tables provide examples and a quick guide to the subjects outlined in the text. At the end of most chapters, a section entitled "Commonly Asked Questions" is included to help the clinician field some of the more difficult patient inquiries.

Our ultimate goal in writing this book is to improve the communication between women and their health care providers. Women need to be told when their breasts are normal and when suspicion exists. They must understand when and why mammography and other imaging modalities are important and why physical examination alone is insufficient screening as one ages past 40 years. They should be provided with detailed descriptions of planned procedures in order to alleviate their fears. They need help to comprehend results of imaging or histologic testing. Finally, women need to feel that their concerns are being addressed with compassion and understanding by a knowledgeable caregiver. We hope this book provides useful information to help the clinician reach these objectives.

ACKNOWLEDGMENTS

Sincere thanks are extended to Ruth Ann Klockowski for her assistance in the preparation of this manuscript. In addition to performing numerous literature searches, editing, and proofreading, she kept the lines of communication open throughout the entire process. Thanks also to Patricia Abbitt, M.D.; Scott Lind, M.D.; Patrick Duff, M.D.; and Hollis Caffee, M.D.; for supplying some of the mammograms and photographs displayed in this book.

BREAST DISEASE
FOR CLINICIANS

ANATOMY, PHYSIOLOGY, AND EMBRYOLOGY OF THE BREAST

INTRODUCTION

The breasts, or mammary glands, are modified sebaceous glands whose function is to secrete milk for the nourishment of offspring. The possession of breasts classifies humans as mammals. This chapter describes the anatomy and physiology of the breast from embryologic development through menopause. It also discusses the endocrine environment that stimulates the breast to perform its ultimate function of lactation.

ANATOMY OF THE BREAST

In adult women, normal breast size and shape vary considerably. While a woman is standing, the breasts typically occupy a position between the second and seventh ribs, with the nipple at the fourth intercostal space. Although the breasts visibly span from the lateral edge of the sternum to the anterior axillary line, a portion of breast tissue extends into each axilla. This tissue is known as the axillary tail of Spence. The breasts lie on the pectoral fascia and the serratus anterior muscles, between deep and superficial layers of the subcutaneous fascia. Only the axillary tail penetrates this fascia. The breasts are supported by fibrous connective tissue septae, known as Cooper's ligaments, that attach the deep layer of subcutaneous fascia to the dermis. The pigmented skin surrounding the nipple—the areola—contains numerous sebaceous glands that lubricate the nipple during lactation. Beneath this skin lie the smooth muscle bundles that cause nipple erection when the breast is stimulated. The adult breast consists of a radially arranged system of 12 to 20 lobes.

Skin puckering or retraction associated with a developing breast mass may result from involvement of Cooper's ligaments.

1

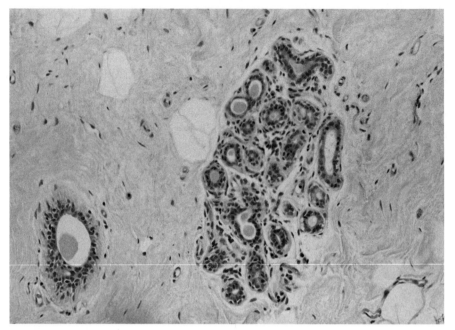

FIGURE 1-1 Normal inactive breast lobule.

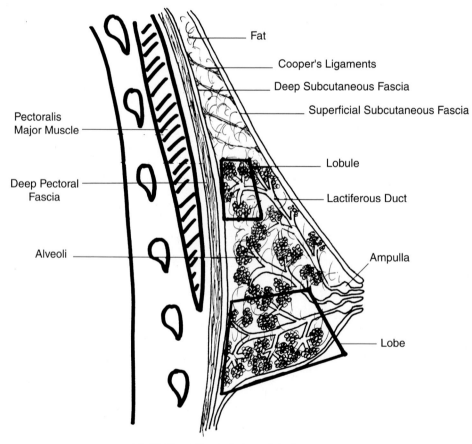

FIGURE 1-2 Sagittal view of the breast.

Each lobe contains numerous lobules that are made up of clusters of alveoli (Fig. 1-1). The low columnar epithelial cells of the alveoli are the milk-producing units, and the lumen of each alveolus empties into an intralobular duct. These ducts join to form a single lactiferous duct that is connected to a minute orifice in the nipple. Just beneath the areola, the lactiferous ducts dilate to form ampullae for milk storage. Stratified squamous epithelium lines the ampullae, whereas the ducts are lined with one to two layers of columnar epithelium. The ducts do not have muscle fibers, but the surrounding matrix of myoepithelial cells and elastic fibers responds to hormonal stimuli, resulting in transport of milk to the nipple. Each lobe is invested in adipose tissue, which is largely responsible for the contour of the breast. Figure 1-2 shows a sagittal view of breast anatomy.

Myoepithelial cells surrounding the alveoli and ducts are responsible for transport of milk to the nipple.

The breast receives its blood supply from three major sources: the internal thoracic artery and the lateral thoracic and thoracoacromial branches of the axillary artery. Venous return begins in an anastomotic circle around the nipple, the circulus venosus, and continues via branches throughout the breast tissue that lead to the axillary and internal thoracic veins.

Lymphatic channels originate alongside the ducts in the interlobular spaces. The subareolar plexus receives lymphatics from the central breast parenchyma, the areola, and the nipple. From there, most of the lymphatic drainage of the breast is to the pectoral group, the subscapular group, and the apical group of axillary lymph nodes. Lymphatics from the medial portion of the breast may pass to the parasternal nodes, which then follow the path of the internal thoracic vessels. Other routes include intercostal, diaphragmatic and abdominal lymphatics and channels from the contralateral breast. Figure 1-3 shows the arterial and venous supply of the breast and its lymphatic drainage.

EMBRYOLOGY

Breast development begins during the sixth week of intrauterine life, when a downgrowth of epidermis along each mammary ridge forms the two primary mammary buds. These primordial structures give rise to secondary buds, which develop into the main lactiferous ducts. By the time of birth, a breast consists of a shallow skin surface depression, the mammary pit, which communicates with the lumina of rudimentary ducts. After birth, the nipple everts and the newborn breasts, responding to maternal hormonal stimuli, may hypertrophy and secrete "witch's milk." This cloudy fluid disappears within 2 to 4 weeks. The breasts remain in a rudimentary state throughout life in males. In females, hormonal stimuli during puberty result in further differentiation of the glandular and ductal system. Fat is deposited, and the connective tissue matrix is constructed.

CONGENITAL ABNORMALITIES

In fetal life, the mammary ridge initially extends from the axilla to the inguinal area. Failure of regression of the caudal portion of this ridge may lead to the formation of breast buds along this "milk line." Supernumerary nipples (polythelia) often are misdiagnosed as moles. Supernumerary breasts (polymastia) occur most commonly in the axilla and may not be recognized until enlargement oc-

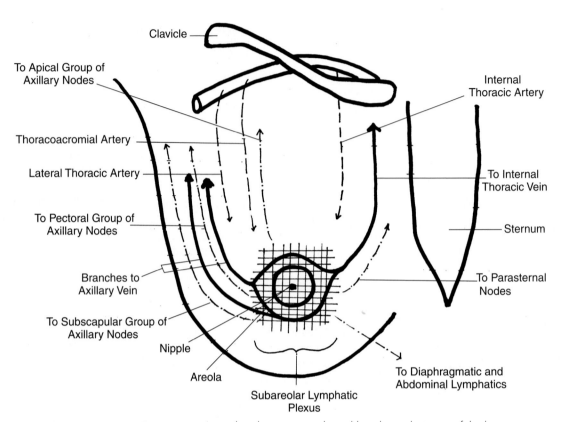

FIGURE 1-3 Arterial and venous supply and lymphatic drainage of the breast.

curs with pregnancy and lactation. Accessory nipples or breasts may be rudimentary or functional, and the optional treatment of these conditions consists of excision.

Although there is nearly always some degree of breast asymmetry, true underdevelopment of one breast, or anisomastia, is uncommon. This condition may be due to variation in the rapidity of breast growth or earlier breast bud development on one side. In extreme cases, the cosmetic defect may be treated surgically by augmentation or reduction.

Mammary hyperplasia, or macromastia, is seen most commonly in adolescent girls and women between 35 and 50 years of age. In the younger group, excessive glandular hypertrophy is responsible, whereas fat deposition usually causes the increase in size in the older group. Surgical reduction is indicated to improve a woman's self-image and treat or prevent back pain.

Failure of the mammary pit to elevate postnatally results in nipple inversion. This condition may resolve spontaneously during pregnancy, and its only clinical significance is potential difficulty with breast-feeding. Acquired nipple inversion later in life may signal an underlying cancer.

Congenital absence of one or both breasts or nipples is exceedingly rare and results from disappearance or developmental failure of the mammary ridges.

PHYSIOLOGY OF THE BREAST

PUBERTY

The primary stimulus for breast growth and development at puberty, or thelarche, is ovarian hormone secretion. In response to estrogen stimulation, the ductal epithelium proliferates, leading to ductal branching. This change is followed by the development of the terminal lobuloalveolar system, which requires both estrogen and progesterone for normal progression. The stroma and myoepithelial cells of the breast also respond to these hormones, but the presence of prolactin, insulin, cortisol, thyroxine, and growth hormone is necessary for full differentiation of the breast. Hereditary factors and variation in environmental conditions (e.g., alteration of the hormonal milieu as a result of regular strenuous exercise during adolescence) also affect the timing of thelarche and final breast size and shape.

Estrogen, progesterone, prolactin, insulin, cortisol, thyroxine, and growth hormone are necessary for full differentiation of the breast.

Thelarche begins at 10 to 11 years of age and is usually the first physical sign of puberty. The progression of breast development to the adult form has been divided into five stages, which are called Tanner stages after the British physician who first described them (Fig. 1-4). The infantile state is Tanner stage 1. Stage 2 corresponds to el-

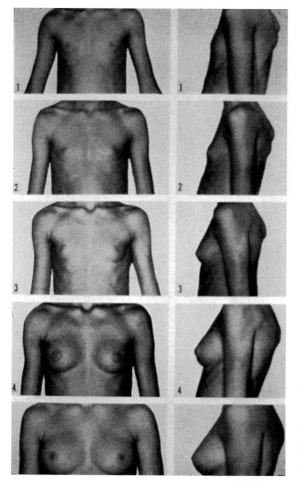

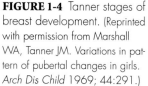

FIGURE 1-4 Tanner stages of breast development. (Reprinted with permission from Marshall WA, Tanner JM. Variations in pattern of pubertal changes in girls. *Arch Dis Child* 1969; 44:291.)

evation of the breast and nipple to form a small mound, or "breast bud," and an increase in the diameter of the areola. During stage 3, the breast and areola continue to enlarge and a continuous contour is maintained. Stage 4 is marked by a change in contour that causes the areola and nipple to form a secondary mound. This secondary mound becomes confluent with the breast again, forming the adult contour in stage 5. Progression through these stages to the adult form usually spans 3 to 4 years.

Premature thelarche is characterized by unilateral or bilateral breast development before age 8 in the absence of other signs of puberty. It may occur at birth or later in childhood, often varies over time, and is usually self-limited.

MENSTRUAL CYCLE CHANGES

The breast returns to its smallest size by day 8 of the menstrual cycle, making this time ideal for breast self-examination, clinical examination, and mammography.

An adult breast responds to the cyclic changes in hormone levels that occur during the menstrual cycle. During the follicular phase, the ducts in the breast parenchyma proliferate. Subsequent dilation of the lumina of the ducts, increased alveolar and ductal secretory activity, interlobular edema, and vascular engorgement result in a premenstrual increase in breast volume of up to 30 mL. With the onset of menses, the secretory activity and lobular size decrease, engorgement wanes, and the breast returns to its smallest size by day 8 of the cycle.

PREGNANCY AND LACTATION

Although the breast matures greatly during puberty, it remains inactive until pregnancy, when complete differentiation of the terminal alveolar cells into milk-producing units occurs. Breast enlargement is one of the first physical symptoms of pregnancy and results from glandular proliferation and vascular engorgement. Clusters of lobuloalveolar units replace adipose tissue, and the stromal tissue becomes less prominent (Fig. 1-5). As the alveoli enlarge during late gestation, the central cells undergo fatty degeneration and are sloughed. These cells, as well as leukocytes, make up the first milk, or colostrum. After delivery, final maturation of the secretory apparatus occurs (Fig. 1-6), and the alveoli become distended with true milk. True milk follows the secretion of colostrum by 3 to 4 days postpartum and is composed of products of alveolar cell exocytosis, apocrine secretion, diffusion, and paracellular transport.

The nipple and areola become more prominent and more darkly pigmented during pregnancy, and the areolar glands (glands of Montgomery) begin to secrete a lubricating substance to protect the nipple during suckling.

HORMONAL CONTROL OF LACTATION

Prolactin promotes breast growth and lactation, but its action on the milk-producing alveolar cells is blocked during gestation by the high estrogen and progesterone levels.

Numerous hormones act in a complex, integrated fashion to promote lactogenesis. Prolactin is the key hormone, but growth hormone, thyroxine, insulin, cortisol, and the sex steroids also play a role in coordinating the control of lactation. The role of human placental lactogen is uncertain.

The serum prolactin concentration begins to rise by the eighth week of gestation and continues to rise until term. This change accompanies an increase in serum estrogen levels, as estrogen stimulates prolactin production and release from the pituitary. Prolactin promotes breast growth and lactation, but its action on the milk-

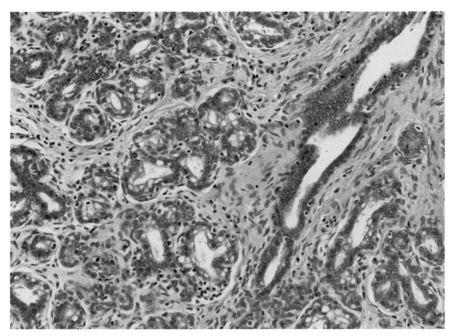

FIGURE 1-5 Secretory changes in pregnancy (early).

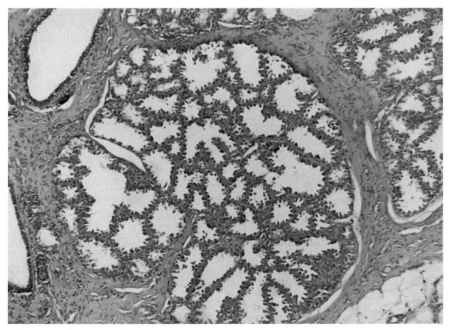

FIGURE 1-6 Secretory changes in pregnancy (late).

producing alveolar cells is blocked during gestation by the high estrogen and progesterone levels. Progesterone antagonizes the action of prolactin at the level of the alveolar cell receptor, preventing casein production and milk secretion during pregnancy. The rapid decline in serum estrogen and progesterone concentrations postpartum releases this inhibition, and milk production ensues. Clearance of the sex steroids may require 3 to 4 days, corresponding with the observed onset of milk flow.

Even in women who breast-feed, prolactin levels fall postpartum. However, they remain higher than basal levels for many weeks. The suckling stimulus causes episodic increases in prolactin that promote further milk production. However, the overall trend is for prolactin levels to decline toward normal and for the pulses of prolactin to be smaller over time. Generally, as a woman breast-feeds less, the prolactin peak is smaller and less milk is produced. Slow cessation of breast-feeding, or weaning, allows regression of the milk-producing apparatus, and prolactin levels normalize.

The transport of milk from the alveolus to the nipple requires contraction of the myoepithelial cells that surround the alveoli. This contraction may occur as a result of direct mechanical stimulation or because of the effects of oxytocin. The myoepithelial cell oxytocin receptors peak in number during the week after delivery. Oxytocin, originating from the supraoptic and paraventricular nuclei of the hypothalamus, is released from the neurohypophysis in response to nipple and areolar stimulation by suckling or by auditory or visual stimuli. Oxytocin then binds to the myoepithelial cell receptors, and the resultant contraction causes the ejection of milk into the ducts and subareolar ampullae. This process is called letdown. The infant's tongue then expresses the milk through the nipple during suckling.

In women who do not breast-feed after delivery, the tactile stimulus for prolactin secretion is absent and prolactin levels return to normal within weeks. In the absence of suckling, engorgement with milk flattens the low columnar alveolar cells, and their secretory activity ceases. Decreased capillary flow, along with autophagic activity, results in regression of the alveoli. The visible and often painful breast engorgement subsides spontaneously after several days. Support of the breasts with a tight-fitting bra, the application of ice, and the administration of analgesics offer symptomatic relief. After 2 to 3 months, the breast is remodeled by regression of glandular tissue and deposition of fat. The administration of bromocriptine, a dopamine agonist, is no longer recommended for the suppression of postpartum lactation because of an increased risk of severe hypertension, seizures, and stroke in puerperal patients. Its use should be reserved for the treatment of the most severe cases of engorgement.

MENOPAUSAL CHANGES

After menopause, the glandular tissue of the breast progressively involutes, leaving only scattered lobules, collecting ducts, and dense connective tissue interspersed with fat. The result is a smaller, fatty, less dense breast without secretory activity.

SUGGESTED READING

Beller F. Development and anatomy of the breast. In: Mitchell GW, Bassett LW, eds. *The Female Breast and Its Disorders.* Baltimore: Williams & Wilkins; 1990:1–12.

Birkenfeld A, Kase NG. Functional anatomy and physiology of the female breast. *Obstet Gynecol Clin North Am* 1994; 21(3):433–444.

Gray H. The urogenital system: Mammary gland. In: Clemente CD, ed. *Anatomy of the Human Body,* 30th ed. Philadelphia: Lea and Febiger; 1985:1581–1586.

Kaplan CR, Schenken RS. Endocrinology of the breast. In: Mitchell GW, Bassett LW, eds. *The Female Breast and Its Disorders.* Baltimore: Williams & Wilkins; 1990:22–44.

2

CLINICAL EVALUATION OF THE BREAST

HISTORY

The initial evaluation of any patient begins with the recording of a thorough history. A patient who presents with breast complaints requires a detailed interview, especially with regard to factors that may influence the risk of breast disease. The historical review for all women seen for health maintenance should include age, complaints, results of previous mammograms, performance of breast self-examination, history of prior breast lumps or surgery (including breast augmentation or reduction), medications, personal or family history of breast cancer (including age at diagnosis), and personal or family history of other gynecologic or gastrointestinal malignancies. Age at menarche, age at first full-term pregnancy, and age at menopause, as well as the history of breast-feeding, are also pertinent.

The most common breast complaints include the presence of a palpable mass, breast pain, and nipple discharge.

The most common breast complaints include the presence of a palpable mass, breast pain, and nipple discharge, and further questioning should focus specifically on the patient's problem. If the presence of a lump is the complaint, note should be made of whether the patient discovered it during routine self-examination or was guided to it by pain. Most breast cancers are painless, whereas fibrocystic changes commonly cause cyclic discomfort. Other important data are the duration of the presence of the lump, the patient's menopausal status, changes in lump size over time or during the menstrual cycle, the presence of skin changes, and a history of chest trauma. A long-standing lump that has not changed over time most likely represents a benign process, whereas continued growth may signal malignancy. Fibrocystic changes tend to be accentuated in the week before menses. Skin dimpling or retraction associated with a mass is suspicious for cancer. Chest trauma can cause fat necrosis with palpable fibrosis and associated skin changes. The evaluation of a breast lump is discussed in further detail in Chap. 4.

TABLE 2-1 COMPONENTS OF A BREAST-DIRECTED HISTORY

GENERAL HISTORY	Age; complaints; prior mammograms; self-examination; prior lumps, excisions, or biopsies; medications
BREAST CANCER RISK FACTORS	History of breast cancer or atypical hyperplasia, breast cancer in first-degree relative, early menarche, late first full-term pregnancy, late menopause, personal or family history of gastrointestinal cancer
SPECIFIC FOR COMPLAINT OF MASS	Duration, location, change over time, cyclicity, chest trauma
SPECIFIC FOR COMPLAINT OF PAIN	Duration, location, quality, severity, cyclicity, radiation, factors affecting pain
SPECIFIC FOR COMPLAINT OF DISCHARGE	Duration, unilateral or bilateral, spontaneous versus provoked, color of discharge, volume, visual changes, headaches

If pain is the patient's presenting complaint, information should be elicited about the duration, location, quality, and severity of the pain as well as alleviating and aggravating factors and any associated problems. Breast pain caused by fibrocystic changes commonly is exacerbated in the premenstrual period whether the pain is localized or diffuse. The evaluation and treatment of breast pain, or mastalgia, are addressed in Chap. 5.

The clinician should determine the duration of time during which any nipple discharge has been present and whether it is spontaneous or provoked, unilateral or bilateral. The color and volume of the discharge, the time since the most recent breast-feeding (if applicable), a history of chest wall trauma or irritation, and the medication history also are of particular relevance. A search for underlying cancer must be undertaken in a patient with unilateral, spontaneous nonmilky discharge. A pituitary adenoma must be excluded in a patient with nonpuerperal milky discharge, especially if visual disturbances or headaches are reported. The evaluation and treatment of nipple discharge are discussed in detail in Chap. 6. The individual components of a breast-directed history are outlined in Table 2-1.

PHYSICAL EXAMINATION

Physical examination of the breasts requires careful inspection and palpation. During the examination, questions that might have been neglected during the initial interview should be asked. The patient should be queried about whether she performs self-examination and should point out the location of any pain or lumps. It may be useful to have her demonstrate her technique for breast self-examination, especially if abnormal nipple discharge is a complaint. The time of the examination should be used for instruction as well as information gathering. Although it is surprisingly controversial, most clinicians believe that breast self-examination is a worthwhile endeavor. Advocates of breast self-examination cite the intuitive benefit of earlier detection of breast cancer as the most attractive feature and the low cost of training,

Physical examination includes inspection and palpation of the breasts and node-bearing areas.

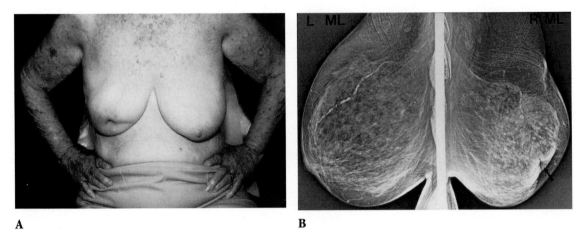

A

B

FIGURE 2-1 *A.* This patient has overt nipple inversion and skin retraction associated with extensive underlying invasive cancer. *B.* A mediolateral oblique film-screen mammogram demonstrating right nipple retraction associated with invasive lobular carcinoma.

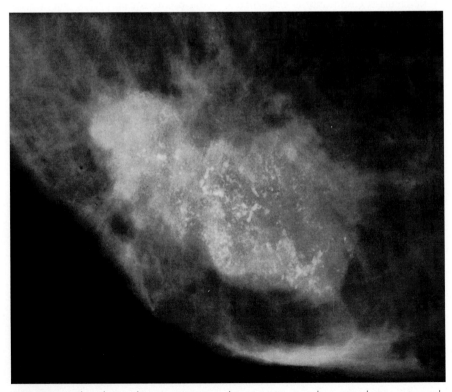

FIGURE 2-2 This obvious breast carcinoma demonstrates stranding, spiculation, microcalcifications, and associated skin retraction.

ease of performance, and noninvasiveness as further benefits. Studies have shown that after proper instruction and periodic reinforcement, patients are capable of performing reasonably accurate self-examination. However, many women never receive instruction or neglect to perform the examination on a regular basis. Opponents of breast self-examination note the frequency with which costly and invasive studies are prompted only to uncover benign disease, especially in younger women. Also, there are conflicting data in the literature about whether survival outcome is improved by its performance. Despite the lack of consensus, it generally is held that there is no compelling reason to change the standard practice of breast self-examination instruction and encouragement. A truly prospective, randomized study comparing breast self-examination to no breast self-examination probably would be impossible to carry out. Therefore, the clinician should explain each step of the breast examination while it is being performed so that the patient understands the technique to perform at home. The follicular phase of the menstrual cycle is the optimal time for this monthly evaluation.

Inspection of the breasts with the patient erect is the first step in self-examination or clinical breast examination. Size, symmetry, and skin changes are noted. Inverted or deviated nipples (Fig. 2-1), erythema, venous prominence, irregularity in contour, skin retraction (Fig. 2-2) or edema, ulceration, and other dermatologic problems may signal underlying pathology. Particular attention should be paid to the skin of the areola and nipple, where flaky or erythematous skin may be a sign of Paget's disease (Fig. 2-3). The Tanner stage (see Chap. 1) should be noted in an adolescent patient.

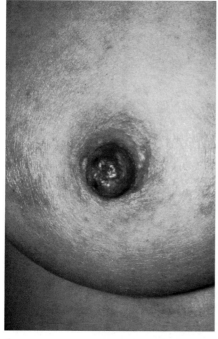

A

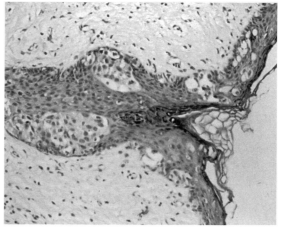

B

FIGURE 2-3 A. The red, eczematous skin on this woman's nipple represents Paget's disease. The intense pruritis often associated with this disease leads to excoriation and crusting in many cases. **B.** Note the surface crust of desquamated epithelium. The squamous epithelium is infiltrated by individual cells and small nests of adenocarcinoma. These cells are differentiated from the benign squamous cells by their abundant cytoplasm, creating a halo appearance.

To detect skin retraction, the patient's arms initially should dangle at her sides. Then the patient should be instructed to press the hands firmly onto the hips, contracting the pectoralis muscles. Finally, the arms should be elevated over the head. The presence of a mass may prevent the overlying skin from moving freely, resulting in an indentation in the skin or areola or nipple inversion. If retraction is suspected, especially in a patient with large breasts, having the patient lean far forward may accentuate the retraction. Also, compressing the entire breast gently toward the chest wall with the examiner's cupped hand may demonstrate skin retraction.

Palpation of the supraclavicular and axillary areas for adenopathy follows. Examination of the axilla is best performed with the patient's arm abducted 30 degrees at rest. This position allows the pectoralis muscle to relax and facilitates palpation deep into the axilla. Nodes less than 1 cm in diameter are normal, while larger nodes may represent infection or another pathology in the hand, arm, breast, or thorax. If adenopathy is present, an explanation must be sought. Most clinicians do not teach patients to palpate for lymph nodes during self-examination because these nodes often are difficult to feel.

Next, palpation of the breasts in the upright and supine positions should be performed. Patients should be instructed to palpate in the shower, using soap as a lubricant, and in the supine position, using skin lotion. With lubrication, the examining fingers are able to slide on the breast skin, moving from one area to the next without omitting any breast tissue. Some experts advocate the "triple touch" technique, in which the examination is repeated three times to compensate for variation in the degree of pressure exerted by the examining fingers.

Depending on the size of the patient's breasts and the level of suspicion of a mass, clinical palpation of the breast with the patient in both the sitting position and the supine position may be indicated. In the supine position, the ipsilateral hand should be placed behind the patient's head to allow access to the entire breast. The placement of a pillow behind the ipsilateral shoulder also helps distribute the breast tissue more evenly over the chest wall. This maneuver is especially useful in a patient with pendulous breasts. With the pads of the middle three fingers, the examiner should compress the breast tissue against the chest wall in small, circular movements, using variable degrees of pressure. The entire breast, including the axillary tail, must be examined. The stripwise pattern is used by many clinicians, but as long as no areas are omitted, any uniform pattern of palpation is acceptable. Characteristics of a mass that are suspicious for malignancy include irregular or poorly defined borders, fixation to the skin or chest wall, and the coexistence of adenopathy, nipple discharge, or skin retraction.

Characteristics of a mass that are suspicious for malignancy include irregular or poorly defined borders, fixation to the skin or chest wall, and the coexistence of adenopathy, nipple discharge, or skin retraction.

Palpation is completed by examination of the areola and nipple. The patient should be discouraged from aggressive nipple manipulation during self-examination because this may elicit a normal physiologic discharge. Most types of clinically significant discharge, whether bloody or serous, can be provoked by pressing on the areola with one finger without pinching or elevating it. However, if a patient reports a discharge that is not readily apparent, a more aggressive examination may be necessary. The breast ducts are stripped by gently stroking the skin from the periphery toward the nipple, using the lateral surface of the thumb. Compression and elevation of the areola between two fingers should express any discharge. The color of the discharge and the number of ducts involved should be noted, and the discharge should be collected for analysis if that is clinically indicated. The individual components of a breast-directed physical examination are outlined in Table 2-2.

TABLE 2-2 COMPONENTS OF A BREAST-DIRECTED PHYSICAL EXAMINATION

INSPECTION	Arms at sides, pressed on hips, and over head Size, shape, symmetry Skin changes (ulceration, erythema, retraction) Nipple inversion, deviation, flaky skin Tanner stage
PALPATION	Seated and supine positions Supraclavicular and axillary nodes Clavicle to bra line, midline to axilla Uniform pattern (stripwise versus circular) Press on areola to elicit discharge
MASS	Location Size, shape, consistency Mobility Tenderness Border definition
NIPPLE DISCHARGE	Unilateral versus bilateral Number of ducts involved Color of discharge Consistency of discharge Test for blood (guaiac) Microscopy for fat globules

DOCUMENTATION

After completion of the physical examination, the physician must document the findings in writing. If no abnormality was detected, the chart should reflect the fact that there was normal symmetry, no adenopathy, no visible skin changes, no dominant masses palpable, and no nipple discharge present. If a lump was detected, a simple drawing may add clarity to the note. The description of the mass should include the location (using quadrant or clock face), size, shape, consistency, mobility, tenderness, and regularity of borders (see Chap. 4). If a nipple discharge was present, the physician must document whether it was unilateral or bilateral, from a single duct or multiple ducts, the color and consistency of the discharge, and whether blood was present as detected by a standard card test or dipstick (see Chap. 6). Serous or sanguineous discharge from a single duct is suspicious for cancer. A useful form for documentation of clinical findings is shown in Table 2-3.

FINE NEEDLE ASPIRATION

If a dominant mass is palpated on physical examination, the next step in the evaluation depends on the examiner's preference and level of expertise. In the setting of a busy office practice, the clinician may decide to refer all patients in whom a breast mass is palpable to a general surgeon for further evaluation. However, some referrals can be avoided if one is skilled in the performance of fine needle aspiration (FNA) (Table 2-4).

TABLE 2-3 CLINICAL BREAST EVALUATION FORM

CC: ○ Lump ○ D/C ○ Pain ○ Abnormal mgm

History: Age: _____ yrs Parity: ___-___-___-___ LMP: ___ /___ /___

Previous mgm? Y/N   Normal? Y/N   Describe: _____
Performs BSE? Y/N   Normal? Y/N   Describe: _____
Prior breast bx? Y/N   Results: _____
Mammoplasty? Y/N   ○ Augmentation   ○ Reduction
Hx Breast Ca? Y/N   ○ Patient   ○ Mother   ○ Sister   ○ Aunt
     Age at Dx?:   _____   _____   _____   _____
GI or Gyn Ca? Y/N   ○ Patient   ○ Parent   ○ Sibling
Menarche: _____ yrs   Menopause: _____ yrs   First term birth: _____ yrs
OCP use?:   Y/N   HRT use? Y/N   Did patient breast-feed? Y/N

Breast Lump History:

Duration: _____ months   Location: ○ Left   ○ Right   ○ Bilateral
Size: _____   Change over time? _____
Discovered by: ○ Patient   ○ Clinician   ○ Mgm   ○ Other

Breast Pain History:

Duration: _____ months   Cyclic?   Y/N   If yes, _____days/month
Severity: 0 1 2 3 4 5 6 8 9 10   Location: ○ Left   ○ Right   ○ Bilateral
Quality: _____
Medications: _____

Nipple D/C History:

Duration: _____ months   Location: ○ Left   ○ Right   ○ Bilateral
Color: _____   Spontaneous: Y/N
Recent breast-feeding?   Y/N
Chest wall trauma?   Y/N
Breast implants?   Y/N
Visual disturbance?   Y/N
Headaches?   Y/N
Medications: _____

(continues)

A dominant breast mass in an older woman or a mass suspicious for malignancy should first be evaluated by mammography because hematoma formation with FNA may temporarily impair mammographic interpretation.

FNA is an office procedure in which a needle is introduced into a mass to allow aspiration of fluid or cellular material. It is indicated as an initial step in the evaluation of a dominant breast mass, particularly in a young patient without obvious signs of malignancy. In this situation, FNA may determine that a mass is a simple cyst, precluding any radiologic study. A dominant breast mass in an older woman or a mass suspicious for malignancy should first be evaluated by mammography because hematoma formation, an uncommon complication of FNA, may temporarily impair mammographic interpretation. Mammography in this setting is used both to evaluate the breasts for concurrent nonpalpable pathology and to characterize the mass itself.

FNA may be performed without the use of local anesthesia. The clinician cleanses the skin with betadine or alcohol and dons sterile gloves. The mass is localized between two fingers of the nondominant hand and stabilized with firm pressure. A 22-gauge needle attached to a syringe is introduced slowly so that penetration of the mass can be appreciated. A pistol-grip syringe holder or thumb-hole

(CONTINUED)

Physical Examination:

Inspection:	Normal symmetry?	Y/N	Describe: _____			
	Skin changes?	Y/N	Describe: _____			
	Inverted nipples?	Y/N		○ Left	○ Right	○ Bilateral

Palpation:	Adenopathy?	Y/N	Describe: _____			
	Mass present?	Y/N		○ Left	○ Right	○ Bilateral
	Describe:	(size, shape, consistency, mobility, tenderness, borders),				

_____

_____

Nipple D/C?	Y/N	○ Left	○ Right	○ Bilateral
Describe:	(no. ducts, color, consistency, guaiac)			

_____

Assessment:

Plan:

type of plunger may afford better control. Then, with 2 to 3 mL of negative pressure from the syringe, the mass is aspirated. If fluid is encountered, total evacuation of the cyst should be attempted. If no fluid is present, several passes into the mass should be made. Negative pressure should be released before removal of the needle from the breast.

To retrieve the cells filling the needle lumen and hub, a few milliliters of air must be present in the syringe. The air may be drawn into the syringe either before the beginning of the procedure or after the needle is withdrawn from the skin. If the latter time is chosen, the syringe must be disconnected from the needle first, or the cellular material will be lost into the syringe. The needle is then reattached, and the cells present in the needle lumen and hub are blown onto a glass slide. Using a second (and possibly a third) slide, the cellular material is spread out, and the slides then are fixed. The fixed slides are submitted for cytologic evaluation. The cytopathologist interpreting the slides may prefer a particular technique of slide

TABLE 2-4 PROCEDURE FOR FINE NEEDLE ASPIRATION OF A BREAST MASS

❑ Review patient's history and obtain informed consent
❑ Prepare slides (label with name, place on towel), fill out cytology requisition form, open fixation bottle (preferably 95% alcohol, but Papanicolaou fixative is acceptable)
❑ If possible, arrange to have cytotechnician present
❑ Cleanse skin with betadine or alcohol and let dry while donning sterile gloves
❑ Attach 22-gauge needle to pistol-grip or control syringe and draw back a few mL of air
❑ Locate and stabilize mass between two fingers of nondominant hand
❑ Introduce needle into mass and aspirate
❑ If cyst fluid is encountered, try to drain cyst completely and test fluid for blood (hemoccult)
   ❑ If positive, send to cytology in sterile container
   ❑ If negative, discard fluid
❑ If no fluid is obtained, maintain negative pressure with syringe and pass needle through mass several times until material is seen in needle hub
❑ Release negative pressure and withdraw needle from skin
❑ Touch needle, bevel side down, to slide and eject material onto slide
❑ Cover first slide with a second slide and then separate the slides as if opening a book

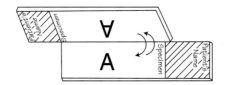

❑ Immediately drop slide into 95% alcohol or spray with Papanicolaou fixative
❑ Repeat aspiration several times if possible, then apply pressure to the breast

SUPPLIES	Alcohol, 22- to 23-gauge needle, control syringe, glass slides, fixative, gloves, bandage
PREPARATION	Cleanse skin, don gloves, localize mass with nondominant hand
PROCEDURE	Introduce needle; aspirate fluid or pass needle several times; release negative pressure; remove needle; apply pressure to breast
SPECIMEN PROCESSING: **(+) Fluid:**	Test for blood: (–) → discard, (+) → cytology
(–) Fluid:	Blow contents of needle and hub onto slide; fix with 95% ethanol or Pap fixative (ask lab)

preparation and fixation, and so communication before the procedure is essential. After the needle is withdrawn, firm pressure is applied to the breast for at least 3 minutes to minimize bleeding. A dressing then is applied to the site.

An experienced clinician may be able to predict the cytologic results on the basis of the texture of the mass as transmitted via the needle during the FNA procedure. For example, a gritty texture may denote the presence of calcifications, as is seen commonly in association with cancer. Fibroadenomas have a rubbery, firm texture that is difficult to penetrate with the needle; the needle pushes the mass away before it enters the capsule. Lymphomas and mucinous tumors have a soft, easily penetrable texture.

The immediate FNA findings can be helpful in the formulation of management plans. For example, withdrawal of fluid from a cystic mass may allow the cyst to collapse and become nonpalpable. If this is the case and the fluid that is obtained is not bloody, no further intervention is required and the patient may simply be followed for recurrence. If the mass does not disappear, the fluid is bloody, or the cyst recurs, FNA of the remaining mass and/or referral for excision to rule out cancer are in order.

An FNA sample obtained from a solid mass can be analyzed for cytologic evidence of malignancy. If it is positive, this advance notice of the presence of cancer gives the surgeon an opportunity to counsel the patient and plan a treatment strategy preoperatively.

A negative FNA result may be helpful if the physical examination and mammographic findings also suggest that a mass is benign (see Chap. 4). However, even when properly performed, FNA carries a 20 percent false-negative rate. In other words, cancer may be present despite a negative FNA in 20 percent of patients. Some forms of breast cancer, such as lobular carcinoma, are especially difficult to detect with FNA. An FNA sample must contain ductal epithelium to be considered adequate for interpretation. An inadequate or marginally adequate specimen should not be considered negative.

Even when properly performed, FNA carries a 20 percent false-negative rate.

Complications of FNA are rare and include infection, hematoma formation, and pneumothorax. Mammography should be delayed for 2 weeks after FNA to ensure that clarity is not obscured. Pneumothorax can be avoided totally by inserting the needle parallel to the chest wall. Contraindications to FNA include the presence of cellulitis, an ill-defined mass, and known metastatic disease. Breast ultrasound, core biopsy, and needle-localization biopsy are discussed in Chaps. 4 and 12.

SUGGESTED READING

Austoker J. Screening and self examination for breast cancer. *Br Med J* 1994; 309:168–174.

Bates B. The breasts and axillae. In: *A Guide to Physical Examination,* 3d ed. Philadelphia: Lippincott; 1983:210–227.

Hindle WH. Contemporary management of breast disease: I. Benign disease—the diagnostic evaluation. *Obstet Gynecol Clin North Am* 1994; 21(3):499–517.

Kaufman Z, Shpitz B, Shapiro M, et al. Triple approach in the diagnosis of dominant breast masses: Combined physical examination, mammography, and fine-needle aspiration. *J Surg Oncol* 1994; 56:254–257.

O'Malley MS, Fletcher SW. Screening for breast cancer with breast self-examination. *JAMA* 1987; 257(16):2197–2203.

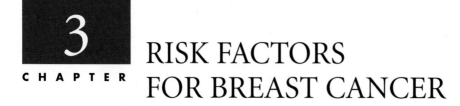

RISK FACTORS FOR BREAST CANCER

Breast cancer is the most common cancer and the second most common cause of cancer death in American women. When breast cancer is detected in the earliest stages through the use of physical examination and mammography, a woman's overall chance of survival is improved. With a lifetime risk of approximately one in nine, breast cancer is a serious concern: One of every two women will consult her physician for a breast complaint, and one in four will undergo breast biopsy. An understanding of the risk factors for breast cancer helps the physician determine the appropriate level of suspicion warranted for an individual patient and guides clinical decision making.

Breast cancer is most often a disease of peri- and postmenopausal women; however, it occurs with surprising frequency in young women as well. The female-to-male ratio is approximately 100:1 in developed countries. Several risk factors have been recognized that when identified individually or together increase a woman's likelihood of developing breast cancer (Table 3-1). These risks include increasing age; genetic and family traits; hormonal and reproductive influences; diet, lifestyle, and environmental factors; and certain pathologic breast findings and premalignant lesions. Unfortunately, many women who develop breast cancer have no known risk factors; therefore, the absence of risk factors should not prevent evaluation or biopsy of a suspicious breast lesion.

Unfortunately, many women who develop breast cancer have no known risk factors; therefore, the absence of risk factors should not prevent evaluation or biopsy of a suspicious breast lesion.

AGE

Carcinoma of the breast is usually a disease of older women. The frequently quoted incidence of one in nine women represents an average lifetime risk that is skewed

TABLE 3-1 RISK FACTORS FOR BREAST CANCER

STRONG	MODERATE	SLIGHT
Female gender	Early menarche	Exogenous hormones
Older age	Late menopause	High-fat diet
Hereditary breast and ovarian cancer	Nulliparity	Obesity
BRCA1 and/or BRCA2 gene mutation	Radiation exposure	
Breast cancer in family	Hyperplasia on breast biopsy	
Previous breast or ovarian cancer		

toward the older population. In postmenopausal women, any new breast mass should be evaluated thoroughly.

The risk in women less than 20 years old is virtually zero, and the risk in women less than 30 years old is very small. However, missed cancer in young women represents a major source of malpractice litigation for gynecologists. Even though most breast masses in young women are benign, any change in character or increase in the size of a mass should prompt a biopsy because breast cancers in young patients tend to demonstrate very aggressive behavior. Women 30 to 35 years of age with a family history of breast disease should consider annual mammography screening and clinical breast examinations. The American Cancer Society recommends initial mammography for all women 40 to 45 years of age and annual screening thereafter.

GENETIC AND FAMILY FACTORS

Familial breast cancer occurs in women who have first- and second-degree relatives with the disease but in whom no pedigree pattern of transmission can be identified. Hereditary breast cancer, by contrast, displays an autosomal dominant genetic expression in families. Among all breast cancers reported, about 67 percent are sporadic, 23 percent are familial, and 10 percent are hereditary.

Hereditary breast cancer has been associated with two intensively studied genes: *BRCA1* and *BRCA2*. The *BRCA1* gene is located on chromosome 17 of the human genome and was cloned 5 years after epidemiologic evidence and linkage analysis implicated its association with early-onset breast and ovarian cancers. *BRCA1* codes for a protein that has a tumor suppressor function. Loss of this function confers an increased susceptibility to both breast and ovarian cancer. Mutations in *BRCA1* are responsible for 50 percent of inherited breast cancers and more than 80 percent of inherited breast and ovarian cancers.

The *BRCA2* gene is on chromosome 13. It also codes for a protein with a tumor suppressor function such that a mutation results in increased susceptibility to breast cancer. *BRCA2* is associated with breast cancer in males. Linkage analysis of 15 high-risk breast cancer families showed that *BRCA2* was not linked to the *BRCA1* locus.

Familial breast cancer occurs in women who have first- and second-degree relatives with the disease but in whom no pedigree pattern of transmission can be identified. Hereditary breast cancer displays an autosomal dominant genetic expression in families.

In addition to these two genetic foci, other DNA mutations may confer susceptibility to many types of cancer, including breast cancer. Examples of these mutations include the tumor-suppressor *P53* gene and the *AT* (ataxia-telangiectasia) gene.

Commercial testing for the *BRCA1* and *BRCA2* genes using DNA sequence analysis requires only a 4-mL sample of blood. Both mutations are relatively rare but are associated with a high risk of breast cancer in young women: an 80 percent probability of breast cancer by age 70 and a 50 percent risk of bilateral disease. The current challenge is to identify women who would benefit from genetic testing and counsel them effectively. Only patients at high risk should be tested: those with a blood relative known to have a *BRCA1* or *BRCA2* mutation, those with a strong family history of breast or ovarian carcinoma, and those with a dignosis of premenopausal breast cancer.

A positive BRCA result in a patient with numerous affected family members may prompt an increase in surveillance, prophylactic surgery, alteration of risk factors, or the institution of chemoprophylaxis (e.g., tamoxifen).

Pretest education, including a discussion of the risks and benefits of genetic testing, should be undertaken by a professional genetics counselor. A positive result that shows that the patient has inherited an altered *BRCA1* or *BRCA2* gene does not define whether or when cancer will develop, only that the woman's risk for cancer is increased. A positive *BRCA* result in a patient with numerous affected family members, however, may prompt an increase in surveillance, prophylactic surgery, alteration of risk factors, or the institution of chemoprophylaxis (e.g., tamoxifen). An important point to address is how a positive or negative result will change the management of an individual already diagnosed with breast cancer. Provision of psychological support for that individual and her family is essential. Testing is entirely voluntary, and the results are confidential. However, recording of positive results in the medical record may affect a patient's ability to obtain medical, life, or disability insurance (Table 3-2).

Increased surveillance for breast and ovarian cancer includes monthly breast self-examination, annual clinical breast examination, and annual mammography screening beginning at age 30. Blood testing for Ca-125, a tumor marker found in patients with ovarian cancer, also may be used as a screening tool. Transvaginal ultrasound is recommended every 6 to 12 months, and a rectovaginal pelvic examination is recommended yearly beginning at age 25.

Surgical options for the reduction of hereditary breast and ovarian cancer risk include bilateral prophylactic mastectomy and oophorectomy at age 35 or after the completion of childbearing. In a woman with a newly discovered breast cancer who is a known *BRCA1* or *BRCA2* carrier, mastectomy is probably a better treatment option than is breast conservation therapy since her risk for recurrence and bilateral disease is very high. She also may want to consider contralateral prophylactic mastectomy with bilateral reconstruction.

TABLE 3-2 ADVANTAGES AND DISADVANTAGES OF *BRCA* GENETIC TESTING

ADVANTAGES	DISADVANTAGES
Positive result may prompt increased surveillance and earlier detection	Positive result does not indicate whether or when cancer will actually develop
Positive result may prompt prophylactic surgery, risk factor reduction, and/or chemoprophylaxis	Positive result may affect ability to obtain or retain insurance
Negative result may decrease anxiety	Testing can be costly

Familial breast cancer, in which breast cancer seems to "run in the family" but does not follow the autosomal dominant inheritance pattern of hereditary breast cancer, also is a strong risk factor for the development of early-onset breast disease. Genetic testing is not yet possible for these women, but prompt biopsy of any suspicious breast lesion is recommended.

REPRODUCTIVE AND HORMONAL FACTORS

Most large epidemiologic studies demonstrate an association between early menarche and an increased risk of breast cancer. This effect decreases with age and is small after menopause. High parity (more than four births) lends some protective effect and reduces breast cancer risk, as does young age at the first term birth. The effect of incomplete pregnancies on breast cancer risk is not clear. Two recent studies have suggested that a first-trimester abortion before the first full-term pregnancy increases the risk of future breast carcinoma. However, other studies have not substantiated this finding. Prolonged breast-feeding is no longer thought to have a protective effect. Infertility and nulliparity increase the risk of breast cancer; the effect of fertility drugs is not known.

Natural menopause before age 45 confers a twofold risk reduction compared with menopause after age 55. Surgically induced menopause also reduces the risk of breast cancer, and this protection is lifelong; early surgical menopause lowers the risk even further.

The effect of hormone supplementation on the risk of breast cancer has been the subject of much debate. Most studies show that combination oral contraceptive pills have no effect on breast cancer risk when used by women in the middle of their reproductive lives (ages 25 to 39). Prolonged use of oral contraceptives may increase the risk of breast cancer slightly, especially when the hormones are administered at an early age and before the first full-term pregnancy. These data are controversial, however, and other studies have failed to show this effect. Early studies of the effect of injectable contraceptives such as medroxyprogesterone (Depo-Provera) have shown no increase or decrease in breast cancer risk.

The effect of hormone replacement therapy given to women after surgical or natural menopause on breast cancer risk has been the subject of much controversy. It is known that estrogen supplementation in postmenopausal women prevents osteoporosis and decreases the incidence of heart disease and colon cancer. In most women, these beneficial effects of estrogen therapy probably outweigh any small increase in breast cancer risk. However, in patients with other risk factors for breast cancer, such as a prior breast cancer, a strong family history, or biopsy-proved atypical proliferative breast disease, hormonal supplementation should be used with caution. Unfortunately, little is known about the effects of products that combine both estrogen and progesterone. Because the latent period for breast cancer development is 10 to 20 years, it may take some time before conclusive data become available. In the absence of such data, it is logical to withhold hormone replacement therapy from women at high risk for breast cancer.

Tamoxifen is a compound that originally was developed as a contraceptive. It blocks the uptake of estrogen at estrogen receptors in a number of tissues, including the breast. In patients with node-negative breast cancer, tamoxifen has reduced the incidence of contralateral primary breast cancer and recurrence of breast cancer in the ipsilateral breast. The National Surgical Adjuvant Breast Project (NSABP) Breast Cancer Prevention Trial is a prospective, randomized clinical trial comparing tamoxifen to placebo in patients at high risk of breast cancer. Early results have shown a 45 percent reduction in the incidence of breast cancer in high-risk women taking tamoxifen. Thus, the role of tamoxifen and other antiestrogen receptor compounds probably will be expanded for breast cancer treatment and prevention. The long-term results of tamoxifen therapy in high-risk women with no medical history of breast cancer are unknown. Tamoxifen may delay rather than prevent the development of breast cancer, and its use as a preventive agent may select for estrogen-receptor-negative tumors.

DIET AND LIFESTYLE FACTORS

Obesity is associated with a twofold increase in the risk of breast cancer. This effect does not seem to result from greater breast volume, as lean women with large breasts have no increase in breast cancer risk compared to lean women with small breasts.

High dietary fat intake and obesity go hand in hand for many patients, and both factors increase the risk of breast cancer.

Dietary fat intake also may influence the incidence of breast cancer. High dietary fat intake and obesity go hand in hand for many patients, and both factors increase the risk of breast cancer. Data from large population studies show that both the quantity and the quality of dietary fat may be important. Native Japanese women have a low incidence of breast cancer, and the fat in their diet, primarily from seafood, has a high content of omega-3 fatty acids. As the Japanese diet has become more westernized, increased processed fat and saturated fat intake has been associated with a doubling of the incidence of breast cancer in Japan. Environmental and dietary factors also are implicated in comparisons of Japanese women living in the United States with those living in Japan: Those living in the United States have a breast cancer incidence similar to that of American women.

Cigarette smoking increases the risk of cancer of all types, including oral, lung, colon, and breast cancers. No data are available about the change in risk for women who have stopped smoking.

Alcohol consumption also has been identified as a possible risk factor for breast cancer. In some studies, breast cancer risk was proportional to the amount of alcohol consumed.

ENVIRONMENTAL FACTORS

Many environmental factors have been studied in relation to breast cancer incidence. Most of them show no correlation. High-voltage wires, water and soil contaminants, and hair dyes have shown no association with breast cancer risk.

Radiation as an environmental factor has been shown to induce primary cancers in some populations. Epidemiologic evidence has documented radiation-induced breast cancer in women exposed during the atomic bombing of Hiroshima in 1945 and in individuals exposed to occupational ionizing radiation.

Patients with a history of Hodgkin's disease should be evaluated carefully for breast carcinoma. Radiation therapy has been very effective in eradicating Hodgkin's disease, but the long-term sequelae include many secondary cancers. The risk of breast cancer within the field of radiation is 75 times greater than the risk among the general population. Young age at the time of mantle irradiation increases the risk further, and bilateral breast disease is common in these patients.

The effect of radiation exposure during diagnostic studies such as chest x-rays and mammograms has been shown to be minimal with respect to breast cancer risk. In the case of mammography, any small increase in risk is far outweighed by the benefit of improved survival associated with the detection of early-stage treatable tumors.

Postoperative radiation in conjunction with breast conservation therapy is known to reduce the incidence of recurrent carcinoma and has not been associated with an increased incidence of contralateral disease.

PREMALIGNANT LESIONS

Many women who undergo breast biopsy are found to have a benign diagnosis upon histologic examination of the excised tissue. However, along the pathologic spectrum between normal breast tissue and frank carcinoma, many of the intermediate diagnoses confer an increased risk of breast cancer. To prove that a benign lesion increases a woman's breast cancer risk, a temporal relationship between the occurrence of the benign lesion and breast cancer should be established. Studies of this type are difficult, as the benign lesion could be a true precursor of cancer, a marker of risk elevation, or a consequence of breast malignancy.

Biopsies containing proliferative lesions are associated with increased breast cancer risk. Mild hyperplasia is excluded from the proliferative disease category because it confers no additional risk. Proliferative disease, including moderate and florid hyperplasia (Fig. 3-1), sclerosing adenosis (Fig. 3-2), and papillomas (Fig. 3-3), approximately doubles the risk of future breast carcinoma.

Proliferative lesions with cytologic atypia meet some but not all of the criteria needed for a diagnosis of carcinoma in situ. The two types of atypical hyperplasia— atypical ductal hyperplasia and atypical lobular hyperplasia—both increase the risk of breast cancer fourfold to fivefold (Fig. 3-4). Atypical hyperplasia usually is diagnosed in perimenopausal women.

The two types of atypical hyperplasia (ductal and lobular) increase the risk of breast cancer fourfold to fivefold.

Lobular carcinoma in situ (LCIS) and ductal carcinoma in situ (DCIS) are discussed in Chap. 7. LCIS is a marker rather than a true precursor of invasive breast carcinoma and is associated with a probability of future malignancy of about 30 percent. The incidence of invasive disease coexisting at the time of diagnosis of LCIS is about 5 percent. DCIS is a precursor of invasive ductal carcinoma, and if untreated, it implies a 50 percent chance of future carcinoma.

BREAST CANCER RISK REDUCTION

The clinical and preclinical evidence accumulated to date has indicated important risk factors for the development of breast cancer. Among these factors, some can be manipulated to reduce risk. Obviously, age and genetic predisposition cannot be changed. However, older women and those with a family history of breast cancer can be encouraged to perform monthly breast self-examination, obtain yearly mammograms, and undergo clinical examination at 6-month intervals.

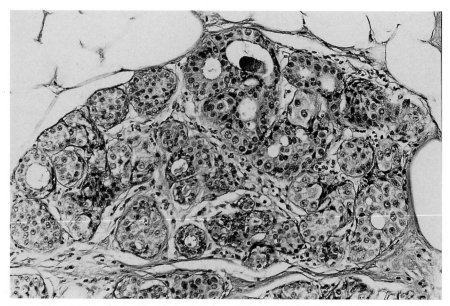

FIGURE 3-1 Hyperplasia. The duct epithelium seen here (200X) is proliferative and forms papillary projections. The cells in the lower right corner demonstrate apocrine metaplasia, which is characterized by abundant pink granular cytoplasm without nuclear enlargement.

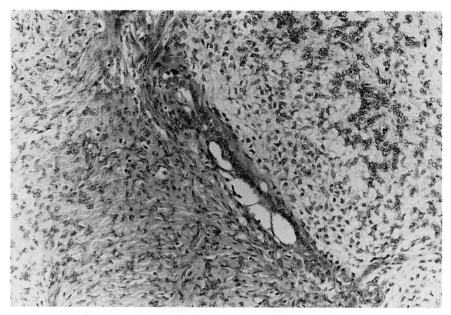

FIGURE 3-2 Sclerosing adenosis. The benign-appearing stroma of the breast lobule is expanded, compressing the epithelium so that the terminal lobuloalveolar units lose their familiar rounded architecture and instead take on a staghorn or pointed appearance. (200X)

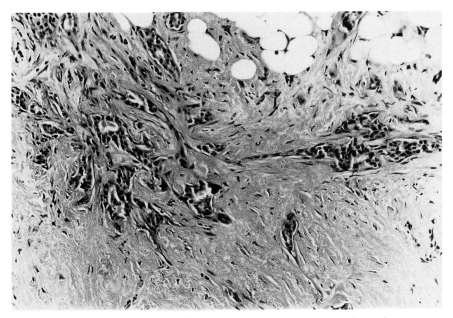

FIGURE 3-3 Intraductal papilloma. This dilated breast duct contains a luminal mass composed of a papillary proliferation of ductal epithelium. (*200X*)

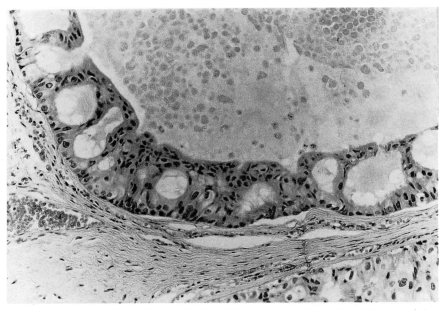

FIGURE 3-4 Atypical hyperplasia. This breast duct contains a luminal proliferation of ductal epithelial cells. Because of the interspersed normal epithelium, the breast duct is insufficiently involved to merit a diagnosis of carcinoma in situ. (*200X*)

Reproductive factors affect the relative risk of breast cancer and potentially can be manipulated. For example, women with a strong family history of breast disease may want to consider early completion of their families. Women at a particularly high risk for developing breast cancer may consider prophylactic mastectomy, which results in a 90 percent or greater reduction in risk.

A postmenopausal woman with known breast cancer or a strong family history of breast cancer probably should avoid estrogen therapy and consider an alternative such as tamoxifen or raloxifene.

Hormonal factors such as age at menarche and menopause are predetermined, but exposure to exogenous estrogens is voluntary. At the present time, a postmenopausal woman with known breast cancer or a strong family history of breast cancer probably should avoid estrogen therapy and consider an alternative such as tamoxifen or a selective estrogen receptor modifier (SERM) such as raloxifene in consultation with her physician.

Sensible eating habits including lower dietary fat intake can be recommended for all women, not just those at high risk for breast cancer. A number of testimonials advocate dietary supplements such as melatonin, beta carotene, vitamin E, zinc, selenium, B-complex vitamins, flax seed, vitamin C, and various minerals for the prevention of breast cancer. In the absence of double-blind, randomized clinical trials, however, support for these supplements is lacking. Success in increasing the survivability of breast cancer has been due to early detection with mammography screening and improving awareness of risk factors. See Table 3-2 for a summary of risk factors for breast cancer.

COMMONLY ASKED QUESTIONS

1. **My mother was diagnosed with breast cancer at age 40. When should I begin to have mammographic screening?** Because the increase in risk is greater when the first-degree relative was premenopausal at diagnosis, screening generally is recommended to commence at age 30. Keep in mind that young women have denser breasts; therefore, the mammographic images may be more difficult to interpret. Any clinically suspicious mass should be biopsied regardless of its mammographic appearance.

2. **I have a cousin and an aunt with breast cancer. Am I at increased risk?** Yes. The risk of breast cancer is increased even when the affected family member is a second-degree relative. However, one cannot be sure whether this patient's second-degree relatives represent unfortunate sporadic cases or if there is a familial tendency toward breast cancer development. Close follow-up with clinical breast examinations every 6 to 12 months, a baseline mammogram at age 35, and annual mammographic screening after age 40 is a reasonable approach.

3. **My mother had premenopausal breast cancer. Should I undergo genetic testing?** The implications of a positive test for *BRCA1* or *BRCA2* are far-reaching, and patients at risk for a genetic abnormality should undergo extensive counseling before considering genetic testing. A positive result affects not only the patient but her female family members as well. If a genetic abnormality is detected, an increase in surveillance as well as prophylactic surgical or pharmacologic treatment may be offered.

4. **I have been on "the pill" off and on for over 15 years. Lately I've heard it could increase my risk of breast cancer. Should I discontinue taking oral contraceptives (OCPs)?** For most patients who take OCPs, the benefits (e.g., lighter, shorter, more regular menses and a decrease in ovarian and endometrial cancer risk after more than 5 years of use) far outweigh any risk from their use. The data regarding OCPs and breast cancer risk are controversial, but no compelling evidence exists to suggest that OCPs should be discontinued after a certain number of years.

5. **I've been told that I have fibrocystic changes in my breasts. Am I at increased risk for breast cancer?** In young reproductive-age women, the breasts are composed primarily of

dense glandular tissue and relatively less fat. The breasts may feel more firm on examination before menses because of the effects of cyclic hormonal changes on the dense parenchymal tissue. The resultant "lumpy-bumpy" texture is commonly called fibrocystic change by clinicians and is a normal finding. However, if biopsy is prompted by examination findings of asymmetry or the presence of a discrete lump, proliferative histologic changes are associated with an increase in cancer risk. Moderate to florid hyperplasia, sclerosing adenosis, and papillomata increase the risk twofold, while atypical hyperplasia increases the risk fourfold to fivefold.

SUGGESTED READING

American Institute of Cancer Research, eds. *Diet and Breast Cancer.* New York: Plenum; 1994.

Atiba J, Meyskens F. Chemoprevention of breast cancer. *Semin Oncol* 1992; 19:220–229.

Beral V, Reeves A. Childbearing, oral contraceptives use and breast cancer. *Lancet* 1993; 341: 1102.

Goss P, Sierra S. Current perspectives on radiation-induced breast cancer. *J Clin Oncol* 1998; 16(1):338–347.

Marcus J, Page D, Watson P, et al. Hereditary breast cancer: BRCA1 and BRCA2 pathobiology and prognosis. *Cancer* 1996; 77:697–709.

4

ETIOLOGY, EVALUATION, AND MANAGEMENT OF A BREAST MASS

INTRODUCTION

The presence of a breast lump, whether self-detected or discovered on clinical breast examination, is an anxiety-provoking problem for the patient and her physician. Even though at least 75 percent of palpable lumps are benign, the patient and physician share concern about the possibility of cancer. Numerous diagnostic procedures often are performed, only to discover that the mass is benign. The physician's goal in his or her attempt to "first do no harm" is to assess the mass properly on examination and perform the fewest and least invasive procedures that will allow an accurate diagnosis. This chapter discusses the most common causes of a palpable or nonpalpable mass and outlines a diagnostic strategy to accomplish that goal.

PATHOLOGY OF BREAST MASSES

The numerous entities that may present clinically as a palpable breast lump can be grouped into physiologic causes and neoplasms (Table 4-1). Physiologic causes and benign neoplasms are discussed briefly below.

PHYSIOLOGIC CAUSES

Inflammation   Acute mastitis is usually a problem only in lactating women and is caused by the ascent of bacteria, most commonly *Staphylococcus aureus,* from the neonate's oropharynx into the duct system through a duct opening or a fissure in the nipple. It also may result from foreign bodies (e.g., nipple rings, implant place-

TABLE 4-1 ETIOLOGY OF BREAST MASSES

PHYSIOLOGIC CAUSES	Inflammation (mastitis, abscess), duct ectasia (plasma cell mastitis), fat necrosis, superficial thrombophlebitis (Mondor's disease), galactocele, fibrocystic changes
BENIGN NEOPLASMS	Fibroadenoma, intraductal papilloma, cystosarcoma phyllodes, granular cell tumor
MALIGNANT NEOPLASMS	Paget's disease, ductal carcinoma in situ, infiltrating ductal carcinoma, lobular carcinoma in situ, infiltrating lobular carcinoma

ment, implant leakage) or trauma. Mastitis usually presents as a unilateral, localized area of erythema, induration, edema, and tenderness (Fig. 4-1). The progression to abscess formation may be rapid if the infection is not treated aggressively with antibiotics. Uncomplicated postpartum mastitis is best treated with oral dicloxacillin 500 mg every 6 h for 10 days and continuation of breast-feeding. Abscess formation must be suspected if clinical improvement does not occur within 48 to 72 h. In that case, hospitalization, administration of intravenous antibiotics (nafcillin or oxacillin 2 g every 4 h or vancomycin 1 g every 12 h for penicillin-allergic patients), and incision and drainage of the abscess are required (Fig. 4-2). In a nonlactating patient, an acute abscess must be distinguished from inflammatory carcinoma (Fig. 4-3, Plate 1), especially if it is associated with nipple discharge. Breast biopsy at the time of incision and drainage is required, and the antibiotic selected should have coverage for anaerobic

Uncomplicated postpartum mastitis is best treated with oral dicloxacillin 500 mg every 6 h for 10 days and continuation of breast-feeding.

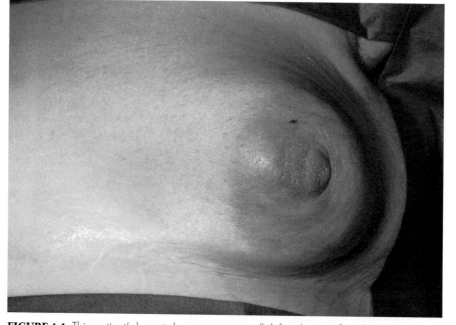

FIGURE 4-1 This patient's breast demonstrates a well-defined area of erythema commonly seen with acute postpartum mastitis. The area is exquisitely tender and somewhat indurated. (Courtesy of Patrick Duff, MD, University of Florida College of Medicine.)

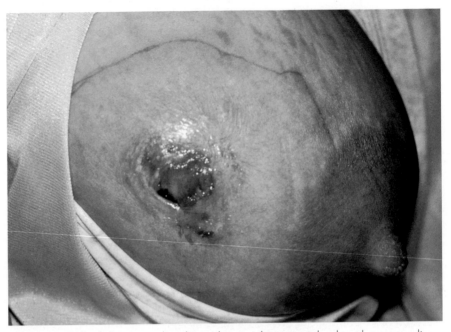

FIGURE 4-2 After failure on oral antibiotic therapy, this patient developed an expanding area of erythema, tenderness, and fluctuance. Treatment with incision and drainage of the abscess and administration of intravenous antibiotics led to resolution of the infection. (Courtesy of Patrick Duff, MD, University of Florida College of Medicine.)

bacteria, such as clindamycin or metronidazole. After the resolution of an abscess, scarring may cause skin or nipple retraction.

Granulomatous inflammation is extremely rare in the breast but may be caused by tuberculosis, mycotic infection, or sarcoidosis. Chronic ductal inflammation, or plasma cell mastitis, is associated with mammary duct ectasia or dilation (see Fig. 13-35), although it is unclear which problem actually occurs first. Duct ectasia is more common in older, multiparous women and may be associated with nipple discharge and pain. Although duct ectasia is not always palpable, the fibrosis that results from subareolar inflammation can cause induration and nipple or skin retraction. The application of warm soaks may alleviate the nipple discharge associated with duct ectasia.

Fat Necrosis   Traumatic injury to the breast is often difficult for a patient to recall. The healing process involves several stages, and fibrosis may be the end result. The healed area can simulate a mass that is painless, firm, and well localized. Adherence of the mass to the skin and mammographic detection of calcification may lead to confusion of this entity with carcinoma and prompt an excisional biopsy (Fig. 4-4, Plate 2).

Superficial Thrombophlebitis   Also known as Mondor's disease, this rare condition may occur spontaneously or in association with breast surgery or pregnancy. It presents as a tender, erythematous cylindrical area of induration, usually along the upper outer quadrant of the breast. Associated skin dimpling or retraction may evoke concern about cancer, but biopsy usually is not necessary. Treatment with warm

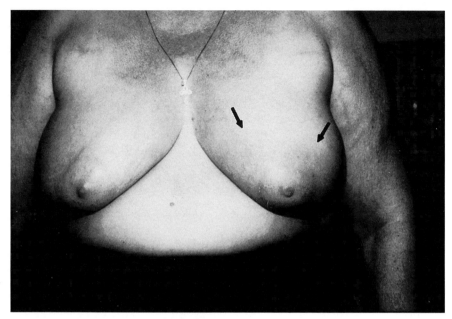

A

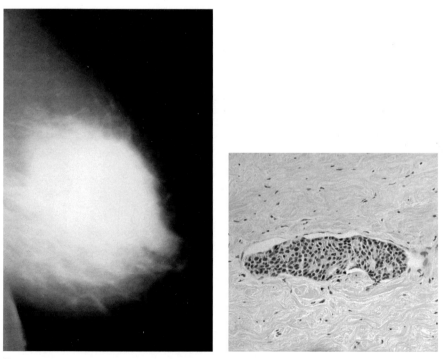

B   **C**

FIGURE 4-3 A. (Plate 1) This postmenopausal woman developed asymmetric erythema of the left breast. No mass was palpable despite the presence of extensive inflammatory carcinoma. **B.** Mammographic evaluation demonstrated a very large, nearly opaque density involving much of the left breast. **C.** Histologic evaluation of the excised mass revealed inflammatory carcinoma. Note the malignant cells within dermal lymphatic channels.

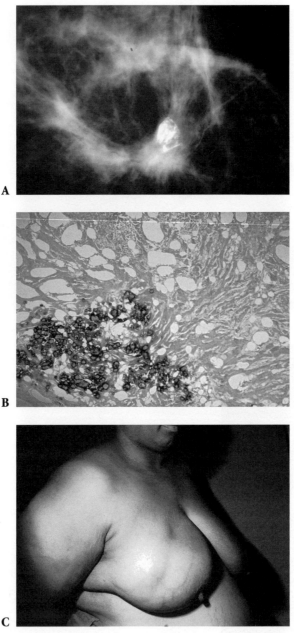

FIGURE 4-4 A Calcifications, ill-defined density, and skin retraction are common mammographic findings after breast trauma and subsequent fat necrosis. This patient had a previous breast biopsy and is now noted to have all these findings.

FIGURE 4-4 B This biopsy taken from the bed of the lump excision in *(A)* demonstrates calcifications within an area of fat necrosis as seen on the mammogram.

FIGURE 4-4 C (Plate 2) Skin retraction after breast trauma is caused by fibrosis within the area of healing. This patient was involved in a motor vehicle accident and sustained an injury to the breast from the shoulder restraint portion of her seat belt. (Courtesy of Scott Lind, MD, University of Florida College of Medicine.)

compresses and nonsteroidal anti-inflammatory agents allows resolution within a few weeks.

Galactocele   Ductal obstruction in a lactating patient may result in the formation of a milk-filled cyst, or galactocele (Fig. 4-5). Rarely, a galactocele may develop in a patient with nonpuerperal galactorrhea, in which case the diagnosis is less obvious. Needle aspiration is diagnostic and therapeutic and may have to be repeated if the problem recurs.

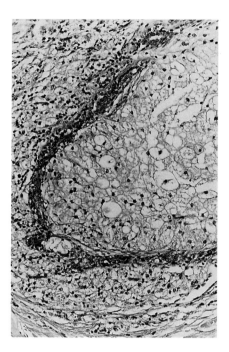

FIGURE 4-5 The appearance of an obstructed breast duct, or galactocele (*200X*). The lumen is enlarged and filled with vacuolated histiocytes called "foamy" histiocytes. Surrounding the duct is an inflammatory stromal reaction.

Fibrocystic Changes   Over the years, terms such as *fibrocystic disease, mammary dysplasia,* and *cystic mastitis* have been replaced with the term *fibrocystic changes* to denote the spectrum of conditions associated with lumpy, often tender breasts. *Fibrocystic changes* seems to be the appropriate term to describe these findings, since they are benign and affect at least half of all women age 20 to 50 years.

The natural history of fibrocystic changes typically involves progression through three stages, each spanning a decade, beginning in a woman's twenties. The first stage, known as *mazoplasia,* is characterized by cyclic mastalgia and an increase in breast density, especially in the upper-outer quadrants. Stromal fibrosis is the predominant histologic change (Fig. 4-6). When it is localized or asymmetric, this palpable induration may raise concern about cancer. The second stage, *adenosis,* involves alveolar and/or ductal proliferation (Fig. 4-7), which may be clinically apparent as multiple small palpable nodules. In the final *cystic* stage, microcysts (< 1 mm), or macrocysts (> 3 mm) may arise from dilation and unfolding of the lobules (Fig. 4-8). Microcysts are nonpalpable, may be multiple and bilateral, and should be considered normal. Macrocysts are often palpable and tender. A tense cyst may simulate a solid mass.

In an attempt to stratify these histologic alterations to reflect the subsequent cancer risk, fibrocystic changes may be classified as nonproliferative, proliferative without atypia, or proliferative with atypia. Nonproliferative changes are not associated with an increase in cancer risk. Such changes include duct ectasia, cysts, mild hyperplasia, and apocrine metaplasia. Proliferative changes without atypia include papillomas, sclerosing adenosis, and moderate to florid hyperplasia; these changes are associated with a 1.5-fold to twofold increase in risk. Atypical ductal or lobular hyperplasia is associated with a fourfold to fivefold increase in the subsequent risk of breast cancer. These risks are doubled if the patient has a first-degree relative with breast cancer.

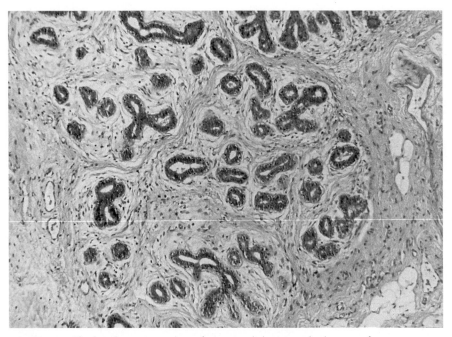

FIGURE 4-6 The histologic equivalent of increased density in the breasts of young women with clinical fibrocystic changes is benign stromal hyperplasia.

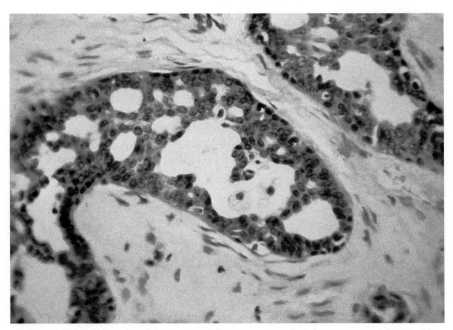

FIGURE 4-7 Later ductal proliferation may become clinically apparent as small palpable nodules.

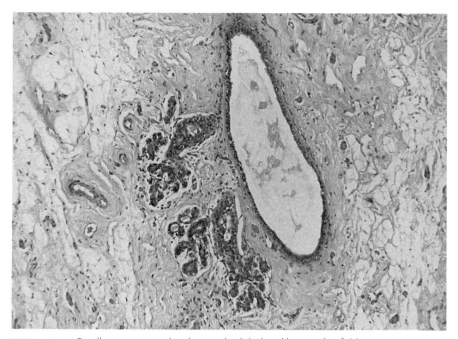

FIGURE 4-8 Finally, microcysts develop as the lobules dilate and unfold.

BENIGN NEOPLASMS

Fibroadenoma   These hormone-sensitive solid tumors are the most common benign breast neoplasms (Fig. 4-9). They are particularly common in women 20 to 40 years of age, in whom they may increase, decrease, or remain stable in size over time. Most fibroadenomas grow slowly and then regress after menopause. A fibroadenoma often presents as a palpable nodule that is detected by the patient on self-examination. Alternatively, the clinician will discover a firm, mobile, well-circumscribed mass on physical examination. These encapsulated tumors are easily excised, but because they are not considered precancerous, a patient with a fibroadenoma can be managed conservatively in some situations, as is discussed below.

Intraductal Papilloma   Exuberant proliferation of ductal epithelium may lead to the development of a fragile frond, or papilloma, within a duct (see Fig. 3-3). Portions of a papilloma may dislodge into the duct lumen and result in serosanguineous or sanguineous nipple discharge. Occasionally, the patient or her physician will detect a small (several millimeters) subareolar nodule on breast examination. Cytologic evaluation of the bloody nipple discharge may disclose the presence of malignant cells, but negative cytology is not completely reassuring. Excision of the duct is always required to exclude the possibility of cancer. As is discussed in Chap. 6, contrast mammography, or ductography, can define the ductal location and architecture, allowing excision of only the involved duct. Intraductal papillomas may be solitary or multiple. Multiple papillomas are more often peripheral in location and are more likely to be associated with carcinoma.

Cytologic evaluation of bloody nipple discharge may disclose the presence of malignant cells, but negative cytology is not completely reassuring. Excision of the duct is always required to exclude the possibility of cancer.

Cystosarcoma Phyllodes or Phyllodes Tumor   These rapidly growing tumors usually occur in older women, are larger at diagnosis, and behave more aggressively than do

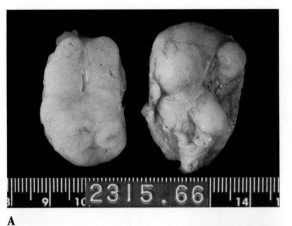

A

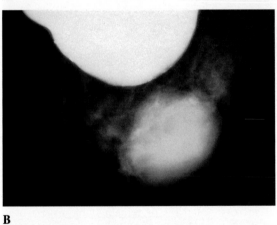

B

FIGURE 4-9 *A.* The gross appearance of a bisected fibroadenoma. Note that the tumor is well encapsulated and has a rubbery appearance. *B.* This patient was found to have two palpable masses in her breast. Her mammogram demonstrates a subglandular breast implant and a large, well-circumscribed fibroadenoma. *C.* Histologically, the bland stromal proliferation causes compression of the epithelial element.

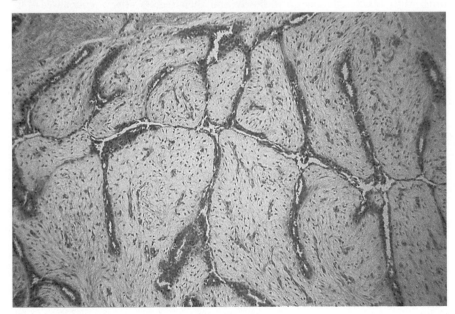

C

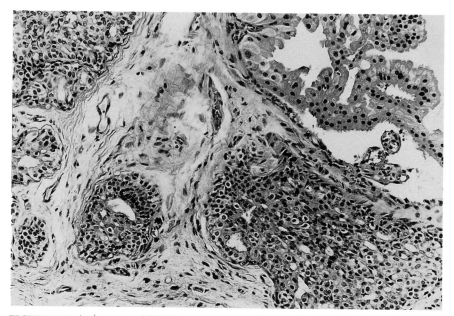

FIGURE 4-10 In the center (200X) is a compressed breast duct lined by benign-appearing epithelium. The accompanying stroma is remarkable for hypercellularity and nuclear atypia, characteristic findings with cystosarcoma phyllodes. This appearance is contrasted with that of a fibroadenoma, which demonstrates benign epithelium and a benign stroma.

typical fibroadenomas (Fig. 4-10). Benign cystosarcomas are treated with wide local excision and may recur if they are not totally excised. Malignant phyllodes tumors may invade locally or metastasize, most commonly to lung or bone, and simple mastectomy is the usual initial treatment.

Granular Cell Tumors   These rare tumors are of Schwann cell origin and are found more commonly in the tongue (Fig. 4-11). They may mimic cancer because of poorly defined borders, firmness, and skin retraction. Excision is diagnostic and therapeutic.

CLINICAL EVALUATION

HISTORY

The first step in the evaluation of any complaint is a thorough historical review, as was outlined in Chap. 2. This detailed interview should determine whether the patient has any risk factors for breast cancer: previous breast cancer or atypical hyperplasia, a history of breast cancer in a first-degree relative (especially if premenopausal at diagnosis), early menarche, late age at first full-term pregnancy (>35 years), late menopause, and uterine cancer. If self-discovery of a mass has brought the patient to seek medical attention, the physician should inquire about how long the mass has been present, whether the mass is tender, and whether it has changed in size over time or with the menstrual cycle.

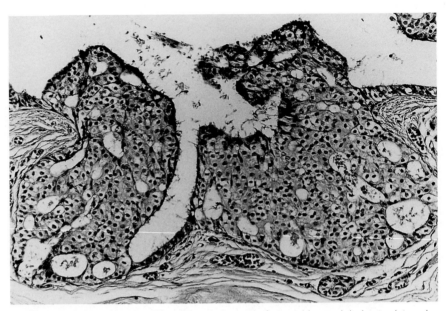

FIGURE 4-11 This granular cell tumor is composed of normal breast lobules (*right*) and monotonous, bland-appearing stromal proliferation (*200X*). The stromal cells are called granular cells because of the expansion of the cytoplasm with a grainy texture.

PHYSICAL EXAMINATION

The complete examination of a patient reporting a breast lump is described in Chap. 2. The examination should be performed with the patient in the sitting and supine positions and should include palpation of the node-bearing areas. The clinician should attempt to identify the lump, and if it is not apparent, the patient should be asked to locate it herself. If it cannot be delineated, further evaluation should follow routine guidelines for screening mammography. If the patient or physician remains concerned, a repeat examination in 2 to 3 months may be warranted. A mass found by the patient but not evaluated properly by the physician is a very common source of malpractice litigation.

If a dominant mass is palpable, its location, size, shape, mobility, tenderness, and border definition should be noted. The clinician should attempt to discern whether the mass is cystic or solid, and the presence of lymphadenopathy should be noted. Characteristics usually associated with a benign breast mass include regular borders, free mobility, cystic texture, and pain with palpation. Malignant masses tend to be hard, painless, and fixed to the skin or chest wall and to have indistinct or irregular borders.

Characteristics usually associated with a benign breast mass include regular borders, free mobility, cystic texture, and pain with palpation. Malignant masses tend to be hard, painless, and fixed to the skin or chest wall and to have indistinct or irregular borders.

DIAGNOSTIC EVALUATION

Fine Needle Aspiration The technique used to perform fine needle aspiration (FNA) is described in detail in Chap. 2. To summarize, the mass is immobilized, and a 22- to 23-gauge needle with an attached syringe is used to aspirate its contents. If it is fluid-filled, the cyst should be completely drained. If it is solid, several passes are made into the mass with the needle, maintaining negative pressure with the syringe.

The vacuum is released before the needle is removed from the breast, and the cellular material from the needle and hub is fixed for cytologic evaluation. FNA is seldom falsely positive but may be negative in up to 20 percent of patients with a malignant mass.

Mammography In a patient with a palpable breast lump, mammography serves two purposes. It is used as a "screening" study to detect coexisting nonpalpable pathology such as asymmetric density (Fig. 4-12) or clustered microcalcifications (Fig. 4-13). It also is used as a "diagnostic" study to identify characteristics that classify a mass as "probably benign" or "suspicious" for malignancy. Benign characteristics include distinct edges, certain calcification patterns [e.g., "popcorn" calcifications (Fig. 4-14) and secretory calcifications (Fig. 4-15)], and stability over time. Spiculated, indistinct, or stellate mass borders (Figs. 4-16 and 4-17) or the presence of clusters of microcalcifications (Fig. 4-18) is suspicious for malignancy.

Unfortunately, mammography may show no worrisome features in up to 15 percent of patients with a palpable cancer. Thus, mammographic interpretation allows a presumptive, not definitive, diagnosis and must be viewed as an adjunct to physical examination and tissue sampling.

Ultrasonography Ultrasound evaluation of the breast is used primarily to define whether a mass is cystic (Fig. 4-19), solid (Fig. 4-20), or complex. It is especially helpful in young women because their breast tissue density impairs adequate mammographic imaging (Figs. 4-21 and 4-22). In a young patient with a palpable mass, the risk of malignancy is low, and the finding of a benign-appearing cyst on ultra-

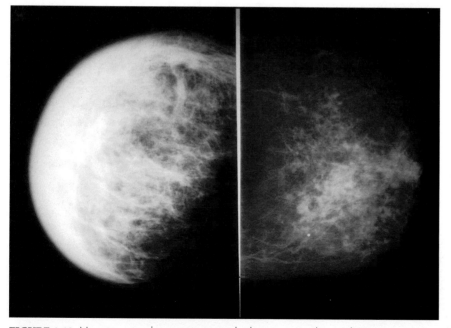

FIGURE 4-12 Mammogram demonstrating marked asymmetric density that was associated with an extensive inflammatory carcinoma.

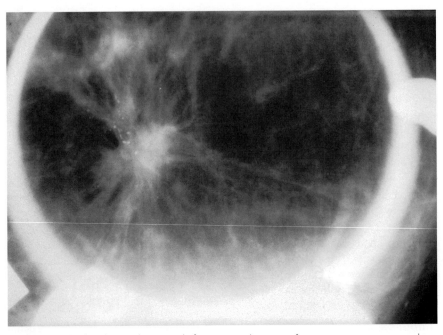

FIGURE 4-13 The clustered microcalcifications in this magnification view were proved to represent invasive carcinoma on biopsy.

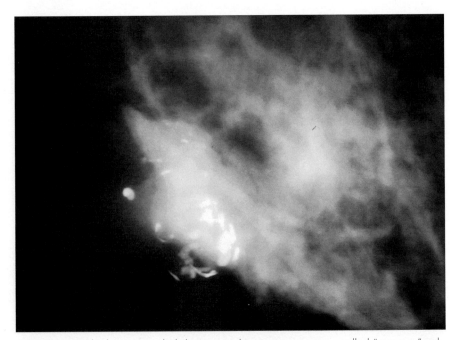

FIGURE 4-14 The large, rounded densities in this mammogram are called "popcorn" calcifications and are classic findings in degenerating fibroadenomas.

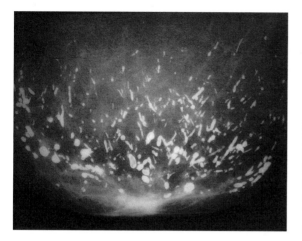

FIGURE 4-15 The numerous linear calcifications here are benign secretory calcifications. They are located within the ducts and appear to be directed toward the nipple. This finding is common in older women.

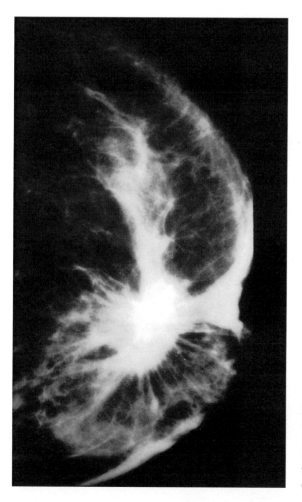

FIGURE 4-16 This obvious breast carcinoma is very large and demonstrates a stellate appearance. Stranding with attachment to the skin also is apparent.

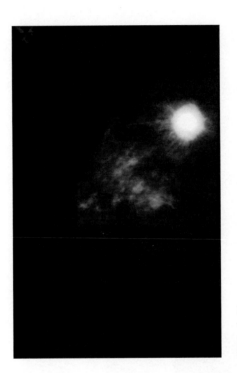

FIGURE 4-17 This high-density mass is very well defined but demonstrates spiculations extending from it into the surrounding tissue.

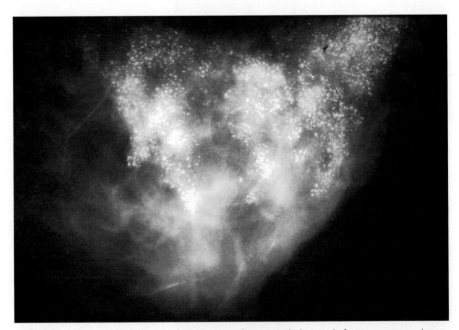

FIGURE 4-18 This mammogram demonstrates the ground-glass calcification pattern that is seen commonly with comedocarcinoma. This patient was only 35 years old, and her very large cancer was not palpable.

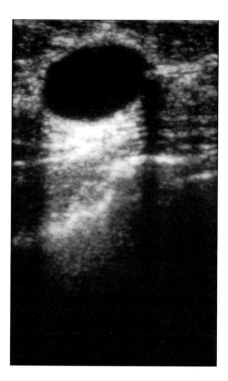

FIGURE 4-19 Ultrasound demonstrating the findings classically seen with a simple cyst: well-defined borders, homogeneous lucency within the mass, and posterior acoustic enhancement.

sound makes mammography unnecessary. However, ultrasound is not always accurate in distinguishing between benign and malignant solid masses, and further evaluation is required.

Stereotactic Procedures   Many breast abnormalities cannot be identified on physical examination but may be detected by screening mammography. The evaluation

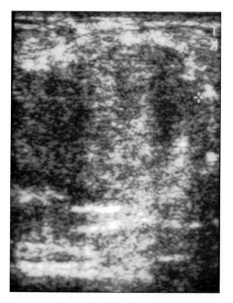

FIGURE 4-20 Ultrasound examination of this solid mass reveals a hypoechogenic texture, less well-defined borders, and distal shadowing.

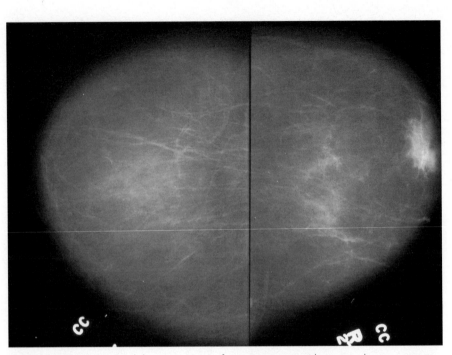

FIGURE 4-21 Craniocaudal mammogram of a postmenopausal woman demonstrating the lucency associated with fatty replacement of glandular tissue.

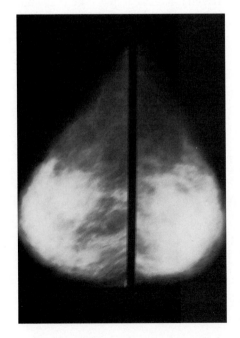

FIGURE 4-22 A mediolateral oblique mammogram from a 30-year-old woman demonstrating the opacity associated with dense fibroglandular tissue.

of these nonpalpable areas requires mammographic or ultrasonographic guidance of biopsy instruments, as is discussed below.

Needle-Localized Biopsy This technique is considered the gold standard for the evaluation of a nonpalpable, suspicious mammographic finding. Using a compression plate containing a grid of holes and routine mammographic views, a hollow needle is guided into the abnormal area. Through the needle, a fine wire barb is advanced and anchored in the breast tissue. After correct placement of the barb has been confirmed mammographically, the needle is removed, the wire is secured with a dressing, and the patient is transported to the operating room. The surgeon uses the wire as a guide to the target area and excises the surrounding tissue. The specimen is immediately examined mammographically to ensure that it includes all of the affected area (Fig. 4-23). This excisional technique allows histologic evaluation of the entire suspicious area (Fig. 4-24), as opposed to tissue "sampling."

Core Biopsy Core biopsy is a relatively new technique that is gaining acceptance as radiologists become increasingly adept at and experienced with interventional procedures. It is an outpatient procedure that is performed under local anesthesia in the radiology suite. Computer-assisted mammography is used to direct the 14-gauge needle of a biopsy gun into the abnormal area (Fig. 4-25). Several samples are taken of the target area, and the specimens are submitted for histologic evaluation.

The goal of core biopsy is to allow tissue diagnosis while avoiding the cost and invasiveness of an operative diagnostic procedure. The technique has been shown to be much more reliable than FNA, allowing histologic instead of cytologic interpretation, as well as typing and grading of malignancies in many cases. When com-

The goal of core biopsy is to allow tissue diagnosis while avoiding the cost and invasiveness of an operative diagnostic procedure. It is more reliable than FNA, allowing histologic instead of cytologic interpretation.

FIGURE 4-23 Specimen mammogram demonstrating microcalcifications halfway between the barb and the tip of the wire.

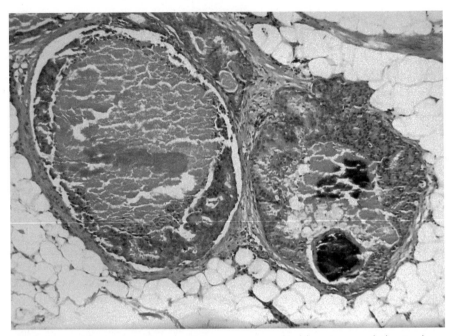

FIGURE 4-24 Histologic evaluation of the tissue surrounding the wire revealed comedo-carcinoma with calcifications seen within the ducts.

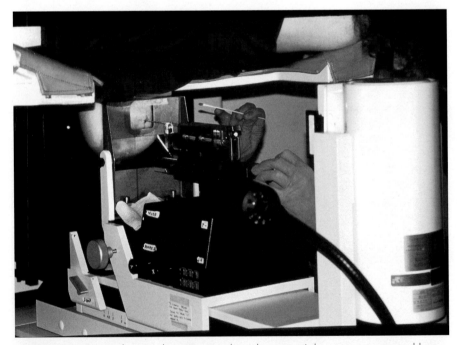

FIGURE 4-25 During the core biopsy procedure, the patient's breast is compressed between two plates. Computer-assisted mammography is used to direct the 14-gauge biopsy needle into the abnormal area.

pared to the accuracy of needle-localized biopsy, the results of the core biopsy technique are likely to be somewhat institution-dependent, at least until training becomes uniform. Percutaneous biopsy is generally reliable and reproducible although slightly less accurate than surgical biopsy, especially in evaluating areas of microcalcifications. Some clinicians believe that as experience with the procedure is gained, it will replace operative biopsy in many, if not most, situations. Currently, settings in which core biopsy already is preferred include assessment of a mammographically suspicious, nonpalpable mass; evaluation of a minimal mammographic abnormality when the patient or her physician prefers the reassurance of tissue sampling over mammographic follow-up; and evaluation of suspicious mammographic changes seen in a tumor bed after radiation therapy.

Ultrasound-Guided Cyst Aspiration   In most cases, breast cysts can be stabilized between two fingers to allow needle drainage. However, ultrasound guidance occasionally may be required to allow the drainage of a deep-seated cyst.

MANAGEMENT

PALPABLE SOLID MASS

A dominant breast lump in the presence of adenopathy should be considered cancer until proved otherwise. In this situation or in any woman over age 35 with a palpable mass, mammography followed by tissue sampling should be performed. The mammogram is performed first since its interpretation may be obscured if a sampling procedure causes hematoma formation. As was mentioned above, mammography is necessary to exclude concurrent nonpalpable pathology. Ultrasonography often is performed in conjunction with mammography to determine whether a mass is cystic, solid, or complex. If a mass is solid or complex, FNA and/or excision are required to exclude the possibility of cancer. Referral to a general surgeon usually occurs at this point in the evaluation.

If a mass that is not associated with adenopathy is found in a young woman, FNA may be performed first. This procedure will be diagnostic as well as therapeutic if the mass is cystic, and imaging studies may not be needed. If no fluid is obtained on FNA, ultrasonography is the preferred imaging study in women under age 30 because it can identify whether the mass is solid or is cystic but was missed by FNA. Then FNA may be repeated under sonographic or mammographic guidance, or excisional biopsy may be performed.

The cellular material extracted by FNA of a solid mass should be submitted for cytologic evaluation because malignant histologic findings will guide the discussion of options and surgical planning. If the aspirate is adequate for evaluation (i.e., contains ductal epithelium) and only benign-appearing cells are seen, further management is somewhat controversial. An aggressive option is to excise any palpable mass, ensuring that no cancer is missed because of false-negative FNA cytology. Alternatively, a strategy incorporating the collective results of the clinical examination, FNA, and imaging studies may be utilized. In this scenario, excision will be performed if the patient desires it or if any of these results are at all suspicious. Otherwise, close follow-up with imaging studies and/or examinations should be sufficient. The role of core biopsy in the evaluation of a palpable mass has not been defined. Certainly, histologic evaluation may further reassure the physician and patient that a mass is benign.

There is no consensus regarding the optimal protocol for the management of a solid breast mass. A sample management protocol is shown in Fig. 4-26. Consideration must be given to the skill and experience of the health care team, including the clinician performing the examination and FNA, the cytologist, the radiologist, and the surgeon to whom the patient is referred. The patient's input must be sought, as he or she may have a strong preference for or against excision. These factors must be weighed, and an individualized management plan must be devised. The patient's age and particular circumstances may dictate the aggressiveness of the approach.

CYSTIC MASS

The management of a mass found on FNA to be cystic depends on the character of the fluid and whether the mass disappears with aspiration. Nonsanguineous fluid removed from a cystic mass may be discarded since it is very rarely associated with malignancy. Bloody fluid should be evaluated cytologically because a diagnosis of malignancy made at that early stage in evaluation may prevent an unnecessary diagnostic biopsy and allow the planning of a therapeutic surgical procedure. Unfortunately, even if a sanguineous aspirate from a cyst is negative for malignant cells, excision must be performed to exclude malignancy. Mammography is indicated before excision to evaluate for coexisting nonpalpable pathology.

If the fluid removed from a cystic mass is nonsanguineous and the mass is no longer palpable after aspiration, the patient should return in 2 to 3 months for reex-

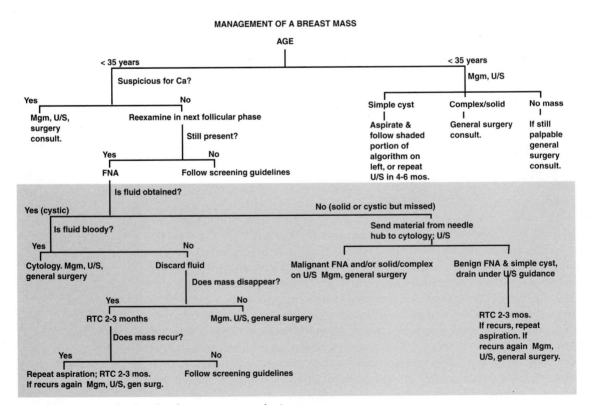

FIGURE 4-26 Sample algorithm for management of a breast mass.

COLOR PLATES*

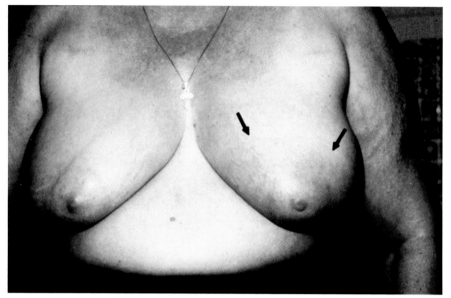

Plate 1 (Fig. 4-3A) This postmenopausal woman developed asymmetric erythema of the left breast. No mass was palpable despite the presence of extensive inflammatory carcinoma.

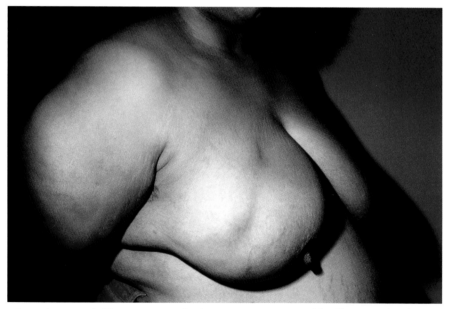

Plate 2 (Fig. 4-4C) Skin retraction after breast trauma is caused by fibrosis within the area of healing. This patient was involved in a motor vehicle accident and sustained an injury to the breast from the shoulder restraint portion of her seat belt. (Courtesy of Scott Lind, MD, University of Florida College of Medicine.)

*The figures in parentheses following the plate numbers have been double-numbered in order to indicate the chapter in which they are discussed and the order of their citation therein.

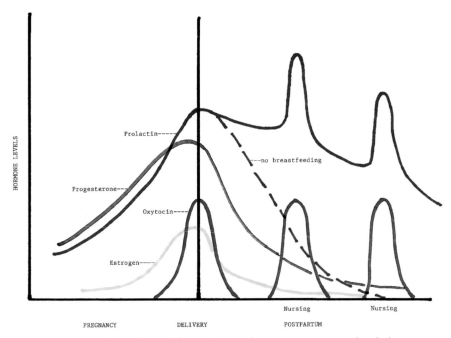

Plate 3 (Fig. 10-1) Pre- and postdelivery hormonal variations associated with the initiation and maintenance of lactation.

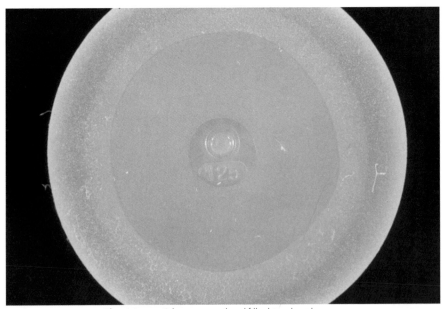

Plate 4 (Fig. 14-14) This Mentor Siltex textured gel-filled implant has an opaque appearance. A relatively large patch covers the majority of the back of the implant. In the center of the back is a circle containing a central raised gel fill point with the size marked in an oval.

amination. If the cyst has not recurred, routine screening guidelines may be followed. However, if the mass is still palpable after drainage, mammography is indicated in most cases, and the mass should be excised to rule out intracystic carcinoma. This entity is very rare but must be considered if a mass persists or recurs repeatedly after two or three aspirations. The biochemical composition of cyst fluid varies, depending on whether the cyst is lined by flattened epithelium or apocrine cells. Unfortunately, determination of the composition of cyst fluid has not been helpful in predicting cancer risk.

Ultrasound may be performed as a primary study in a young patient with a palpable mass or may be performed to define the character of a mass seen on mammography. In either case, the ultrasound appearance of a cyst may help determine further management. If a cyst is simple with well-defined margins, posterior acoustic enhancement, and no internal echoes, no further diagnostic studies are necessary and drainage is optional. If these criteria are not met, aspiration should be performed.

REFERRAL

The timing of the referral of a patient with a breast lump to a general surgeon differs dramatically from physician to physician. Some gynecologists prefer to manage breast complaints themselves unless or until mastectomy is required. Others refer the patient immediately after finding a lump. It is common practice to perform FNA in the gynecologist's office if the mass presents benign characteristics on examination. If there is suspicion of cancer or if the mass is solid, most patients are referred.

The decision about when to refer depends greatly on the clinician's interests and experience. Although surgically capable, most gynecologists have not been trained to perform ductal excisions, open (excisional) biopsies, or needle-localized biopsies. Such training is not likely in residency and must be gained through preceptorship with a gynecologic or general surgeon who is experienced in these techniques. The gynecologist also must be granted privileges to perform these procedures in his or her hospital. The decision to grant privileges may depend on the relationship between general surgeons and obstetrician–gynecologists at a particular institution and the perceived boundaries between the specialties.

COMMONLY ASKED QUESTIONS

1. **I've noticed a lump in my breast that waxes and wanes in size with time. Sometimes I can find it, and sometimes I can't. Should I be worried?** No. As long as a palpable lump gets smaller at times, it probably represents fibrocystic change and is not of great concern. Generally, neoplasms do not regress in size even when benign. An exception might be a fibroadenoma that gets slightly smaller postpartum. In a young woman in whom a lump is unlikely to be cancer, follow-up over a few menstrual cycles often is warranted before aggressive evaluation begins. In a woman over 35 years of age, however, any lump deserves analysis.

2. **I've had mastitis three times so far, and I'm only 4 months postpartum. How can I prevent it from coming back again?** Most commonly, mastitis is associated with milk stasis. Complete, regular evacuation of milk from the ducts may help prevent bacteria from having a chance to multiply and cause infection. The patient should vary the breast-feeding positions and/or employ a breast pump to ensure that all portions of the breast are drained consistently. Also, she should not stop taking antibiotics before a 10-day course is complete.

3. **I had a breast biopsy a few years ago that was benign. Since then, it seems like there's a lump right next to my scar. Should I be worried?** Depending on how much tissue was removed with the biopsy, examination may reveal skin retraction, a firm area under or near the scar, a depression beneath the scar, and even an area adjacent to the biopsy site that feels like a lump. All these findings may result from fat necrosis in the surrounding breast tissue. Imaging studies may or may not be helpful because calcification also commonly occurs. Several months after the biopsy, once the healing process is complete, any further changes in the patient's self-examination or clinical examination warrant evaluation. If any suspicion for cancer exists, a core biopsy may be indicated.

4. **I've had a breast lump since I was 25 years old and am told it's a fibroadenoma. It keeps growing slowly, and now that I'm 35, I wonder if I should have it removed.** Fibroadenomas are benign solid tumors that are hormone-sensitive. They typically grow until menopause and then shrink a bit. Factors that favor excision when a fibroadenoma is first detected include proving the diagnosis histologically, preventing further growth that may lead to breast asymmetry, assuring the patient that she is healthy, and removing an obstacle to complete breast examination. Excision causes a skin scar and possible fat necrosis of the breast tissue that could obscure future examinations. Some clinicians consider excision unnecessary when the clinical suspicion for cancer is extremely low. The patient should be included in the decision-making process.

SUGGESTED READING

Bianchi S, Palli D, Galli M, Zampi G. Benign breast disease and cancer risk. *Crit Rev Oncol Hematol* 1993; 15:221–242.

Connolly JL, Schnitt SS. Clinical and histologic aspects of proliferative and non-proliferative benign breast disease. *J Cell Biochem Suppl* 1993; 17G:45–48.

Feig SA. Breast masses—mammographic and sonographic evaluation. *Radiol Clin North Am* 1992; 30(1):67–92.

Galea M, Blamey RW. Diagnosis by team work: An approach to conservatism. *Br Med Bull* 1991; 47(2):295–304.

Kaufman Z, Shpitz B, Shapiro M, et al. Triple approach in the diagnosis of dominant breast masses: Combined physical examination, mammography, and fine-needle aspiration. *J Surg Oncol* 1994; 56(4):254–257.

Lindfors KK, Rosenquist CJ. Needle core biopsy guided with mammography: A study of cost-effectiveness. *Radiology* 1994; 190:217–222.

Love SM, McGuigan KA, Chap L. The Revlon/UCLA breast center practice guidelines for the treatment of breast disease. *Cancer J* 1996; 2(1):2–13.

Masood S. Recent updates in breast fine-needle aspiration biopsy. *Breast J* 1996; 2(1):3–12.

Page DL, Simpson JF. Benign, high-risk, and premalignant lesions of the mamma. In: Bland K, Copeland T, eds. *The Breast: Comprehensive Management of Benign and Malignant Diseases.* Philadelphia: Saunders; 1991:113–134.

Parker SH, Burbank F, Jackman RJ, et al. Percutaneous large-core breast biopsy: A multi-institutional study. *Radiology* 1994; 193:359–364.

Ramzy I. Pathology of benign breast disease. In: Mitchell GW, Bassett LW, eds. *The Female Breast and Its Disorders.* Baltimore: Williams & Wilkins; 1990:82–99.

BREAST PAIN

INTRODUCTION

Breast pain, also known as mastalgia or mastodynia, is second only to the presence of a lump as the most common breast complaint for which a woman seeks evaluation. Mastalgia may be mild and insignificant or may be so severe that it interferes with a woman's activities of daily living. Only 10 to 20 percent of women with this problem have sufficiently debilitating symptoms or concern about cancer to prompt a physician consultation. This chapter describes the various causes of breast pain (Table 5-1) and reviews the evaluation and treatment of affected patients.

ETIOLOGY

CYCLIC MASTALGIA

Mastalgia can be classified as cyclic or noncyclic, and this distinction guides evaluation and management. Mild premenstrual breast pain that lasts less than 7 days is considered normal; cyclic pain of greater severity or duration is considered abnormal. Most women with cyclic mastalgia are 30 to 40 years of age when the symptoms begin, and the problem usually waxes and wanes for years. It may resolve spontaneously in some patients, but more often it persists until menopause. The patient may state that her breasts feel "full, heavy, lumpy, and tender," especially in the upper outer quadrants. The symptoms are usually bilateral and may be severe enough to preclude intimate contact.

Cyclic breast pain is usually worst in the luteal phase of the menstrual cycle and

Mild premenstrual breast pain that lasts less than 7 days is considered normal; cyclic pain of greater severity or duration is considered abnormal.

TABLE 5-1 POSSIBLE CAUSES OF MASTALGIA

CYCLIC MASTALGIA	Hormonal imbalance or hypersensitivity, prolactin hypersensitivity, fibrocystic changes, nerve root irritation, breast cancer (rare)
NONCYCLIC MASTALGIA	Inflammation (mastitis, duct ectasia), thrombophlebitis, galactocele/engorgement, costochondritis, trauma/musculoskeletal pain, breast implants, angina, cervical radiculopathy, hiatal hernia/gastroesophageal reflux disease/ulcer, breast cancer (rare)

diminishes rapidly after the onset of menses. This close temporal relationship with the menstrual cycle and the effectiveness of medications that disrupt the normal hormonal milieu (e.g., danazol, tamoxifen) have suggested an endocrine basis for cystic mastalgia and/or fibrocystic changes (see Chap. 4).

Another proposed etiologic theory for cyclic mastalgia is hypersensitivity of the breast to the effects of steroid hormones. The mechanism of this sensitivity may be alteration of cell membranes in response to a relative deficiency of essential fatty acids. This theory is supported by the success of therapy with evening primrose oil, a rich source of linolenic acid.

The role of prolactin in cyclic mastalgia is unclear. Basal prolactin levels are often normal in these patients, but peak physiologic levels and the prolactin response to thyrotropin-releasing hormone stimulation may be increased. Bromocriptine, as is discussed below, is significantly more effective than placebo in relieving breast pain.

The early theory that breast pain in the luteal phase is due to the relative estrogen excess seen with inadequate progesterone production by the corpus luteum has lost favor. Luteal serum progesterone concentrations are not consistently low in these patients, and progesterone supplementation in the luteal phase has been no more successful than has placebo in relieving pain.

Cyclic mastalgia often is thought of as synonymous with fibrocystic changes, and indeed, many women with fibrocystic changes have cyclic pain. Rapid expansion of a single cyst may cause point tenderness in one breast, whereas fibrosis or adenosis may cause more generalized tenderness. However, not all women with cyclic pain have histologic evidence of fibrocystic changes. For example, enlargement of a hormone-sensitive fibroadenoma may cause pain. Nerve root irritation caused by inflammation or breast engorgement in the luteal phase may be the underlying cause of the pain. Uncommonly, cyclic breast pain may be a symptom of an occult malignancy.

NONCYCLIC MASTALGIA

Noncyclic pain is much less common than its cyclic counterpart and usually presents later in life. It may be unilateral or bilateral and constant or intermittent and may resolve spontaneously in approximately 50 percent of patients. Noncyclic pain specific to the breast may be caused by an inflammatory process such as periductal mastitis, duct ectasia, mammary abscess, or thrombophlebitis. In a lactating woman, noncyclic mastalgia may be due to a galactocele, breast engorgement, or mastitis. Fewer than 10 percent of patients with noncyclic mastalgia as the only symptom have an underlying cancer, and most of these cancers are detected by clinical and mammographic examination.

Chest irritation caused by breast implants may be associated with noncyclic pain. Chest wall disorders can cause pain that is perceived by the patient as originating in the breast. The pain of costochondritis usually is confined to the upper medial aspect of one or both breasts. Traumatic injury and muscle strain are usually self-evident and resolve spontaneously. Angina may be misinterpreted by the patient and physician as breast pain because of a perceived superficial location. Cervical radiculopathy may be associated with chronic, nagging breast pain as well as physical signs of nerve root compression. Gastrointestinal problems such as hiatal hernia, gastroesophageal reflux, and peptic ulcer disease also may cause pain in the chest.

Fewer than 10 percent of patients with non-cyclic mastalgia as the only symptom have an underlying cancer, and most of these cancers are detected by clinical and mammographic examination.

EVALUATION

The first step in evaluating a patient with breast pain is the recording of a thorough history. The pain should be characterized in an effort to determine its cause. Specific location, duration, cyclicity, radiation, alleviating and aggravating factors, and prior treatment may help narrow down the possible etiologies. For example, unrecognized trauma to the breast may cause acute-onset continuous localized pain that may improve with the intake of nonsteroidal anti-inflammatory agents. Cyclic pain is more likely to be due to fibrocystic changes. The severity of the pain, including its effect on activities and lifestyle, should be described to determine whether it warrants pharmacologic treatment. Particular interest should be paid to related symptoms, medication use, a personal and family history of breast disease, recent lactation or nipple discharge, and caffeine and chocolate intake.

The physical examination should be careful and detailed. Ideally, clinical examination should be performed in the follicular phase of the menstrual cycle, when the breasts are least dense and tender. In addition to its importance in excluding palpable pathology, the examination may be viewed by the patient as an acknowledgment that her symptoms are being taken seriously. The presence of a dominant mass or nipple discharge should be evaluated thoroughly, using protocols such as the ones described in Chaps. 4 and 6. If a patient with mastalgia is 35 years of age or older, a normal physical examination should be followed by screening mammography.

To assist with further management, a symptom diary form (Table 5-2) and instructions on its completion should be provided to the patient. Daily recording of the occurrence and severity of pain as well as the days of menstrual bleeding may be useful if pharmacologic therapy is requested, as is discussed below.

TREATMENT

The patient's initial visit for evaluation of breast pain should be used as an opportunity to instruct her in the technique and timing of breast self-examination as well as the normal cyclic changes she can expect to discover during those examinations. Simple reassurance that her current breast examination is normal often will give the patient considerable relief.

A discussion of the possible benefits of noninvasive management options also should be undertaken. For example, continuous use of a well-fitting support bra

TABLE 5-2 MASTALGIA SYMPTOM DIARY

MONTHLY MASTALGIA/MENSTRUAL DIARY

MONTH																														
DAY OF CYCLE	1	2	3	4	5	6	7	8	9	10	11	12	13	14	15	16	17	18	19	20	21	22	23	24	25	26	27	28	29	30
DATE																														
BLEEDING (X)																														
BREAST EXAM																														
PAIN RATING 5																														
4																														
3																														
2																														
1																														
TREATMENT																														

GRADING OF BREAST PAIN (ASSESSED AT END OF DAY):
1. Not a problem today.
2. Noticed pain briefly today.
3. Manageable pain present several times today.
4. Pain present; interfered with activities.
5. Severe, disabling pain today.

may lessen discomfort. Avoidance of coffee, tea, colas, and chocolate, which contain methylxanthines, may alleviate symptoms in some women. Vitamin supplementation, especially vitamins A, E, and B complex, and decreased dietary fat intake (to < 15 percent of total calories) may benefit some women. Keep in mind that vitamins A and E are fat-soluble vitamins and that megadoses are not excreted readily. Women of childbearing age should avoid exceeding the recommended dietary allowance of vitamin A (2700 IU of preformed vitamin A or 8000 IU of beta-carotene) unless they are using contraception because megadoses of vitamin A can be teratogenic.

After sufficient discussion, many women decide to try to manage their pain without pharmacologic intervention. A repeat examination should be scheduled for 2 to 3 months unless the patient's symptoms have abated. For the 15 percent of patients who go on to request treatment, review of the completed symptom diary is helpful in defining the cyclicity of pain and its impact on the patient's lifestyle. This review allows the clinician to counsel the patient about the risks and expected success of various treatment options. Maintenance of the diary during treatment also will allow the physician to better gauge the efficacy of treatment.

For the 15 percent of patients who request treatment of mastalgia, review of the completed symptom diary is helpful in defining the cyclicity of pain, and its impact on the patient's lifestyle.

PHARMACOLOGIC OPTIONS

Pharmacologic treatment of cyclic mastalgia is usualy reserved for patients who have experienced severe pain for several months and in whom the pain lasts at least 7 days per month. In general, hormonal medications are more successful in the treatment of cyclic than noncyclic mastalgia. Their clinical effect is usually noticeable during the first month of use, and the need for them should be reassessed 3 to 6 months after therapy is initiated. The effect of dietary (fat reduction, caffeine avoidance) or nutritional (vitamin supplementation) modification may take 3 to 4 months to be achieved or may not be noticeable at all.

Mastalgia is often an intermittent problem of variable severity, and it frequently responds to treatment with placebo. Thus, the efficacy of medications used for the treatment of mastalgia should be analyzed in double-blind, placebo-controlled studies. Thus far, only danazol, bromocriptine, tamoxifen, and evening primrose oil have been proved to be more effective than placebo for the treatment of mastalgia. Birth control pills, nonsteroidal anti-inflammatory agents, diuretics, progesterone, vitamins, and fat restriction have not been consistently effective. The selection of a particular medication must be individualized on the basis of the timing and severity of symptoms, the likelihood of success, and the acceptability of side effects. The dosing and cost of the most effective pharmacologic treatments for mastalgia are listed in Table 5-3.

Only danazol, bromocriptine, tamoxifen, and evening primrose oil have been proved to be more effective than placebo for the treatment of mastalgia.

Danazol   Danazol is a synthetic steroid that suppresses the pituitary–ovarian axis and has weak androgenic activity. It is U.S. Food and Drug Administration (FDA)-approved for the treatment of fibrocystic breast disease and has been the most effective drug used to treat severe mastalgia. It may be prescribed in a dose of 50 to 200 mg twice daily, but rarely is a dose over 100 mg twice daily required. If therapy is successful, titration of the medication to a substantially lower dose over time is usually possible. After 2 months, a decrease to 100 mg every other day in the follicular phase and 100 mg per day in the luteal phase may be tried. After 6 months, therapy should be discontinued and the patient should be followed for recurrence of symptoms. If reinstitution of therapy is necessary, the dose of 100 mg daily may again be decreased over time. Some patients may require only 400 to 600 mg per month to control symptoms, and even this dose should be discontinued periodically to reassess the symptoms. Unfortunately, the use of danazol often is limited by androgenic side effects. The possibility of weight gain, oily skin, acne, and hirsutism should be discussed with the patient before treatment. The rare but potentially significant problem of deepening of the voice may not be reversible after treatment ceases. Danazol can cause androgenic effects on a female fetus and at the doses listed above may not prevent ovulation. Therefore, nonhormonal contraception is required in these patients.

Bromocriptine   Bromocriptine is an ergot derivative with dopamine agonist activity. It has been shown to reduce cyclic breast pain both during and up to 3 to 6 months after treatment. The serum prolactin concentration declines during treatment even if the baseline level is in the normal range before treatment. Using an

TABLE 5-3 DOSING AND COST COMPARISON FOR PHARMACOLOGIC TREATMENT OF MASTALGIA

MEDICATION	DOSE, MG	ROUTE	FREQUENCY	COST*
Danazol	50	PO	bid	$54
Bromocriptine	2.5	PV	q HS	$45
Tamoxifen	10	PO	qd	$36
Evening primrose oil	1000	PO	tid	$36

*Approximate cost for 30-day supply of medication.

oral dose of 2.5 mg twice per day, 75 percent of patients are able to tolerate the side effects of nausea, vomiting, and dizziness. Therapy should begin at a dose of 1.25 to 2.5 mg at bedtime and increased gradually. Intravaginal administration of the tablets allows better absorption of the drug with avoidance of gastrointestinal side effects. The once-daily dosing schedule associated with vaginal administration makes this the preferred route.

Tamoxifen   Tamoxifen is a nonsteroidal drug that competes with estrogen for breast receptor sites. It is FDA-approved for adjuvant treatment of breast cancer and is being studied for usefulness in the treatment of cyclic mastalgia. In a dose of 10 to 20 mg per day, its efficacy has been encouraging and the side effects of nausea, hot flashes, irregular bleeding, and vaginal discharge generally have been tolerable. The use of tamoxifen for the treatment of mastalgia should be regarded as experimental.

Evening Primrose Oil   Evening primrose oil has recently received attention as an effective nonhormonal treatment for mastalgia. This supplemental source of gamma-linolenic acid reverses the relative deficiency of essential fatty acids proposed to be present in these patients. It is available at natural-food and nutrition stores in the form of soft gel-caps. When the drug is taken in a dose of 1000 mg three times per day, up to half of patients with cyclic mastalgia and a quarter of those with noncyclic mastalgia may find relief. Evening primrose oil is well tolerated, and the side effects are minimal. It is an excellent option for patients who are expected to require long-term therapy, those who are not candidates for hormonal therapy, and those who do not wish to discontinue taking oral contraceptive pills. Unfortunately, evening primrose oil therapy can be fairly expensive, with a 1-day supply costing approximately $1.50. Therapeutic efficacy may not be achieved until 3 to 4 months after the initiation of treatment.

Up to half of patients with cyclic mastalgia and a quarter of those with noncyclic mastalgia find relief by taking evening primrose oil 1000 mg three times per day.

GnRH Agonists   The pseudomenopause induced by gonadotropin-releasing hormone (GnRH) agonists consistently improves the symptoms of cyclic mastalgia. However, their use should be avoided in the management of mastalgia for several reasons. GnRH agonists are expensive (approximately $300 per dose), cause menopausal side effects such as vasomotor instability and vaginal dryness, and, when used for more than 6 months, have undesirable effects on lipids and bone mineral density.

TREATMENT OF NONCYCLIC MASTALGIA

As was mentioned above, noncyclic mastalgia frequently resolves spontaneously and often improves with placebo alone. These factors make it difficult to define the frequency of success of various treatment regimens. The medications discussed above may be helpful but generally are less effective than they are when used to treat cyclic pain. A search for the specific cause of noncyclic mastalgia may allow a focused treatment plan to be devised.

Duct ectasia, which may be the end result of chronic periductal inflammation, occurs most commonly in women in the late premenopausal years. Warm compresses may hasten the resolution of this problem, but if bacterial infection is present, antibiotics effective against staphylococcal organisms are required. Nonsteroidal anti-inflammatory drugs (NSAIDs) also may be helpful. Mondor's disease, or superficial thrombophlebitis of the breast veins, may cause upper outer quadrant breast pain associated with a palpable cord. The problem usually resolves spontaneously, but NSAIDs may be of value.

In a lactating woman, breast engorgement usually subsides within 2 to 3 weeks of the onset of breast-feeding. If a postpartum patient does not wish to breast-feed, she should wear a snug-fitting support bra. The use of bromocriptine for postpartum lactation suppression is no longer recommended by the manufacturer because of concern about the risk of severe hypertension, seizure, and stroke. Its use should be reserved for only the most severe cases of engorgement.

Puerperal mastitis usually is associated with unilateral localized breast pain, erythema, and induration. Systemic symptoms also may be present. Antibiotic treatment (see Chap. 4) must be timely to prevent abscess formation, and breast-feeding should continue during treatment. Occasionally, burning or shooting breast pain after feedings or persistent nipple pain is associated with candidiasis. Treatment consists of oral nystatin or local miconazole application.

Breast pain is an uncommon complaint after menopause unless the patient is taking exogenous hormones. Then, depending on the hormone replacement regimen prescribed, a woman may experience cyclic or noncyclic pain. A woman who initiates hormone replacement therapy and then experiences pain may be concerned about the possibility that the pain is being caused by cancer. With reassurance that the examination and mammogram are normal, many women agree to continue hormone replacement therapy.

> *Breast pain is an uncommon complaint after menopause unless the patient is taking exogenous hormones.*

COMMONLY ASKED QUESTIONS

1. **My breasts get so sore before my period that it hurts to take my bra off. I was told to eliminate caffeine and chocolate intake, but it doesn't seem to help. What can I do?** Many woman notice improvement in cyclic mastalgia when they curtail their methylxanthine intake, but for others, no change in the symptoms occurs. If the discomfort is brief, wearing a "sports bra" at bedtime may be all that is needed. If the symptoms are severe or last longer than a few days, the patient may want to try taking evening primrose oil, 1000 mg three times daily throughout the month. Most women find relief within a few months.

2. **When I take the pill for birth control, I notice that I have more breast pain before my period. Should I try something else?** Oral contraceptive pills have not been shown to affect cyclic mastalgia any more than placebo does. However, for women who experience premenstrual breast pain, an alternative form of contraception that may be of benefit is intramuscular injection of depot medroxyprogesterone acetate 150 mg every 3 months. Ovulatory cycles generally cease, and most women become amenorrheic by the third injection. Mastalgia usually improves.

3. **Ever since I started taking hormone replacement therapy 3 months ago, I have experienced severe tenderness in my breasts. Should I stop taking it?** A common side effect of hormone replacement therapy in postmenopausal women is noncyclic mastalgia. Many women stop taking the medication because of the pain or out of fear that the pain represents cancer. Reassurance that the pain typically diminishes with time is all that many women need in order to continue their therapy. An alternative is to recommend raloxifene therapy. Raloxifene is a selective estrogen receptor modulator (SERM) that does not affect the breast or endometrium. It has similar effects to estrogen for the prevention of osteoporosis and adverse changes in lipid levels after menopause. However, raloxifene does not prevent hot flashes or urogenital atrophy.

SUGGESTED READING

BeLieu RM. Mastodynia. *Obstet Gynecol Clin North Am* 1994; 21(3):461–477.

Drukker BH. Fibrocystic change of the breast. *Clin Obstet Gynecol* 1994; 37(4):903–915.

Gately CA, Mansel RE. Management of the painful and nodular breast. *Br Med Bull* 1991; 47(2):284–294.

Gately CA, Mansel RE. Management of cyclical breast pain. *Br J Hosp Med* 1990; 43:330–333.

Mansel RE, Dogliotti L. European multicentre trial of bromocriptine in cyclical mastalgia. *Lancet* 1990; 335:190–193.

NIPPLE DISCHARGE

INTRODUCTION

Nipple discharge in a nonlactating woman is an uncommon presenting complaint and is usually of benign etiology. However, it may be the harbinger of breast or central nervous system disease and therefore warrants evaluation. Unexpected nipple discharge may be spontaneous or provoked, unilateral or bilateral, and may egress through one or many duct openings. On breast self-examination, many nonlactating women are able to express a small amount of milky, gray, or even dark-colored sticky discharge from numerous ducts, and this is considered normal. More of a concern is spontaneous discharge, especially if it is watery, serous or serosanguineous, unilateral, or from a single duct opening.

This chapter discusses the most common causes of abnormal nipple discharge and proposes a strategy for its evaluation.

ETIOLOGY

GALACTORRHEA

Galactorrhea is persistent milky nipple discharge that is not related to pregnancy or lactation. Usually, it is bilateral and involves numerous ducts (Fig. 6-1). The discharge does not contain blood or pus, and low-power microscopic examination of the discharge reveals copious fat droplets (Fig. 6-2). Galactorrhea typically comes to the attention of the physician after the patient notices spontaneous discharge or discharge that is present during breast self-examination. The condition is caused by an excessive level of bioactive prolactin.

Galactorrhea does not contain blood or pus, and low-power microscopic examination of the discharge reveals copious fat droplets.

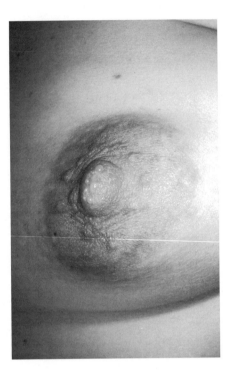

FIGURE 6-1 Photograph depicting milky discharge, or galactorrhea, emanating from numerous ducts.

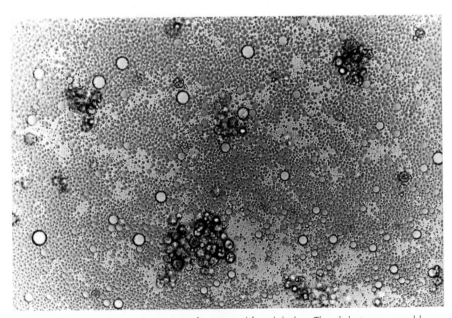

FIGURE 6-2 Low-power microscopy of unstained fat globules. The slide is prepared by placing a drop of discharge on a clean glass slide and covering it with a coverslip. Characteristic features include perfectly round fat globules suspended in a granular-appearing fluid. Scattered groups of cells represent foamy macrophages.

Prolactin is the pituitary hormone that is responsible for milk production. Control of prolactin secretion is due primarily to the negative effect of the hypothalamic prolactin inhibitory factor (PIF) dopamine. Thus, prolactin secretion occurs when dopamine release is decreased. Inhibition of dopamine release may be due to decreased production, depletion of dopamine stores, or blockade of dopamine receptors. In addition, thyrotropin-releasing hormone, serotonin, and other substances may be direct stimulators of prolactin release.

Hyperprolactinemia has many possible secondary causes (Table 6-1), most of which are reversible. Numerous medications have the potential to affect prolactin secretion. For example, the estrogen in oral contraceptives has a direct stimulatory effect on lactotrophs in the anterior pituitary. Phenothiazines, metoclopramide, diazepam, tricyclic antidepressants, and reserpine deplete dopamine or block its receptors. Discontinuation of the causative medication usually results in the return of prolactin levels to normal and the cessation of galactorrhea within 3 to 6 months.

Suckling causes milk production by suppressing PIF formation. Chest wall irritation as may occur with herpes zoster, breast implants, scarring, trauma, and aggressive foreplay or breast self-examination can activate the same afferent arc that suckling activates and result in galactorrhea. Primary hypothyroidism can cause galactorrhea as a result of the prolactin-stimulating effect of thyrotropin-releasing

TABLE 6-1 CAUSES OF HYPERPROLACTINEMIA AND GALACTORRHEA

HYPOTHYROIDISM	Thyroid releasing factor (TRF) causes prolactin release
MEDICATIONS	Estrogen/oral contraceptives Phenothiazines Metoclopramide Diazepam Tricyclic antidepressants Reserpine
SIMULATION OF SUCKLING REFLEX	Breast-feeding Shingles Breast implants Scarring Trauma Aggressive foreplay Frequent and/or aggressive self-examinations
STRESS	Trauma Surgery
CENTRAL CAUSES	Empty sella syndrome Lactotroph hyperplasia Prolactinoma Sellar impingement (central nervous system tumors) Hypothalamic tumors
DECREASED PROLACTIN CLEARANCE	Renal failure

hormone. Stress, surgery, and trauma also may inhibit PIF and lead to galactor-rhea.

Central causes of hyperprolactinemia include the empty sella syndrome, lactotroph hyperplasia, a prolactin-secreting pituitary tumor, and impingement of the pituitary stalk by other masses, such as a craniopharyngioma. The critical location of the pituitary gland transforms a "benign" tumor into a dangerous entity. The most significant problems caused by pituitary expansion are visual impairment (bitemporal hemianopsia) and headaches, but hyperprolactinemia also may cause anovulation. Tumors of the hypothalamus and stress may affect hypothalamic dopamine secretion and cause hyperprolactinemia. Renal failure also may cause hyperprolactinemia as a result of decreased prolactin clearance.

OTHER CAUSES OF NIPPLE DISCHARGE

The differential diagnosis of nipple discharge includes galactorrhea, fibrocystic change, intraductal papilloma, duct ectasia, mastitis, and cancer.

The differential diagnosis of nipple discharge includes galactorrhea, fibrocystic change, intraductal papilloma, duct ectasia, mastitis, and cancer (Table 6-2). The color of the discharge and the number of ducts involved help distinguish these problems from galactorrhea. As was mentioned above, the milky discharge of galactorrhea usually emanates from many ducts and is usually bilateral. Discharge that is other than white in color, is unilateral, or comes from one or a few ducts may be caused by one of these other conditions. Maceration of the skin of an inverted nipple also may cause a discharge that resolves with meticulous hygiene.

Cystic changes in the breast may wax and wane in response to hormonal variation. A cyst that maintains ductal communication may resolve after an episode of nipple discharge that is often green in color. Intraductal papillomas are usually asymptomatic, but the patient may present with a spontaneous serous or bloody discharge. A subareolar thickening or mass may be palpable on examination. Duct ectasia caused by chronic inflammation is associated with an increase in glandular secretions that often is seen as a colored nipple discharge. Nonpuerperal mastitis is uncommon, but inflammation of the periareolar area may cause a multicolored discharge. Bilateral sanguineous nipple discharge in pregnancy is typically benign and is caused by damage to the fragile ductal epithelium. Mammary duct fistulas are uncommon and occur in response to chronic inflammation or abscess formation. Cancer typically does not present with nipple discharge in the absence of a mass, but if the discharge is clear, serous, serosanguineous, or sanguineous, cancer risk is

Discharge in the presence of a mass should be considered to represent cancer until proved otherwise.

TABLE 6-2 CAUSES OF NONMILKY NIPPLE DISCHARGE

Fibrocystic changes

Intraductal papilloma

Duct ectasia

Mastitis

Skin maceration with inverted nipple

Mammary duct fistulas

Cancer

increased. Discharge in the presence of a mass should be considered to represent cancer until proved otherwise.

EVALUATION

The first step in establishing the etiology of nipple discharge is the recording of a thorough history. As was discussed in Chap. 2, a historical review is helpful in identifying risk factors for breast disease, current medications, and characteristics of the discharge. The patient should be asked about the duration of the problem, the quantity of discharge, and characteristics of the discharge (spontaneous versus provoked, unilateral versus bilateral).

Physical examination of the breasts should follow the algorithm outlined in Chap. 2. If the discharge is not easily expressed, the patient may be able to assist. The number of involved ducts should be noted, and the discharge should be tested for the presence of blood with a Hemoccult card or dipstick. It then may be examined microscopically for the presence of fat. White color, absence of blood, and presence of fat globules are diagnostic of galactorrhea. If the discharge is confirmed to be milk, as was defined above, the next step in the evaluation is measurement of serum prolactin and thyroid-stimulating hormone levels. The serum prolactin concentration may be normal or elevated in a patient with galactorrhea. If it is elevated, a search for confounding causes should begin. A prolactin level below 100 ng/mL may be attributable to medication use or chest wall irritation, but these factors rarely cause an elevation greater than 100 ng/mL. In any patient without an obvious cause of hyperprolactinemia, radiographic evaluation of the sella turcica is indicated. Computed tomography (CT) scan has replaced a coned down view of the sella as the most commonly performed study. Magnetic resonance imaging (MRI) is much more expensive but is now the gold standard for the diagnosis of sellar pathology (Fig. 6-3).

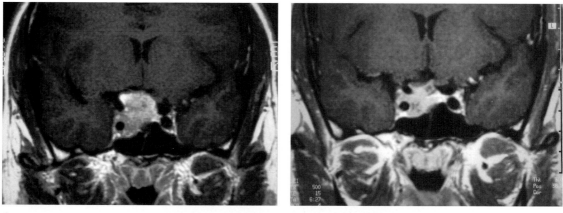

A   **B**

FIGURE 6-3 *A.* MRI of the head demonstrating a pituitary macroadenoma before treatment with bromocriptine. Note the convexity of the sella. *B.* After bromocriptine administration, MRI demonstrates dramatic shrinkage of the prolactinoma. The previous area of convexity has become concave.

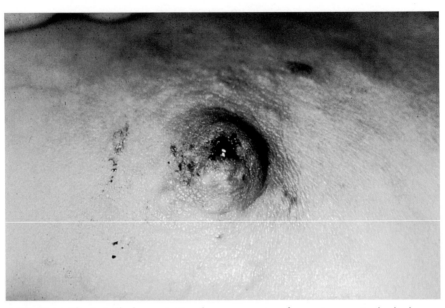

FIGURE 6-4 Photograph demonstrating the appearance of sanguineous nipple discharge. This finding could be associated with an intraductal papilloma or a malignancy.

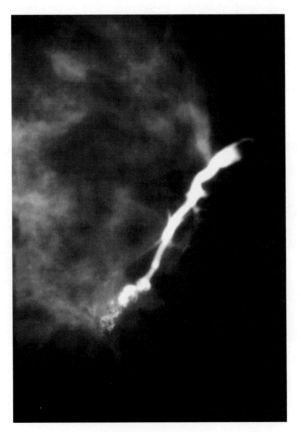

FIGURE 6-5 Contrast mammogram, or ductogram, demonstrating abrupt cessation of contrast flow within a duct. This patient was found to have invasive cancer.

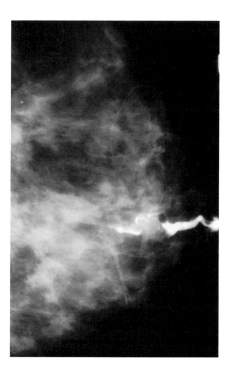

FIGURE 6-6 This ductogram also shows an abrupt cutoff of contrast flow. This patient had an intraductal papilloma.

Historically, cytologic evaluation of nipple discharge was recommended. However, the overall high false-negative rate led to controversy regarding its cost-effectiveness. Sanguineous (Fig. 6-4) or watery discharge is more highly associated with cancer than is colored or sticky discharge, making cytologic evaluation warranted in these cases. Positive results may influence further management plans.

If the discharge is not milk and is heme-negative and no mass is palpable, the next step should be mammography. If the results are negative, the patient should be reexamined in 3 months. If the discharge is heme-positive, ductography may be able to demonstrate the location of an abnormality or allow staining of the duct for easier surgical identification.

Ductography, or contrast mammography, involves examination of the nipple under magnification to allow the introduction of a 30-gauge catheter or needle into the affected duct or ducts. Contrast material is injected, and magnified mammographic images are obtained (Figs. 6-5 and 6-6). Ductography may demonstrate the classic appearance of duct ectasia or fibrocystic changes, in which case surgical excision of a duct may be avoided. More commonly, an abnormality on ductography is nonspecific, and excision is required to rule out malignancy. Duct cannulation also allows the instillation of methylene blue dye to aid the surgeon in localizing excision to only the duct in question. If a poorly visualized cyst is seen communicating with a duct, air can be injected to improve contrast and allow better delineation of the features of the cyst wall.

If a breast mass is palpable in a patient with nipple discharge, tissue sampling by fine needle aspiration (FNA) or biopsy is necessary for diagnosis. If cytology of the FNA is positive for malignancy, definitive management may be planned. However, a negative FNA does not exclude malignancy, and excision of the mass is required. Mammography is still necessary to rule out a concurrent nonpalpable abnormality.

If a breast mass is palpable in a patient with nipple discharge, tissue sampling by FNA or biopsy is necessary for diagnosis.

TREATMENT

GALACTORRHEA

A sample management protocol for galactorrhea and nonmilk nipple discharge is presented in Figure 6-7. If hyperprolactinemia and galactorrhea result from hypothyroidism, thyroid hormone supplementation will allow serum prolactin levels to return to normal. In a patient with normal prolactin and thyroid-stimulating hormone levels, treatment is not required unless the discharge is significantly bothersome. Bromocriptine (see below) is effective in eliminating galactorrhea in the face of normal or elevated prolactin levels. If the prolactin level is mildly elevated (<100 ng/mL) and no overt etiology can be found, baseline sellar imaging and periodic follow-up are indicated. With a normal CT scan or MRI, prolactin measurements may be repeated every 12 months if the levels remain stable. Repeat imaging is indicated if the prolactin level rises. Again, bromocriptine should be used only if indicated for the treatment of symptoms of galactorrhea or oligoovulation.

If the patient has a prolactin level above 100 ng/mL or if sellar imaging demonstrates a pituitary tumor, treatment should be based on symptoms, tumor size, and rapidity of tumor growth. There are several management strategies, each with unique risks and benefits. Although surgical treatment is a safe and initially effective option, tumor recurrence is common. Surgery usually is reserved for the treatment of large or rapidly expanding tumors that are not responsive to bromocriptine. Some tumors regress spontaneously, and most are very slow-growing, making observation a reasonable option in many cases.

Pharmacologic therapy with bromocriptine is useful to shrink or prevent the growth of prolactinomas, allowing close surveillance instead of surgery for most pa-

Pharmacologic therapy with bromocriptine is useful to shrink or prevent the growth of prolactinomas, allowing close surveillance instead of surgery for most patients.

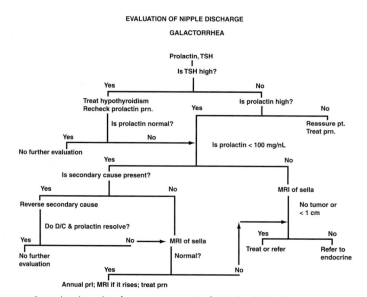

FIGURE 6-7 Sample algorithm for management of nipple discharge.

tients. To avoid the side effects of postural hypotension and dizziness, bromocriptine therapy should begin with a low dose (1.25 to 2.5 mg) at bedtime. After 3 days, a twice-daily regimen may be instituted. The dose is increased every 3 to 7 days until the prolactin level returns to normal. The therapeutic dose ranges from 2.5 to 15 mg per day. Bromocriptine tablets may be administered orally (with food) or intravaginally. The vaginal route has two main advantages: The common side effects of nausea and vomiting are avoided, and drug absorption is improved. The longer serum half-life that results makes once-daily dosing feasible.

Surveillance of patients with microadenomas (< 1 cm) managed conservatively should include a prolactin level every 6 months. Repeat CT or MRI studies should be based on symptoms, examination, and prolactin levels. Patients with macroadenomas (> 1 cm) always require treatment to prevent the serious complication of vision loss. Once the prolactin level returns to normal, it should be reevaluated every 6 months. Imaging studies should be repeated if the prolactin level rises again.

TREATMENT OF OTHER CAUSES OF NIPPLE DISCHARGE

The sticky, often dark discharge seen with cyclic cystic changes in the breast is usually self-limiting and does not require treatment. Intraductal papillomas should be treated by local excision of the involved duct (see Chap. 10). This procedure requires anesthesia in an operating room setting. The discharge associated with chronic inflammation in duct ectasia may resolve with the application of warm compresses several times per day for 2 to 3 weeks. Mastitis can be cured with antibiotic therapy alone unless abscess formation has occurred, in which case incision and drainage are required. Mammary duct fistulas result from recurrent drainage of a subareolar abscess. Treatment requires the administration of a local anesthetic to the nipple and the passage of a probe through the fistulous tract between the involved duct orifice and the skin. Incision of the skin overlying the probe with a scalpel allows drainage; healing then occurs by secondary intention. If evaluation of nipple discharge leads to the diagnosis of cancer, treatment will be determined by clinical indicators.

Even if ductography suggests a benign papilloma, the presence of bloody nipple discharge should prompt excision of the duct.

COMMONLY ASKED QUESTIONS

1. **I stopped breast-feeding my baby over a year ago, but I still sometimes leak milk. Is that normal?** Some normal parous women can elicit a small amount of nipple discharge by stripping the ducts from the periphery toward the nipple and then squeezing the areola below the nipple. However, spontaneous galactorrhea is not normal this long after weaning. Once suckling ceases, prolactin levels should return to normal within weeks and milk should no longer be produced. Spontaneous galactorrhea may be a sign of hyperprolactinemia, and the prolactin level should be checked.

2. **I was diagnosed with a prolactin-secreting pituitary adenoma and am taking bromocriptine. Should I stop the medication before I start trying to conceive?** Many women with hyperprolactinemia do not ovulate regularly and have oligo- or amenorrhea. The administration of a dopamine agonist (e.g., bromocriptine or cabergoline) is indicated in these situations to help the patient resume her ovulatory cycles. Once conception has occurred, the decision about whether to discontinue the drug should be based on the size of the tumor and its response to treatment. Prolactin levels rise during pregnancy,

making them no longer useful for monitoring purposes. Symptoms of headache or visual disturbance and signs of optic chiasm compression (bitemporal hemianopsia on visual fields testing) become more useful indicators of change in tumor size. Bromocriptine and cabergoline are Category B drugs and may be used during pregnancy if needed.

3. **How should hyperprolactinemia be evaluated in a patient with a severe psychiatric disorder that is well controlled on a phenothiazine medication?** Because these drugs commonly are associated with elevations in serum prolactin, the question becomes whether the drug should be discontinued in order to determine whether the prolactin level will return to normal. If the patient has been difficult to stabilize from a psychiatric standpoint, continuation of the medication and evaluation of the sella turcica by magnetic resonance imaging is an alternative.

SUGGESTED READING

Cardenosa G, Doudna C, Eklund GW. Ductography of the breast: Technique and findings. *AJR* 1994; 162:1081–1087.

Conry C. Evaluation of a breast complaint: Is it cancer? *Am Fam Physician* 1994; 49(2): 445–450.

Gulay H, Bora S, Sadik K, et al. Management of nipple discharge. *J Am Coll Surg* 1994; 178(5):471–474.

Speroff L, Glass RH, Kase NG. Amenorrhea. In: *Clinical Gynecologic Endocrinology and Infertility,* 6th ed. Baltimore: Williams & Wilkins; 1999:421–460.

MANAGEMENT OF EARLY BREAST CANCER

Breast cancer usually is an indolent and slow-growing disease. When it is not treated, the median survival is about 3 years from the diagnosis. Metastases usually develop within the first 2 years after surgical treatment but can occur as late as 25 years after the initial diagnosis. The most likely cause of death in a woman with breast cancer 5 to 10 years after treatment is metastatic disease.

The preclinical period, when a tumor is too small to be recognized, may be prolonged. With a doubling time of 100 days, 8 years would be required for a single neoplastic cell to become a 1-cm mass. Current data suggest that metastasis rarely occurs until after a primary tumor reaches 0.5 cm in size. Early detection of breast cancer with mammography screening therefore improves the survival rate of breast cancer patients.

STAGING

Breast cancer staging describes the anatomic extent of disease and thus guides decision making regarding the appropriate therapy. When uniform criteria for staging are employed universally by treating physicians, data on the outcomes of different treatment regimens can be collected and compared. Such retrospective reviews are the source of important prognostic information.

Early-stage breast disease may be eradicated by surgery alone, while late-stage disease requires adjunctive chemotherapy and radiotherapy. The size of the untreated tumor (T) increases progressively. Local invasion probably occurs early in the disease process and is followed by spread to the regional lymph nodes that drain

71

the area of the tumor. Lymph node (N) involvement in breast cancer is a marker of the progression of disease and can be noted on clinical examination of the patient. Finally, distant metastases (M) to the lung, brain, bone, and liver cause death from metastatic disease.

The TNM staging system (Table 7-1) was developed by the American Joint Committee on Cancer (AJCC) in cooperation with the TNM Committee of the International Union against Cancer (UICC). The TNM system incorporates both clinical and pathologic features of breast disease; for the purposes of this discussion, the clinical staging system will be emphasized. Clinical staging includes physical examination with careful inspection and palpation of the skin, breasts, and lymph nodes (axillary, supraclavicular, and cervical). Histologic examinaton of a breast tumor establishes the diagnosis of breast cancer and determines tumor size, the presence or absence of chest wall invasion, and the presence or absence of regional and distant metastases.

Clinical staging includes physical examination with careful inspection and palpation of the skin, breasts, and lymph nodes (axillary, supraclavicular, and cervical).

The clinical T measurement may be based on physical examination of the breast or on mammographic estimation of size, whichever is thought to be more accurate. The breast tumor is described as TX (data not available), T1 (primary tumor ≤ 2 cm), T2 (tumor > 2 cm but ≤ 5 cm), T3 (tumor > 5 cm), or T4 (any size tumor with skin or chest wall invasion). For the purposes of adjuvant therapy after surgery, T1 is subdivided into T1a (primary tumor ≤ 0.5 cm), T1b (tumor > 0.5 cm but ≤ 1 cm), and T1c (tumor > 1 cm but ≤ 2 cm). T4 is subdivided into T4a (chest wall exten-

TABLE 7-1 CLINICAL TNM STAGING FOR BREAST CANCER

T: PRIMARY TUMOR		
TX		Unknown
T0		No evidence of primary tumor
Tis		Carcinoma in situ, intraductal carcinoma
T1		Tumor ≤ 2 cm
	T1a	Tumor ≤ 0.5 cm
	T1b	Tumor > 0.5 cm but ≤ 1 cm
	T1c	Tumor > 1 cm but ≤ 2 cm
T2		Tumor > 2 cm but ≤ 5 cm
T3		Tumor > 5 cm
T4		Tumor involves chest wall or skin
	T4a	Extension to chest wall
	T4b	Extension to skin with edema or ulceration
	T4c	Both chest wall and skin extension
	T4d	Inflammatory carcinoma, involvement of dermal lymphatics

N: REGIONAL LYMPH NODES	
NX	Unknown
N0	No palpable nodes
N1	Palpable ipsilateral nodes
N2	Fixed or matted ipsilateral nodes
N3	Ipsilateral internal mammary nodes

M: DISTANT METASTASES	
MX	Unknown
M0	No distant metastasis
M1	Distant metastasis; includes ipsilateral, supraclavicular, and cervical nodes

sion) and T4b (inflammatory breast cancer documented by dermal lymphatic infiltration by cancer cells).

In the clinical TNM system, the N category is divided into four groups: NX (cannot be assessed), N0 (no palpable axillary lymph nodes), N1 (palpable axillary nodes), N2 (matted or fixed axillary nodes), and N3 (ipsilateral internal mammary adenopathy). Supraclavicular, cervical, and contralateral internal mammary adenopathy are considered to represent distant metastases (M0 absent, M1 present).

Breast cancer staging by the TNM system is accurate and specific but somewhat cumbersome in daily use. The stage groupings have evolved as a clinical shorthand to describe breast disease. Stage 0 (TisN0M0) refers to in situ tumors that have not penetrated the basement membrane of the ductule or lobule. Because there are no lymph node or distant metastases, these tumors have an excellent prognosis. Stage I (T1N0M0) refers to tumors ≤ 2 cm without metastases to the lymph nodes or distant organs. Stage IIA includes nonpalpable (T0N1M0) or small tumors (T1N1M0) with regional lymph node invasion and larger tumors without metastases (T2N0M0). Stage IIB describes a large tumor without metastases (T3N0M0) and carries a prognosis similar to that of stage IIA disease. Stage IIIA refers to any size tumor with fixed or matted lymph nodes (T0–3 N2). Stage IIIB refers to locally advanced disease (T4) and advanced regional metastases (N3). Stage IV refers to cases with documented distant metastases (any T, any N, M1).

The 5-year survival of breast cancer patients can be estimated roughly by the stage of disease at the time of diagnosis (Table 7-2). Stage 0, or preinvasive, disease is essentially curable, while stage IV is lethal.

The evaluation of a woman with newly diagnosed breast cancer begins with a detailed history. Occasionally, symptoms of metastatic disease become apparent. The next step is clinical staging using both physical examination and mammography. Physical examination can identify areas of palpable disease in the breast and regional lymph nodes. Mammography can help determine the size of the cancer, look for satellite lesions in the ipsilateral breast, and screen for disease in the contralateral breast before the planning of definitive surgical therapy.

Other imaging studies, such as magnetic resonance imaging (MRI), bone scan, and computed tomography (CT) scans of the chest, abdomen, or head, are used when a patient's history and physical examination suggest the presence of metastases. Routine CT for patients with early-stage cancer adds cost without conferring much benefit. Many studies have shown that exhaustive screening of asymptomatic women does not improve survival rates compared with testing only patients with

Mammography can help determine the size of the cancer and the presence of satellite lesions in the ipsilateral breast as well as screen for disease in the contralateral breast before the planning of definitive surgical treatment.

TABLE 7-2 BREAST CANCER SURVIVAL BY STAGE OF DISEASE

CLINICAL STAGE	5-YEAR SURVIVAL, %
Stage 0: Carcinoma in situ, no metastases	100
Stage I: Tumor < 2 cm, no metastases	85
Stage II: Tumor < 5 cm (T1 or T2) Nodes, if palpable, not fixed or matted (N0 or N1)	65
Stage III: Tumor > 5 cm (T3) or Tumor with involvement of chest wall and/or skin (T4)	40
Stage IV: Presence of distant metastases	10

symptomatic metastatic disease. Among asymptomatic patients who develop metastases, standard chest x-ray and serum liver function tests, combined with history and physical examination, will identify those who require further evaluation. CT is indicated in the presence of hepatosplenomegaly, abnormal liver function tests, or neurologic symptoms. Chest CT also may be used to determine the extent of disease in a woman with large palpable adenopathy and in planning for postoperative radiotherapy.

The use of bone scans in the staging of breast cancer is controversial. These radionuclide tests are very sensitive but not very specific for the presence of bony metastases. False-positive tests are seen with degenerative joint disease, osteoarthritis, and previous bone fracture. Plain films, CT, or MRI may be required to characterize an abnormal finding on bone scan, and so routine bone scans are not indicated in women with early-stage breast cancer. Bone scans are indicated, however, in patients with bone pain, advanced local disease (T3 or T4 lesions), or known metastatic disease. A baseline bone scan also is useful in patients at high risk for metastatic disease.

SURGICAL MANAGEMENT OF BREAST CANCER

The role of surgery in the treatment of breast cancer is to reduce tumor volume and prevent, or at least delay, tumor metastasis and death. In patients with early-stage breast cancer, surgical removal of the primary tumor prolongs disease-free survival. An improved understanding of the timing of cancer dissemination, along with the emergence of radiotherapy and chemotherapy as treatment adjuncts, has influenced the types of surgical procedures used for the primary treatment of breast cancer. Less disfiguring surgical approaches are now possible when combined with pre- or postoperative chemotherapy and irradiation.

Early-stage breast cancer is locoregional or confined, whereas later-stage disease becomes systemic. Surgical therapy is aimed at locoregional disease before its dissemination. As chemotherapy and radiation therapy become more sophisticated and are better tolerated by patients, wide surgical extirpations will no longer be necessary.

In the early twentieth century, the prevailing theory of cancer dissemination was that breast cancer spreads linearly from the breast to the underlying muscle, lymphatics, and bone. Thus, Halstead's radical mastectomy removed the breast, the pectoralis major and minor muscles, the axillary lymph node basin, and often the rib cage and clavicle as well. The modified radical mastectomy was developed in the mid-twentieth century and includes total mastectomy with removal of the tumor, ipsilateral breast tissue, overlying skin, and axillary lymphatics. However, the pectoralis major and the long thoracic and thoracodorsal nerves were preserved. The modified radical technique has been equivalent to radical mastectomy in terms of disease-free and overall survival in a number of carefully controlled, prospectively randomized clinical trials. The only remaining indication for radical mastectomy is a deep tumor with invasion and penetration of the pectoralis fascia and muscle.

The concept of surgical lumpectomy, or the removal of a palpable breast tumor with a rim of normal breast tissue, evolved from the success of prompt surgical management of early breast cancer. Lumpectomy has many accepted synonyms, including partial mastectomy, segmental mastectomy, segmentectomy, quadrantec-

Lumpectomy is removal of a palpable breast tumor with a surrounding rim of normal tissue. Simple (total) mastectomy is removal of the breast without the axillary contents.

tomy, and tylectomy, as well as wide excision or excisional biopsy to pathologically clear margins. All these terms refer to surgical excision of a breast tumor with normal breast tissue included as a "safe margin" to remove any tendrils of invasive carcinoma. For some early-stage breast cancers, such as small low-grade ductal carcinoma in situ (DCIS), lumpectomy alone constitutes appropriate management.

Breast conservation therapy is the term applied to the regimen of lumpectomy, axillary node dissection, and postoperative radiation therapy. The National Surgical Adjuvant Breast and Bowel Project (NSABP) B-06 trial demonstrated that breast conservation therapy is as effective as modified radical mastectomy in the treatment of stage I and stage II breast cancer. If radiation therapy is omitted after surgery, the recurrence rate is quite high.

Breast conservation therapy is combined lumpectomy, axillary node dissection, and postoperative radiation therapy.

Simple mastectomy, also called total mastectomy, means removal of the breast without the axillary contents. Simple mastectomy is used in stage 0, noninvasive carcinoma, and prophylactic mastectomy. Since pure DCIS and lobular carcinoma in situ (LCIS) do not spread to the lymphatics, removal of the axillary lymph nodes is not necessary. In women with biopsy-proved LCIS and a strong family history of breast and ovarian carcinoma, prophylactic mastectomy may be combined with immediate breast reconstruction.

The skin-sparing mastectomy is a version of the simple mastectomy that is used to remove subareolar tumors or for prophylaxis. It includes removal of the nipple-areolar complex and breast tissue with immediate reconstruction. Proponents of skin-sparing mastectomy note that breast skin is relatively sensate and that preservation of the inframammary fold results in a more cosmetic reconstruction.

Subcutaneous mastectomy is the surgical removal of breast tissue from a periareolar incision, leaving the nipple-areola complex intact. This procedure usually is reserved for the treatment of gynecomastia in men, but its use has been suggested for prophylactic mastectomy in women with a high risk of bilateral breast cancer. However, since breast tissue is left with the areola and nipple, subcutaneous mastectomy cannot be recommended for prophylaxis.

EARLY BREAST CANCER

Early breast cancer, which sometimes is called minimal breast disease, includes three clinical entities that often are confused but for which the treatment paradigms are quite different. Included in the early breast disease category are DCIS, LCIS, and early invasive carcinoma. These three types of early breast cancer can be envisioned as points along a timeline in the development of breast cancer. A long indolent period is represented by LCIS. As normal breast ductal epithelial cells undergo malignant transformation and pile up within the breast ducts, DCIS becomes evident. Finally, as the malignant cells penetrate the duct basement membrane and invade the lobular stroma of the breast, the process becomes infiltrating or invasive ductal carcinoma.

DUCTAL CARCINOMA IN SITU

Ductal carcinoma in situ is probably a true precursor of invasive ductal carcinoma. The average age at diagnosis of DCIS is the same as that for invasive disease: about 55 years. After surgical excision of DCIS, recurrences typically occur in the same site and often display invasive histology. The size and extent of DCIS are directly related to the incidence of multifocal disease and synchronous invasive foci. After treatment, the recurrence rate of DCIS is higher if the surgical margins were positive, and the rate can be decreased by postoperative radiation therapy.

The overall incidence of DCIS is 13 percent, and 50,000 new cases are diagnosed annually in the United States. In women who undergo screening mammography, about 40 percent of all newly diagnosed breast cancers are DCIS. The typical mammographic appearance of DCIS is radiologically dense tissue with multiple punctate calcifications. The disease also may present as a clinically palpable mass.

Histologically, DCIS is characterized by proliferation of the ductal epithelium to form papillary ingrowths into the duct lumen. These ingrowths crowd the lumen until the rounded spaces between papillary stalks produce a cribriform pattern (Fig. 7-1). Pure papillary DCIS has a more orderly appearance and shows nonaggressive biological behavior. Comedo DCIS develops as cells far from the epithelial capillary become anoxic and necrotic. Comedo DCIS is an aggressive subtype and contains more calcification, anaplasia, and possible microinvasion (Fig. 7-2). More recent histologic classifications divide DCIS into comedo and noncomedo subtypes, and this designation is important in making surgical treatment decisions.

The biological aggressiveness of DCIS also may be estimated by histologic assessment. Lesions with a higher nuclear grade, a high S-phase fraction, and aneuploid DNA are farther along the biological path to invasive carcinoma than are lesions with normal nuclei, a low S-phase fraction, and diploid DNA. Like invasive breast cancer, DCIS with a high mitotic rate has a recurrence risk approaching 20 percent.

Size and multifocality of DCIS also must be considered in determining appropriate therapy. Mammography can detect foci of DCIS as small as 0.5 cm in diameter. Larger lesions are associated with greater biological aggressiveness and

The typical mammographic appearance of DCIS is radiologically dense tissue with multiple punctate calcifications.

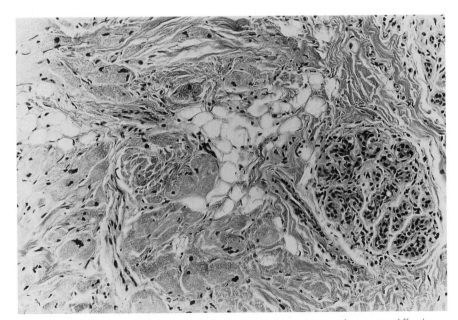

FIGURE 7-1 Ductal carcinoma in situ without necrosis may present diagnostic difficulties because of the absence of microcalcifications. Shown here is a breast duct (*200X*) with epithelial proliferation forming "stiff bridges." The basement membrane is not traversed.

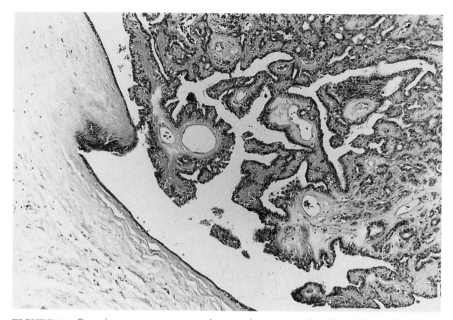

FIGURE 7-2 Ductal carcinoma in situ with comedonecrosis. The dilated breast duct lumen is plugged by carcinoma in situ. Note the central necrosis (comedonecrosis) indicated by smaller, pyknotic nuclei surrounded by cellular detritus.

multifocality. Most comedo lesions are large, aneuploid, and estrogen-receptor (ER)-negative.

Treatment options for DCIS include wide excision alone, wide excision with postoperative radiation, and simple mastectomy. Pure DCIS does not metastasize, and so axillary lymph node involvement is likely to be related to occult invasive disease. Thus, treatment does not include axillary lymph node dissection unless the final pathology report identifies invasive cancer in the specimen.

Few randomized studies have addressed the ideal width of the surgical excision margin for DCIS. Residual disease is found in up to 50 percent of reexcisions for "close" margins. Because of the high recurrence rate with DCIS, the entire breast usually should be treated by mastectomy or radiation. Exceptions to this rule include small cribriform tumors without necrosis and micropapillary variants. These subtypes rarely recur, and excision alone may be sufficient.

The role of postoperative radiotherapy for DCIS after wide excision was examined in the NSABP-17 study. In that trial, DCIS was not stratified according to size or histologic subtype, but the addition of radiation reduced the recurrence rate of DCIS at 4 years from 16.4 to 7.0 percent. The recurrence rate also is related to size (> 2.5 cm) and cribriform or comedo histology.

The risk of recurrence of DCIS after breast conservation (wide excision with postoperative radiation) is higher than that after mastectomy. However, the likelihood of metastasis is low, and recurrences are usually DCIS rather than invasive disease. Thus, wide excision to pathologically clear margins followed by radiation therapy is a reasonable alternative to mastectomy for DCIS.

Mastectomy is indicated for the treatment of large, aggressive, or multifocal DCIS. Retrospective studies of survival after mastectomy for DCIS reported survival

Because of the high recurrence rate with DCIS, the entire breast usually should be treated by mastectomy or radiation.

rates of almost 100 percent. Mastectomy may be favored over breast conservation therapy when the mammogram shows diffuse microcalcifications, the surgical margins show diffuse involvement of DCIS, or other factors, such as family history and previous contralateral breast cancer, are present. Mastectomy also is a reasonable choice for the treatment of lesions with a high nuclear grade, aneuploid DNA, a high S-phase fraction, and extensive necrosis.

Foci of microinvasion through the ductal basement membrane can be seen in some cases of DCIS, and the biological behavior of these lesions approaches that of invasive carcinoma. Wide excision with postoperative radiation therapy probably constitutes adequate treatment, yet with these lesions, axillary node metastases have been found in 5 to 10 percent of axillary dissection specimens. The rationale for breast conservation therapy in these cases is to preserve breast tissue so that salvage mastectomy can be performed if recurrence occurs. However, reconstruction after breast irradiation is problematic, and many surgeons prefer mastectomy with immediate reconstruction. Therapy must be individualized, and the histologic findings of each specific case must be considered. For example, DCIS with an occasional focus of microinvasion is probably a very different lesion from DCIS showing anaplasia, multiple areas of central necrosis, and widespread microinvasion.

LOBULAR CARCINOMA IN SITU

Not truly a premalignant lesion itself, LCIS is a risk factor for the subsequent development of breast cancer.

Not truly a premalignant lesion itself, lobular carcinoma in situ of the breast is a risk factor for the subsequent development of breast cancer. Its actual incidence is not known, but it is present in approximately 5 percent of breast biopsy specimens. Histologically, LCIS is characterized by distended terminal ducts filled with bland homogeneous cells without mitoses or necrosis (Fig. 7-3).

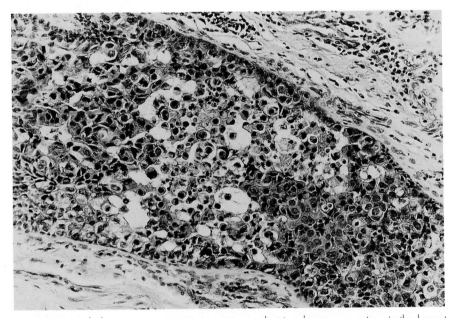

FIGURE 7-3 Lobular carcinoma in situ is a process that involves every acinus in the breast lobule. The tumor plugs the terminal lobuloalveolar units but does not traverse the basement membrane.

Lobular carcinoma in situ usually is diagnosed in premenopausal women around age 45. The fact that women with LCIS are 10 to 15 years younger than those diagnosed with invasive carcinoma lends support to the transition theory of breast cancer development. However, LCIS is now known to be a marker, rather than an anatomic precursor, of subsequent invasive disease. Cancers found 10 or 15 years after a diagnosis of LCIS usually have invasive ductal rather than lobular histology and are outside the area biopsied for LCIS. The relative risk of future invasive carcinoma is about 35 percent, and the risk is equal in both the ipsilateral breast and the contralateral breast. The incidence of simultaneous foci of invasive carcinoma at the time of diagnosis in either breast is around 5 percent. The relative amount of LCIS present in a biopsy specimen or the finding of multifocal LCIS does not predict the incidence or biological behavior of future invasive disease.

Treatment options for a woman diagnosed with LCIS include close follow-up and bilateral simple mastectomy. Negative surgical margins are not necessary with LCIS biopsies because the disease is frequently diffuse. Contralateral, or "mirror-image," biopsy of the contralateral, otherwise normal breast is not advised and would not change management decisions. Close follow-up with biannual physical examination and yearly mammography is reasonable. This expectant management plan also is used for women with increased breast cancer risk because of previous contralateral breast cancer or a positive family history of disease.

Treatment options for a woman diagnosed with LCIS include close follow-up and bilateral simple mastectomy.

Some women, especially young women who have a sister or mother with breast cancer, are unwilling to accept the 10 to 37 percent risk of subsequent invasive carcinoma after biopsy-proved LCIS. For these women, management is directed at both breasts. Treatment of one breast with simple mastectomy and biopsy of the contralateral breast is illogical because the risk of subsequent breast cancer is bilateral regardless of the original biopsy site. The only reasonable surgical option is bilateral simple mastectomy with or without reconstruction. In this case, all breast tissue, including the nipple-areola complex, is removed. A simple mastectomy rather than a modified radical mastectomy is recommended because the risk of axillary node metastases in patients with pure LCIS is less than 2 percent. If the lymph nodes were involved, the metastases would be from occult invasive breast cancer rather than from LCIS.

There is no role for adjuvant chemotherapy or radiation therapy in the treatment of LCIS. In the future, women with biopsy-proved LCIS may be candidates for a chemoprevention regimen such as tamoxifen. The NSABP tamoxifen trial may soon include women with LCIS and/or a family history of breast cancer.

EARLY INVASIVE BREAST CANCER

Randomized clinical trials have demonstrated that in patients with early invasive breast cancer (stage I or stage II), long-term survival is similar whether treatment consists of modified radical mastectomy or the combination of lumpectomy, axillary dissection, and irradiation. In 1990, the National Institutes of Health Consensus Panel on Early Breast Cancer concluded that breast conservation therapy is the preferred option in eligible patients. Of course, that recommendation is based on the definition of *eligible*.

Because multiple factors influence the outcome and prognosis in early-stage breast cancer patients, several centers have advocated a team approach to treatment. The team consists of the patient and her surgeon, a radiation therapist, a medical

In patients with early invasive breast cancer (stage I or stage II), long-term survival is similar whether treatment consists of modified radical mastectomy or the combination of lumpectomy, axillary dissection, and irradiation.

oncologist, and a plastic surgeon. The patient should be actively involved in the decision-making process, weighing the risk of recurrence and metastatic disease against her cosmetic concerns. The surgeon and the radiation therapist develop a plan to accomplish local control of disease, while the medical oncologist's role is the prevention or treatment of systemic disease. The plastic surgeon offers options for breast reconstruction, if necessary.

The goal of breast conservation therapy is to achieve local control of the disease while maintaining an acceptable cosmetic result. The success of this strategy depends on the size, location, and histology of the tumor. Breast conservation therapy generally is recommended for lesions less than 4 cm in diameter. However, the overall size of the patient's breast also must be considered. For example, a very large breast may not receive a uniform dose of radiation, and excision of a large tumor from a small breast may not yield an acceptable result.

In the past, the subareolar location of a breast cancer was considered a contraindication to breast conservation therapy. The recent demonstration that removal of the tumor and the nipple-areola complex can achieve a positive cosmetic result, with preservation of the natural inframammary fold and breast contour, has led to acceptance of this option.

When multiple primary lesions occur in the same breast, treatment with modified radical mastectomy usually is preferred. Occasionally, however, separate excisions with clear margins are possible. Distinct primary lesions within the same breast quadrant are more amenable to lumpectomy than are multiple scattered lesions.

The importance of breast cancer histology in decision making about modified radical mastectomy versus breast conservation therapy is not clear. Early reports of invasive lobular carcinoma suggested that recurrence was unacceptably high after lumpectomy and radiation therapy. Other studies have shown no statistically significant difference in recurrence rates. A recent review of over 1000 breast cancer patients followed for a median of 10.5 years after conservative treatment showed no difference in the relapse rate between any of the histologic subtypes. When excised appropriately, breast cancers of all histologic subtypes have similar recurrence rates, and a recurrence may be treated with salvage mastectomy.

Patient age and the presence of comorbid disease are additional factors to consider in planning breast cancer treatment. Very young and very old patients have higher and lower recurrence rates, respectively. Premenopausal women under age 40 experience a higher local failure rate with breast conservation therapy than do older women. Two obvious explanations for this finding are apparent. First, in the absence of comorbid disease, a young patient with breast cancer has a longer postsurgical life span in which to experience a recurrence. Second, tumors found in younger patients typically display more worrisome histologic features (e.g., high nuclear grade) and aggressive behavior than do tumors found in the elderly. The option of genetic testing should be offered to a premenopausal patient with breast cancer to better define the recurrence risk in the ipsilateral breast as well as the risk of developing a new primary tumor in the contralateral breast.

The option of genetic testing should be offered to a premenopausal patient with breast cancer to better define the recurrence risk in the ipsilateral breast as well as the risk of developing a new primary tumor in the contralateral breast.

Some breast cancer treatment centers do not recommend irradiation for patients over age 70. In the NSABP B-06 protocol, the addition of radiation therapy to surgical lumpectomy did not improve survival in these older patients significantly but did reduce the incidence of breast cancer recurrence. If an elderly patient has a low recurrence risk and a relatively short life expectancy, postoperative radiation for

TABLE 7-3 COMPARISON OF EARLY-STAGE BREAST CANCERS

	LOBULAR CIS	DUCTAL CIS	STAGE I/II
Patient age	45	55	55
Mammographic appearance	No findings	Microcalcification	Microcalcification +/– dense or spiculated mass
Physical examination	+/– Palpable mass	+/– Palpable mass	Palpable mass
Relationship to invasive cancer	Marker	Precursor	Invasive
Treatment options	Expectant: 1. Close follow-up 2. Bilateral simple mastectomy and reconstruction	Definitive: 1. Lumpectomy 2. Lumpectomy and radiation 3. Simple mastectomy +/– sentinel node biopsy and reconstruction	Definitive: 1. Lumpectomy, axillary node dissection, and radiation 2. Modified radical mastectomy and reconstruction

small, low-grade lesions may confer no additional benefit. Consideration also must be given to the presence of comorbid conditions, which may diminish the life expectancy of geriatric patients to a greater extent than does a diagnosis of breast cancer.

Patients who are unable to tolerate chest wall irradiation are not candidates for breast conservation therapy. For example, radiation therapy in patients with collagen vascular disease such as systemic lupus erythematosus and scleroderma may result in an unacceptable fibrotic reaction. Prior radiation to the chest wall is a clear contraindication to additional radiation therapy. Heart and lung diseases are relative contraindications (depending on the severity and the planned radiation field), as is rheumatoid arthritis.

In summary, a number of interrelated factors must be considered in planning the treatment of a woman with stage I or stage II breast cancer. Age, comorbid disease, and personal preference must be weighed against tumor size, location, multifocality, and histology in making the choice between modified radical mastectomy and lumpectomy, axillary dissection, and postoperative radiation therapy. The types of early-stage breast cancer are compared in Table 7-3.

TREATMENT OF THE AXILLA

The most powerful prognostic indicator for survival in patients with breast cancer is the presence or absence of lymph node metastases. Variables such as tumor size, ER status, and ploidy may increase the power of the prognostic model, but only after nodal status is considered. The classic treatment for invasive breast cancer has therefore employed axillary lymph node dissection to provide information on prognosis and aid in the planning of adjuvant therapy. It is difficult to prove that removal of axillary lymph nodes improves survival in node-positive patients; however, axillary node dissection does reduce the rate of recurrence in the axilla.

The most powerful prognostic indicator for survival in patients with breast cancer is the presence or absence of lymph node metastases.

Axillary lymph node dissection carries some inherent risks. Postoperative morbidity is common and includes paresthesia and axillary seroma formation. Less common but problematic postoperative syndromes include lymphocele formation, infection, skin necrosis, and lymphedema of the arm. The dissection requires general anesthesia, hospital admission (usually), and arrangements for nursing and drain care. The current challenge is to identify women with early breast cancer in whom axillary dissection can be omitted without affecting the prognosis.

Initially described as a method of detecting occult lymph node metastases in patients with malignant melanoma, sentinel node biopsy is now recognized as a possible alternative to axillary lymph node dissection. Specific areas of the breast are drained by afferent lymphatics to a "sentinel node" and then to other nodes in the axillary basin. Many recent studies have demonstrated that the sentinel lymph node is a good predictor of the status of metastases in the neighboring lymph nodes; that is, if the sentinel lymph node is negative, the rest of the axillary contents are also negative with a 95 to 100 percent likelihood. Thus, the morbidity of axillary node dissection can be avoided in patients who are unlikely to benefit from it.

The disease status of the sentinel node is a good predictor of the status of neighboring nodes; that is, if the sentinel node is negative, the rest of the axillary contents are also negative with a 95 to 100 percent likelihood.

Sentinel lymph node biopsy in the treatment of early-stage breast cancer has not been accepted as the standard of care, and the procedure is available only at a few university centers. Patients with a very low risk of axillary metastases—those with DCIS, microinvasive carcinoma, or a small pure tubular carcinoma—can be treated adequately without axillary lymph node dissection. Sentinel node biopsy in early stage I or stage II disease has identified metastases even with very small cancers: 15 percent in tumors under 1 cm. Most patients (85 percent) can be spared a full axillary dissection if the sentinel node is negative.

The technique of sentinel node biopsy involves the injection of a vital blue dye, isosulfan blue, and/or a Tc-99 radiolabeled sulfur colloid into the breast tissue adjacent to the tumor. The surrounding lymphatic ducts take up and concentrate the tracer into the sentinel node. The labeled node then is identified by visual inspection of the axillary contents or detected by lymphoscintigraphy and/or a handheld gamma ray detector. A distinct learning curve has been demonstrated by surgeons trained in the technique.

A standard axillary dissection specimen contains 10 to 25 lymph nodes. For routine histologic evaluation, the nodes are bisected and one to nine sections are examined microscopically. With such a small proportion of the node actually seen under the microscope, it stands to reason that some metastases are missed. Sentinel node biopsy involves the study of a single lymph node, and so many additional sections should be processed. Such intensive study of the sentinel node may upstage some early breast cancer patients and provide better information for predicting survival outcome than does a standard axillary lymph node dissection. New developments, including the use of immunohistochemical stains and molecular markers, will improve accuracy further.

CHEMOTHERAPY FOR EARLY BREAST DISEASE

Both premenopausal and postmenopausal women with tumor size greater than 1.0 cm are candidates for chemotherapy regardless of their lymph node status.

Once reserved for use in patients with late-stage breast cancer, chemotherapy is now recommended for women with early-stage disease as well. Both premenopausal and postmenopausal women with tumor size greater than 1.0 cm are candidates for chemotherapy regardless of their lymph node status. Data from the Early Breast

Cancer Trialists' Collaborative Group demonstrated a 23.5 percent reduction in the annual risk of recurrence and a 15.3 percent reduction in the annual risk of death when multidrug chemotherapy was administered to women with early-stage disease. A similar effect was seen in both node-positive and node-negative patients.

Numerous characteristics of the patient and her cancer must be considered before one makes the decision to treat with chemotherapy. Age, menopausal status, general health, cancer stage, the presence or absence of nodal disease, the ER and progesterone receptor (PR) status of the tumor, and the histologic subtype are all weighed to determine the risk of recurrence after local therapy alone. This risk then is compared with the potential risks and benefits of chemotherapy to arrive at a rational plan.

Chemotherapy regimens vary between treating institutions, and evaluation by a qualified medical oncologist is mandatory. Three of the most common protocols are CMF (cyclophosphamide, methotrexate, and 5-fluorouracil), CAF (cyclophosphamide, adriamycin, and 5-fluorouracil), and AC (adriamycin and cyclophosphamide). Adriamycin also is known as doxorubicin. The standard duration of treatment for chemotherapy is four to six monthly cycles. Toxicity and side effects are common and usually are short-lived. They include nausea, vomiting, malaise, amenorrhea, and neutropenia. Mucositis and local infections also are common. Alopecia is expected if the regimen includes doxorubicin. Also, cardiac toxicity causing congestive heart failure occurs in 1 to 2 percent of patients treated with this drug.

Tamoxifen is a nonsteroidal drug that exhibits antiestrogenic properties by virtue of competitive inhibition at the ER. Tamoxifen can inhibit the growth of ER-positive breast tumors. The drug is administered orally every day for 5 years. Although tamoxifen reduces recurrence and improves survival when patients have received therapy for at least 2 years, clinical trials indicate that further benefit is gained when treatment continues for 5 years. After local breast cancer therapy was completed, treatment with tamoxifen for 5 years was shown to reduce the risk of recurrence by 47 percent and the risk of death over 10 years of follow-up by 26 percent. These benefits were seen regardless of age or menopausal status.

Tamoxifen therapy usually is well tolerated. Side effects are relatively mild and include hot flashes, vaginal discharge, and nausea. Thrombophlebitis is a serious but rare adverse effect, and tamoxifen use increases the risk of endometrial cancer twofold to threefold. There has been an association between tamoxifen use and hepatocellular carcinoma in rat studies but not in humans.

In pre- or postmenopausal breast cancer patients with negative axillary lymph nodes and tumor size less than 1.0 cm, survival after local treatment alone is higher than 90 percent and chemotherapy is not recommended. With 1.0- to 2.0-cm tumors, decision making may be guided by histologic assessment of the tumor. Favorable histologic characteristics such as tubular and mucinous subtypes and tumors with a low nuclear grade and low S-phase fraction may not require further treatment. Patients with negative nodes but tumors larger than 2.0 cm should receive multidrug therapy with CMF, CAF, or AC. When node-negative breast cancer is ER- and/or PR-positive, tamoxifen is added to the chemotherapy regimen.

Breast cancer patients who have metastases to the axillary lymph nodes should be considered for systemic chemotherapy regardless of tumor size. Only comorbid cardiac or pulmonary disease and poor general health are reasons to withhold cytotoxic therapy.

Postmenopausal node-positive breast cancer patients are treated with tamoxifen and/or combined chemotherapy without respect to the hormonal status of the tumor. Clinical trials have reported a 20 percent reduction in recurrence and an 11 percent reduction in mortality in postmenopausal women with ER-negative tumors treated with tamoxifen. Premenopausal node-positive patients are treated with multidrug chemotherapy and tamoxifen if the tumor is ER-positive. Chest wall and axillary radiotherapy also may be considered for young node-positive patients even after mastectomy, since recent data have demonstrated a distinct survival benefit. The addition of tamoxifen to chemotherapy results in additional survival benefit over chemotherapy alone, but the tumor marker ErbB2 may indicate tamoxifen resistance.

Chemotherapy for breast cancer is a rapidly evolving field. As new data regarding high-dose, alternating non-cross-resistant chemotherapy and neoadjuvant chemotherapy are analyzed, it is likely that the recommendations cited in this chapter will change. Targeted immunotherapy will soon be available for breast cancer treatment and, it is hoped, will have fewer adverse effects than the standard regimens in current use.

COMMONLY ASKED QUESTIONS

1. **Why is carcinoma in situ (CIS) in other locations in the body (e.g., cervix, vulva) considered to be a precancer while CIS of the breast is called *cancer*?** Carcinoma in situ is defined as neoplasia that involves only the epithelium without penetration of the basement membrane. Spread of disease to the lymph nodes does not occur unless the integrity of the basement membrane has been disrupted, and the lesion is then called invasive carcinoma or cancer. Complete excision of CIS therefore should effect a cure.

   CIS of the skin and cervix often is visible and can be excised completely. Histologic evaluation then determines the status of the basement membrane as well as the surgical margins. With the breast, however, the abnormal epithelium is located beneath the skin and often is difficult to detect. The sheer size of the organ makes discovery of multifocality problematic. Physical examination and mammography detect some but not all abnormalities.

   Ductal CIS by definition should be curable by local excision, and lymph nodes should not be involved. However, recurrence and/or subsequent invasion are common, suggesting that multifocality or occult invasion may be present but undetected. The recommended treatment therefore often includes removal of or radiation to the entire breast.

   Lobular CIS is not thought to be a true precursor to cancer but a risk factor for it. LCIS coexists with cancer in 5 percent of patients, and the presence of LCIS denotes a future risk of cancer of up to 35 percent. The cancer can occur in either breast, and so bilateral mastectomy and very close follow-up are the recommended options for management.

   Because invasion frequently coexists with breast CIS and the treatment options for DCIS and LCIS are comparatively unpalatable, inclusion of CIS under the umbrella term *cancer* is reasonable.

2. **With all the possible options available for the treatment of my breast cancer, how do I know which one is right for me?** For some patients, more than one option probably will yield similar disease-free survival and life expectancy. However, numerous factors influence treatment decisions. From the clinical perspective, tumor size and location, breast size, histologic subtype, nuclear grade, and receptor status, as well as axillary node status, all affect decision making. From the patient's perspective, cosmetic concerns and reconstruction alternatives as well as the future risks associated with radiation versus surgery are

important considerations. Sometimes a second opinion from another experienced surgeon will help the patient come to a final decision.

3. **I have been on tamoxifen therapy since my breast cancer surgery 2 years ago. I had not had any bleeding since menopause, but now I'm having some brownish discharge. What should I do?** Because tamoxifen has been associated with an increased risk of endometrial cancer, any bleeding should be evaluated fully. The ultrasound appearance of the uterus in women taking tamoxifen often includes a thickened endometrial stripe. However, saline infusion sonohysterography may demonstrate a classic pattern of subendometrial cystic change. If no discrete abnormality or polypoid lesions are seen, office endometrial sampling for histologic evaluation will suffice. If the ultrasound appearance is unusual or a polyp is seen, diagnostic hysteroscopy with endometrial curettage may be required.

SUGGESTED READING

Early Breast Cancer Trialists' Collaborative Group. Systemic treatment of early breast cancer by hormonal, cytotoxic or immune therapy: 133 randomized trials involving 31,000 recurrences and 24,000 deaths among 75,000 women. *Lancet* 1992; 339:1–15, 71–85.

Giuliano A, Barth A, Spivack B, et al. Incidence and predictors of axillary metastasis in T1 carcinoma of the breast. *J Am Coll Surg* 1996; 183(3):185–189.

Jacobson J, Danforth D, Conwan R, et al. Ten year results of a comparison of conservation with mastectomy in the treatment of stage I and stage II breast cancer. *N Engl J Med* 1995; 332:907–911.

Silverstein M, Gierson E, Colburn W, et al. Can intraductal carcinoma be excised completely by local excision? Clinical and pathologic predictors. *Cancer* 1994; 13:2985–2989.

MANAGEMENT OF LATE BREAST CANCER

With the currently available treatment strategies of surgery, radiation therapy, and adjuvant chemotherapy, early-stage breast cancer has become a highly curable disease. Unfortunately, the prognosis for late-stage disease is much less favorable. Late breast disease includes metastatic cancer as well as four distinct clinical entities unaccompanied by distant metastases: recurrent disease, inflammatory breast cancer, and stages IIIA and IIIB breast cancer.

LOCALLY RECURRENT BREAST CANCER

Local/regional recurrence refers to a second clinical manifestation of breast cancer in either the primary site or the regional lymphatics. Despite the success of multidisciplinary treatment, local/regional recurrence is documented in 10 to 30 percent of patients after radical or modified radical mastectomy. Chest wall recurrence is related to the extent of disease at the time of primary resection and the response after postoperative radiation therapy.

Some features of breast cancer that are associated with high recurrence rates after surgery and radiation are the presence of gross residual disease after lumpectomy, large tumor size, multiple primary tumors in the same breast, invasion of lymphatic vessels, and lobular histologic findings. Clear surgical margins of resection are critical to decrease the risk of local recurrence. Since microscopically clear margins are technically difficult to achieve in cases of invasive ductal carcinoma with an extensive intraductal component or invasive lobular carcinoma, the high rate of local recurrence in these cases may be related to the presence of residual disease.

Local recurrence must be treated aggressively. From a practical standpoint, the treatment options differ, depending on the therapy the patient has already received. The following discussion compares the treatment of local recurrence after mastectomy, after reconstruction, and after lumpectomy with postoperative radiation.

RECURRENCE IN THE MASTECTOMY SITE

Local recurrence after mastectomy may occur in the residual breast tissue, the chest wall incision, or skin flaps. Commonly, the problem presents as painless cutaneous nodules in close proximity to the patient's scar. These nodules are initially 1 to 2 mm in size, but they eventually coalesce, infiltrate the skin, and cause ulceration. The late manifestations of skin erythema and edema appear to be similar to the skin changes seen with inflammatory breast carcinoma.

Although they often are feared as a harbinger of widely metastatic disease, only one-third of patients with local/regional recurrences have distant metastases. The time interval between the treatment of the primary tumor and the discovery of local recurrence is directly related to the stage of disease at the time of initial treatment. Treated patients with stage I or stage II breast cancer have a longer disease-free interval between diagnosis and recurrence and between recurrence and death than do patients with stage III disease.

Appropriate therapy may permit long-term control of recurrent breast cancer. After a lengthy disease-free interval, patients with minimal recurrence may be treated with surgical excision alone. However, extensive resections often require prosthetic, skin graft, or flap coverage of the chest wall. Control of local recurrence by radiotherapy alone also may be possible, depending on the volume of breast tissue remaining. When surgical resection is combined with radiation therapy, 5-year survival ranges from 20 to 30 percent. Systemic therapy with tamoxifen also produces a significant improvement in 5-year disease-free survival.

Although they often are feared as harbingers of widely metastatic disease, only one-third of patients with local/regional recurrences have distant metastases.

RECURRENCE IN A RECONSTRUCTED BREAST

Immediate breast reconstruction after mastectomy offers the advantages of lower postoperative psychological morbidity and avoidance of a second operation, with its inherent risks (surgical and anesthetic) and cost. Concern that immediate reconstruction would increase the risk of recurrence or delay the diagnosis of recurrence proved unfounded in studies of follow-up after mastectomy and transverse rectus abdominis musculocutaneous flap (TRAM) reconstruction. In fact, a decreased rate of recurrence in the reconstructed breast was demonstrated, but this finding was partly attributable to selection bias.

A problematic contraindication to immediate reconstruction is the need for radiotherapy. The effectiveness of postoperative radiation in preventing local/regional recurrences in women with stage II or stage III breast cancer has been confirmed by two long-term studies. Irradiation after mastectomy significantly improved disease-free survival and overall survival irrespective of tumor size, histology, or the presence of positive lymph nodes. Since control of local recurrence has a significant effect on overall survival and since chemotherapy alone is less effective at controlling residual cancer in premenopausal women than is the combination of chemotherapy and radiotherapy, patients with stage I disease also may benefit from postoperative radiation. Reconstruction after mastectomy and chest wall radiation is a safe alternative to immediate reconstruction in a high-risk patient.

RECURRENCE AFTER BREAST CONSERVATION THERAPY

The results of several randomized trials affirm that lumpectomy combined with axillary node dissection and radiotherapy is as effective as mastectomy in eliminating recurrence in patients with stage I and stage II breast cancer. In an update of the National Cancer Institute data, the rate of cancer recurrence in the treated breast was 18 percent. In this series, salvage mastectomy was effective in eliminating disease. The local control rate and disease-specific survival were affected adversely by advancing stage. Premenopausal status and close surgical margins also were associated with recurrence. The local failure rate was reduced by radiation therapy, a protocol that is now fairly standard in most institutions.

Cancer found in a previously treated breast may represent recurrent disease or a new primary cancer. When cancer recurs in the ipsilateral breast after conservative surgery plus radiation therapy, salvage mastectomy is the most common treatment. Multifocal disease is found in about 20 percent of these patients. Some studies with limited follow-up have reported acceptable results after repeat wide excision for breast cancer recurrence. Reirradiation to limited fields also has been reported.

A special problem related to breast conservation therapy is the development of angiosarcoma after radiation therapy. First reported in 1987, angiosarcoma appears after a latency of 5 to 7 years after radiation, and its appearance does not seem to correlate with the radiation dose. Most patients undergo salvage mastectomy as the primary treatment for angiosarcoma, but among these patients, 50 percent develop recurrent angiosarcoma of the chest wall. Conclusions about the treatment and prognosis of angiosarcoma after breast conservation and radiation therapy are limited by the rarity of the finding (about 1 percent of breast cancer patients treated by irradiation) and the lack of data regarding long-term follow-up.

INFLAMMATORY BREAST CANCER

Frequently mistaken for mastitis, inflammatory carcinoma is characterized by diffuse enlargement of the breast and erythematous and/or edematous skin changes.

Inflammatory breast cancer is an aggressive form of locally advanced disease. Fortunately, it is uncommon, accounting for only about 2 percent of all breast cancers. Frequently mistaken for mastitis, inflammatory breast cancer is characterized by diffuse enlargement of the breast and erythematous and/or edematous skin changes. Obstruction of the dermal lymphatics is common and may give the breast skin a classic "peau d'orange," or orange peel, appearance. An underlying mass may or may not be palpable.

The age group most commonly affected by inflammatory breast cancer is similar to that affected by noninflammatory disease: 45 to 54 years. The disease occurs more often in African-American women. It may be present but is not more common in pregnant or lactating women.

Inflammatory breast cancer is classified as a T4 tumor and is considered to be at least stage IIIB at diagnosis. The poor prognosis of inflammatory carcinoma is evidenced by the early involvement of lymph nodes; most of these patients have clinical evidence of lymph node metastases at the time of diagnosis. Among those patients,

20 percent also have distant metastatic disease. In contrast, only about 5 percent of patients with noninflammatory breast cancer present with metastatic disease.

Inflammatory breast cancer is usually of the invasive ductal type, but it can display lobular or even medullary histology. The diagnosis may be suspected on the basis of clinical findings, but confirmation requires histologic demonstration of dermal lymphatic emboli and/or extensive lymph node involvement. A patient who presents with a rapidly growing tumor but no overt inflammatory skin changes should undergo skin biopsy before receiving treatment.

The symptoms of inflammatory carcinoma include breast heaviness, aching, and an increase in size accompanied by firmness or redness of the breast. On physical examination, the breast appears erythematous and edematous, especially in the dependent portion near the inframammary fold. The breast is warm and tender to palpation, and a discrete mass may or may not be present. Nipple retraction is commonly seen.

The differential diagnosis of a warm, erythematous, and edematous breast includes mastitis, breast abscess, radiation dermatitis, and lymphoma. Mastitis and breast abscess usually are seen in the puerperal period rather than after menopause. However, infection also may occur after injury to the breast, for example, after nipple piercing, mammaplasty, or lumpectomy. Breast infection usually is associated with fever, leukocytosis, and localized tenderness—features that are absent in inflammatory breast cancer. Breast ultrasound may be helpful in defining an abscess. Patients with inflammatory breast cancer often are treated with a course of antibiotics for a presumed infection, delaying the diagnosis.

Radiation dermatitis is an acute inflammatory change that occurs 2 to 4 weeks after breast irradiation. Postradiation fibrosis, which occurs much later, can mimic the appearance of inflammatory breast cancer, but the skin surface is usually brawny rather than erythematous. Lymphoma involving the breast may be clinically indistinguishable from inflammatory breast cancer.

Patients with suspected inflammatory breast cancer should be examined by a surgeon for possible biopsy. The biopsy specimen can be obtained by using a core biopsy needle, a 3-mm punch biopsy trocar, or a scalpel, and a sample of skin should be included.

Management of confirmed inflammatory breast cancer involves combined surgery, radiation, and chemotherapy. Inflammatory breast cancer is likely to be a systemic disease by the time of diagnosis, and so local therapy alone is inadequate. After a staging workup that includes chest x-ray, abdominal and chest computed tomography (CT), and bone scan, patients start a doxorubicin-based chemotherapy regimen. If a good clinical response to primary chemotherapy is demonstrated, a modified radical mastectomy or breast conservation therapy may be considered. Surgery is followed by additional chemotherapy and chest wall radiotherapy. In the absence of a clinical response to primary chemotherapy, a secondary protocol that includes taxol and radiotherapy can be initiated. Finally, a bone marrow transplant may be considered.

Inflammatory breast cancer is likely to be a systemic disease by the time of diagnosis, and so local therapy alone is inadequate.

STAGE IIIA BREAST CANCER

Stage IIIA breast cancer is locally advanced disease that is technically operable. Tumor size in stage III disease is generally large (T1, T2, or T3), and axillary node metastasis (N1 or N2) is present. About 7 percent of women with breast cancer present with stage IIIA disease.

Surgery for stage IIIA breast cancer is technically feasible because mastectomy with primary skin flap closure can be performed without cutting into the gross tumor. Surgery alone, however, constitutes insufficient treatment. The 5-year survival rate of women treated by mastectomy without adjuvant chemotherapy for stage IIIA breast cancer is only about 30 percent. Recurrence after mastectomy for stage IIIA survivors is also about 30 percent.

Chemotherapy for advanced local breast cancer includes CMF (cyclophosphamide, methotrexate, and 5-fluorouracil) or AC (adriamycin and cyclophosphamide). The order of therapy, that is, chemotherapy versus surgery first, offers no clear survival advantage in patients with stage IIIA disease. The maximum response to induction (presurgery) chemotherapy usually is seen after three cycles have been administered. About 70 percent of stage IIIA patients respond to induction therapy, and among these patients, 10 to 15 percent have a pathologically complete response.

Patients with a good clinical response to chemotherapy may be candidates for breast conservation therapy with wide excision of the tumor mass and postoperative radiation. Even after mastectomy, however, patients with stage IIIA disease are at high risk for local recurrence and should consider chest wall irradiation.

STAGE IIIB BREAST CANCER

Stage IIIB breast cancer is technically inoperable at the time of presentation because of direct extension of tumor into the pectoralis muscle or skin of the chest wall (T4). Metastasis to the ipsilateral internal mammary lymph nodes (N3) also defines stage IIIB disease. Initial surgery for these patients is contraindicated.

Since the incidence of distant metastases at presentation is high with stage IIIB disease, a metastatic workup is warranted and includes a bilateral mammogram, a chest x-ray, chest and abdominal CT, and a bone scan.

Pretreatment evaluation of patients with stage IIIB breast cancer includes a complete history and physical examination as well as measurements of any palpable masses. The diagnosis of breast cancer is confirmed by fine needle aspiration or core biopsy rather than excisional or incisional biopsy. Since the incidence of distant metastases at presentation is high, a metastatic workup also is warranted and includes a bilateral mammogram, a chest x-ray, chest and abdominal CT, and a bone scan.

The optimal management of locally advanced breast cancer involves a multidisciplinary approach in which medical oncologists work closely with surgeons and radiation oncologists. Combined-modality treatment can yield optimal disease-free and overall survival as well as adequate local control of the disease. Induction chemotherapy regimens for stage IIIB disease are CMF, cyclophosphamide, adriamycin, and 5-fluorouracil (CAF), and AC. If skin changes or other evidence of inoperable disease resolves with chemotherapy, surgery and radiation therapy maximize the chance of achieving local control. Patients who do not respond to the initial induction chemotherapeutic agents may benefit by changing to a non-cross-resistant regimen of drugs.

METASTATIC BREAST CANCER

Despite improvements in detection and treatment, breast cancer remains the most common cancer in women and is second only to lung cancer as the most common cause of cancer deaths. The age-adjusted death rate for breast cancer is 22 per 100,000 population, and these women die of metastatic disease. While virtually every organ has been reported as a site of breast cancer metastasis, the usual sites are lymph nodes, chest wall, bone, liver, and lung. Metastases to brain, pleura, and pericardium, though less common, may have difficult clinical symptomatology.

The probability of distant metastasis in breast cancer is best predicted by the status of the regional lymph nodes and the maximum tumor diameter in lymph-node-negative patients. Many other prognostic factors have been described, including histologic type, hormone receptors, growth factors, proliferative rate, cathepsin D, and the presence of the *HER-2/neu* oncogene. Detection of micrometastases in bone marrow by immunologic techniques may select some patients at high risk for relapse who could benefit from intensive adjuvant treatment. The presence of *HER-2/neu* expression in some breast cancers may make them amenable to treatment with herceptin.

The duration of disease-free survival is strongly associated with survival after relapse. Most breast cancer recurrences are seen within the first 2 to 3 years after treatment. Visceral (liver and brain) metastases are associated with a short survival, while bone and locoregional recurrences are associated with a longer median survival. An estrogen-receptor (ER)-positive patient is likely to have metastasis to bone, while an ER-negative patient frequently presents with brain or liver metastasis.

Visceral (liver and brain) metastases are associated with a short survival, while bone and locoregional recurrences are associated with a longer median survival.

Treatment for breast cancer metastasis consists of combination chemotherapy (CAF, CMF, or AC) as well as taxane regimens. A number of high-dose regimens are under study at university centers, as are investigational trials with antibodies directed against tumor growth factors. The initial enthusiasm for high-dose chemotherapy with stem-cell rescue (bone marrow transplant) for metastatic breast cancer has waned somewhat. Although most patients die of metastatic disease after bone marrow transplantation, some benefit with prolonged disease-free survival. Patients with metastasis at a single site survive longer than do patients with disease at multiple sites. Patients with hepatic metastasis fare poorly regardless of chemotherapy or bone marrow transplantation. If a complete remission is seen after induction chemotherapy, the prognosis is improved after bone marrow transplantation.

Radiotherapy is very effective in the treatment of localized metastatic disease. The primary goal in this setting is palliation, and this form of therapy is reserved for patients who are symptomatic or are likely to develop irreversible symptoms. The pain caused by bony metastases, for example, can be reduced by radiation therapy. Impending fracture of the long bones or vertebral bodies by metastatic breast cancer can be delayed by radiation treatment and appropriate orthopedic stabilization.

One of the common indications for palliative radiotherapy in patients with metastatic breast cancer is brain metastasis. Stereotactic radiosurgery combined with steroid therapy is used for the majority of patients with this presentation. Some patients with solitary brain metastasis and no clinically evident extracranial disease also may benefit from surgical excision of the lesion. Impending spinal cord compression by metastatic disease represents a true radiotherapy emergency, and treatment can delay paraplegia in these patients.

Malignant pleural effusions are a common presentation of metastatic breast cancer. Pleural disease is associated with mediastinal lymph node metastasis and parenchymal lung metastasis. A new pleural effusion in a breast cancer patient may respond to systemic chemotherapy, but treatment of most malignant effusions is palliative. A patient with metastatic breast cancer may complain of a cough or dyspnea on exertion. Chest x-ray reveals a pleural effusion of up to 1 L of fluid. The diagnostic pleurocentesis also is therapeutic. After confirmation of the diagnosis by cytologic examination of the pleural fluid, most patients are treated with tube thoracostomy. Once the thoracostomy output has decreased to about 100 to 200 mL a day, pleurodesis is performed in an attempt to close the potential space between the parietal pleura and the chest cavity. Sclerosing agents such as tetracycline, bleomycin, and talc are infused via the tube thoracostomy. The ensuing inflammatory reaction of the parietal pleura produces fibrosis, obliterates the pleural space, and prevents further exudate.

Malignant pericardial effusion is seen in 10 to 20 percent of patients with end-stage breast cancer. Metastases are thought to reach the pericardium and heart through involved mediastinal lymph nodes. The severity of the resulting cardiac tamponade is related to the volume of effusion, the rapidity of fluid accumulation, and the patient's underlying cardiac function. Several liters may accumulate when the onset is insidious. A critical point is reached when the decreased cardiac stroke volume caused by external tamponade results in cardiovascular collapse. When the pericardium is thickened by tumor infiltration or radiation fibrosis, compensatory stretching to accommodate the pericardial effusion is limited and the critical point is reached early. When untreated, pericardial metastases are rapidly fatal. Pericardiocentesis may be lifesaving in the acute situation. However, the fluid usually reaccumulates within 48 to 72 h. Some patients benefit from sclerotherapy with the same agents used in pleurodesis. External-beam radiation therapy may be helpful after repeatedly unsuccessful attempts at sclerotherapy. The creation of a pericardial window to drain pericardial fluid into the pleural space is another therapeutic option. In less critical patients, these techniques often are supplemented by systemic antitumor therapy.

SUGGESTED READING

Halverson K, Perez C, Kuskee R. Survival following local regional recurrence of breast cancer: Univariate and multivariate analysis. *Int J Radiat Oncol Biol Phys* 1992; 23:285–291.

Hays D, Henderson C, Shapiro C. Treatment of metastatic breast cancer: Present and future prospects. *Semin Oncol* 1995; 22(2):5–21.

Overgaard M, Hansen P, Overgaard J, et al. Postoperative radiotherapy in high risk premenopausal women with breast cancer who receive adjuvant chemotherapy. *N Engl J Med* 1997; 337:949–955.

Singletary S, Dhinga K, Yu D. New strategies in locally advanced breast cancer. In: Pollack RE, ed. *Advances in Surgical Oncology.* Boston: Kluwer, 1996.

BREAST DISEASE IN PREGNANCY AND LACTATION

INTRODUCTION

Any breast mass that occurs in a woman of childbearing age may present during pregnancy or lactation. In fact, a preexisting mass may become apparent during pregnancy as the patient comes under medical scrutiny for the first time in her life. Many breast masses are hormonally sensitive, and growth during pregnancy may prompt their detection.

Because 70 to 80 percent of breast masses that present during pregnancy are benign and because the youth of pregnant patients promotes a false sense of security on the part of health care providers, the evaluation of a breast mass in a pregnant patient often is deferred. This delay may allow a cancer to progress from a localized to a metastatic state. No woman with a breast mass should be told that the initial diagnostic evaluation can wait until the pregnancy is over. Only whan a consensus in favor of benignity exists among the obstetrician, surgeon, radiologist, and cytologist should postponement of definitive treatment occur.

This chapter describes the most common benign and malignant conditions that affect the breast in pregnant women (Table 9-1). Diagnostic and treatment strategies are outlined.

BENIGN PREGNANCY-ASSOCIATED BREAST CHANGES

PROBLEMS OF MILK STASIS

During the puerperal period, the most common benign breast problems result from milk stasis. When a duct becomes obstructed, backup of milk causes ductal dilation

TABLES 9-1 COMMON CAUSES OF BREAST MASSES DURING PREGNANCY

PROBLEMS OF MILK STASIS	BENIGN NEOPLASMS	BREAST CANCER
Duct obstruction	Lactating adenoma	In situ
Galactocele	Fibroadenoma	Invasive
Mastitis/abscess	Breast hypertrophy	

Ductal obstruction leads to milk stasis and ductal dilation. Unrelieved obstruction results in galactocele formation.

and pain. Continued obstruction may lead to duct rupture, and further collection of milk causes a tender cystic swelling, or galactocele, to develop. Relief of ductal obstruction is achieved by local heat, massage, and continued milk evacuation. The most efficient means of emptying the breast is suckling by the infant, but manual expression and the use of a breast pump also are effective. Occasionally, the plug persists and the clinician must use a hypodermic needle to draw tenacious secretions out of the duct orifice at the nipple. When relief of the obstruction does not result in the resolution of an associated breast lump, fine needle aspiration is warranted. A galactocele may be diagnosed and cured by percutaneous needle drainage. If the lump is not a milk cyst, additional workup is necessary, as is described below.

Mastitis is associated with fever, malaise, and localized erythema, edema, and pain in the breast. Prompt antibiotic therapy and continued evacuation of milk constitute effective treatment.

Breast milk is an excellent medium for bacterial growth. Organisms from the infant's mouth may gain entry into the ductal system through the nipple. These bacteria can proliferate rapidly in an area of stagnant milk, causing a breast infection, or mastitis. The patient usually presents with fever, malaise, and localized erythema, edema, and pain. Treatment with oral antibiotics results in rapid clinical improvement. If the response to therapy is suboptimal, the presence of an abscess should be suspected. The diagnosis is confirmed by palpation of a fluctuant mass. Treatment requires incision and drainage in addition to antibiotic therapy (see Chap. 4).

BENIGN BREAST TUMORS IN PREGNANCY

Lactating adenomas and fibroadenomas are the most common benign breast tumors in pregnancy.

Under the influence of the hormones of pregnancy, the proliferation of ductal and lobular epithelium results in an increase in breast size and weight. At times, well-demarcated nodules of hyperplasia called lactating adenomas are palpable. These benign tumors are unique to the puerperium and are found in the majority of biopsy specimens taken from young lactating women.[1,2] They present as enlarging, nontender, well-circumscribed masses that are firm to palpation.[3,4] On ultrasound, they appear solid, with well-defined borders and posterior acoustic shadowing.[4] Excision is diagnostic and therapeutic.

Another common benign breast neoplasm is the fibroadenoma. Presenting as a solitary, rubbery, firm well-circumscribed mass, these hormone-sensitive tumors may grow during pregnancy. Fine needle aspiration or core biopsy is needed to confirm the diagnosis. Only if the presentation, clinical examination, and needle diagnosis all suggest fibroadenoma should excision be delayed until after lactation. Occasionally, infarction causes a sudden increase in mass size and acute pain.[5] Excision is then necessary to confirm the diagnosis.

BREAST HYPERTROPHY

Gigantomastia, or massive breast hypertrophy, is an uncommon occurrence. The normal physiologic increase in breast size becomes exaggerated, sometimes to the point of causing pressure necrosis of the overlying skin.[5] This condition usually is self-limiting and resolves postpartum. However, gigantomastia may recur with subsequent pregnancy, and reduction mammoplasty sometimes is required.[5]

PREGNANCY-ASSOCIATED BREAST CANCER

INTRODUCTION

Breast cancer is the most common malignancy diagnosed during pregnancy.[6–9] Among the 186,000 breast cancers diagnosed each year, 10 to 20 percent occur in women of childbearing age[10] and 1 to 3.8 percent occur during pregnancy.[5,9,11,12] The incidence of pregnancy-associated breast cancer (i.e., breast cancer diagnosed during or within 1 year after pregnancy) is 1 to 7 per 10,000 pregnancies.[5,8,11,12] The average age at diagnosis during pregnancy is 32 years.[11]

Among the 186,000 breast cancers diagnosed annually, 10 to 20 percent occur in women of childbearing age and 1 to 3.8 percent occur during pregnancy.

The incidence of pregnancy-associated breast cancer is likely to be increasing.[6] Women in this country are delaying childbearing until later in their adult lives in order to complete their education, start a career, and become more financially secure. Childbirth among women older than 30 years more than doubled between 1970 and 1990.[6,10] Because increasing age is a risk factor for breast cancer, the result of postponing childbirth is that more women will be pregnant at the time when breast cancer is diagnosed.

Laboratory data confirm a role of estrogens in the initiation and promotion of breast cancer.[13] Some studies even suggest that surgical treatment during the estrogen-dominant follicular phase of the menstrual cycle has a detrimental effect on the subsequent prognosis.[10,13] Reproductive history, specifically a long duration of ovulatory cycles (i.e., early menarche, nulliparity, late menopause), is an important determinant of risk for breast cancer. Surgical castration before age 35 has been shown to decrease breast cancer risk by 50 percent.[13]

For many years, concern that the hormonal milieu of pregnancy would increase the risk of breast cancer or worsen its prognosis prevented aggressive diagnostic or therapeutic interventions from being offered.[6,7] These concerns were unfounded. In regard to the incidence of breast cancer, studies have shown that 7 to 14 percent of breast cancers in women of childbearing age occur during pregnancy.[7,12] Since most of these cancers occur between the ages of 25 and 40 (a 180-month period) and assuming that a woman will have two children during those years (18 months of pregnancy), one would expect that approximately 10 percent (18 of 180) of breast cancers in this age group would occur during gestation.[7,12]

Breast cancer has not been shown to behave more aggressively in pregnant women than in nonpregnant women of the same age. However, a delay in diagnosis during pregnancy is common and may worsen the prognosis by allowing the cancer to reach a more advanced stage before treatment.[14] When diagnosed during pregnancy, 56 to 90 percent of women with breast cancer have involved regional lymph nodes,[7,12,15] compared with 30 to 50 percent of similarly aged women who are not pregnant.[12]

A delay in diagnosis during pregnancy worsens the prognosis by allowing the cancer to reach a more advanced stage before treatment.

Many factors are responsible for diagnostic delay (Table 9-2). Hormonal stimulation of the breasts during pregnancy causes physiologic changes that may mask the presence of a lump. The breasts become larger, denser, and more nodular as pregnancy progresses, and so a thorough breast examination at the patient's first prena-

TABLE 9-2 FACTORS THAT CONTRIBUTE TO DELAY IN THE DIAGNOSIS OF BREAST CANCER DURING PREGNANCY

PHYSIOLOGIC FACTORS	PHYSICIAN BEHAVIORAL FACTORS
Increased breast size and density hamper detection of mass on physical examination	Low index of suspicion for cancer because of youth of pregnant patients
Mammographic interpretation is impaired by dense or engorged breast tissue	Reluctance to order breast imaging studies during pregnancy
Histologic evaluation is more difficult because of proliferative changes during pregnancy	Reluctance to recommend breast biopsy during pregnancy

tal visit is crucial. Most clinicians harbor a low index of suspicion for cancer when they discover a lump. Both the patient and the practitioner may be reluctant to employ surgery or imaging procedures to evaluate the mass further. Pregnancy-related histologic changes in the breast create difficulty for a radiologist interpreting mammograms and for a pathologist interpreting fine needle aspirates. During the postpartum checkup, breast examination frequently is omitted because engorgement and blocked ducts are expected to prevent optimal palpation.

To avoid delay in diagnosis, breast examination should be performed at both the first prenatal visit and the postpartum follow-up, and every mass should be evaluated fully. Also, the clinician should maintain a relatively high index of suspicion for cancer when a mass is detected during pregnancy. Early intervention can have a major impact not only on the patient but on her entire family.

DIAGNOSIS

Pregnancy-associated breast cancer typically presents as a self-detected painless lump.[7] Less often, the clinician discovers an abnormality on routine screening breast examination. Any of the classic signs of malignancy may be present, including an enlarging mass, skin dimpling or retraction, axillary adenopathy, and bloody nipple discharge. Observation for change in the size of a mass over time is problematic because changes in the density and size of the breast during pregnancy may prevent a persistent lump from being palpable.

Fine needle aspiration and ultrasonography are the most helpful initial studies when a breast mass is found during pregnancy.

When a mass is detected, the clinician may proceed with an ultrasound study of the breast or fine needle aspiration (FNA). Ultrasound is useful in determining whether a mass is cystic or solid but cannot differentiate between benign and malignant solid masses with certainty. Ultrasonography is preferable to mammography as the initial imaging study of choice during pregnancy because patients with a simple cystic mass need no further evaluation and because the increased parenchymal density in pregnancy may obscure mammographic visualization. Some authors exclude mammography from the algorithm for the management of a mass during pregnancy because of its low sensitivity.[12,15,16] However, it may be useful in clinically worrisome cases because calcifications or the presence of a suspicious mass may be seen.[11] The use of a skin marker over the palpable lump may improve mammographic sensitivity.[11] The lack of a worrisome abnormality on mammography should not prevent or delay diagnostic biopsy of a clinically worrisome mass.

Mammography should not be avoided because of concern about radiation exposure. The fetus receives a radiation dose of 0.005 mGy during a shielded bilateral mammographic study with two views of each breast.[11] The threshold of radiation exposure that causes harm to the fetus is not known exactly but is likely to be 0.05 to 0.15 Gy.[7,11]

Fine needle aspiration may be diagnostic and therapeutic when a cyst or galactocele is discovered. If the palpable abnormality disappears after drainage of the cyst, no further study is necessary. FNA of a solid mass during pregnancy is associated with higher false-negative and false-positive rates than is the case in nonpregnant patients.[6,15] FNA is technically more difficult to perform during pregnancy because of nodularity and engorgement of the breasts, and this may cause sampling error.[15] When FNA of a solid mass is performed, the cytologist must be advised that the specimen was taken from a pregnant patient because the cellular atypia and proliferation associated with gestation can otherwise be mistaken for malignant change.[6,17]

Histologic examination of a mass is required for a definitive diagnosis. If FNA and/or ultrasound reveal that a mass is solid or if no abnormality is found on ultrasound despite the presence of a palpable mass, the patient should be referred for histologic sampling (core biopsy) or excision of the mass to exclude the possibility of cancer. Core biopsy is performed in the radiology suite, using a large-bore needle. Several passes through the mass are taken to sample the abnormal area adequately and supply a sufficient quantity of material for histologic interpretation. Core biopsy during pregnancy has not been well studied but is probably preferable to open excisional biopsy in cases where the clinical suspicion for cancer is low. Possible complications include hematoma formation, infection, and milk fistula.

Excisional biopsy is the gold standard for the diagnosis of a breast mass. If a mass is not suspicious and core biopsy and/or FNA show normal glandular epithelium, delay of excision until the postpartum period can be considered. Excision is performed in the operating room under local or general anesthesia. The increased risk of biopsy complications during pregnancy (e.g., milk fistula) and the 70 to 80 percent chance that a biopsy result will be benign contribute to delay in the diagnosis of pregnancy-associated breast cancer.[6] Milk fistula is more likely to occur when the patient continues to breast-feed before and/or after the procedure and when the lump to be excised is central in location. Postoperative infection and hematoma formation also are common complications.

STAGING

Staging of breast cancer in pregnancy involves careful examination of the breasts and axillae (see Chap. 7). A chest x-ray (with abdominal shielding) is indicated, and blood testing for liver function is necessary. Bone scan or computed tomography (CT) of the liver or brain should be performed only if symptoms or blood tests suggest metastatic disease.[15]

TREATMENT

Options for the treatment of breast cancer in pregnancy include surgery, cytotoxic drugs, and radiation therapy. Modified radical mastectomy with axillary lymph node dissection is the mainstay of treatment for breast cancer during the first and second trimesters of pregnancy. An alternative for patients in the middle to late third trimester is breast conservation therapy (lumpectomy and axillary node dis-

Modified radical mastectomy with axillary node dissection is the mainstay of treatment for breast cancer diagnosed during pregnancy.

section), with radiation therapy delayed until after delivery. A lapse of more than 7 weeks between surgery and radiation is associated with an increased risk of local recurrence.[18]

The use of radiation and chemotherapy is limited by their potential deleterious effects on the fetus. The consequences of radiation exposure depend on the stage of gestation and the radiation dose. The fetal effects can be lethal, teratogenic, growth-retarding, or carcinogenic or may alter structure and function.[18] Lethal effects are most common before and just after implantation. During the period of organogenesis, teratogenic and growth-retarding effects predominate. As the pregnancy progresses, teratogenicity declines but the central nervous system is still sensitive to radiation effects and growth retardation is common.[18] After radiation therapy, the breast becomes firm and dense to palpation because of sclerotic and fibrotic changes within the parenchyma.[19] The glandular epithelium becomes atrophic and no longer responds to hormonal stimulation. Therefore, during a subsequent pregnancy, it will not change in size or produce milk.[19]

The standard radiation dose used for the treatment of breast cancer is approximately 50 to 60 Gy. With maximal shielding, phantom measurements of fetal dose can be as low as 4 percent of the tumor target dose, but this still exceeds the threshold of 0.1 Gy associated with fetal abnormalities.[19]

For premenopausal women with early-stage disease but positive lymph nodes, adjuvant chemotherapy has been proved to improve survival.[9,15] Some survival benefit after chemotherapy has been demonstrated even in node-negative women.[15] Because axillary disease is present in 56 to 90 percent[7,12,15] of pregnant breast cancer patients and because the primary tumor often is large, adjuvant chemotherapy often is recommended during pregnancy. The type of drug used and the gestational age of the fetus combine to determine the effect of chemotherapy on the pregnancy. In general, cytotoxic drugs used in the first trimester of pregnancy are more likely to cause teratogenic effects. Antimetabolites (e.g., methotrexate, 5-fluorouracil, cytarabine, 6-mercaptopurine) are the worst offenders and should not be given in the first trimester.[9,15] When administered in the second and third trimesters, antineoplastic drugs are not associated with an increase in congenital defects,[10,13] but prematurity and low birthweight are more common.[10,12] The most frequently used drugs for adjuvant treatment of breast cancer are cyclophosphamide (Cytoxan), methotrexate, 5-fluorouracil, and doxorubicin (adriamycin). When administered after the first trimester, these drugs have not increased the frequency of congenital abnormalities.[15] The timing of delivery should be orchestrated to avoid a hematologic nadir. Breast-feeding is contraindicated in patients receiving chemotherapy.[15]

Because axillary disease and large tumor size are common when breast cancer is diagnosed during pregnancy, adjuvant chemotherapy often is recommended.

ESTROGEN AND PROGESTERONE RECEPTOR STATUS

Hormone receptor status is frequently negative in women with pregnancy-associated breast cancer.

Breast cancers in premenopausal women are more likely to be estrogen-receptor (ER)- and progesterone-receptor (PR)-negative (40 to 66 percent) than are those in postmenopausal women, and this may be related to the observed aggressive behavior of breast cancer in youth.[6] Few data are available in the literature regarding the ER and PR status of breast cancers diagnosed during pregnancy. Most reports describe less than 25 percent ER positivity[2,6,12,14] but this number may be falsely low. During pregnancy, the high levels of circulating estrogen and progesterone may down regulate ER and PR at the tumor level. Also, the ligand binding assay used in most studies to assess receptor status may be limited by saturation of the receptors.[6,12]

SURVIVAL AND PROGNOSIS

The initially held belief that breast cancer during pregnancy or lactation has a worse prognosis than breast cancer in nonpregnant patients has been disproved. Early studies did not take into consideration the patient's age, the stage of disease, and nodal status when making comparisons. Once matched for these variables, survival is similar irrespective of pregnancy status.[6,8,14] However, pregnant patients do more poorly on the whole because they usually present with later-stage disease.[6]

When matched for age, stage, and nodal status, the survival for breast cancer in pregnancy is similar to that in non-pregnant patients.

Involvement of axillary lymph nodes at the time of diagnosis is the most important prognostic indicator for breast cancer.[8] The 5-year survival rate for node-negative patients with pregnancy-associated breast cancer is 60 to 82 percent.[6,12,14] When nodes are positive, the survival rate decreases to 40 to 50 percent.[6,12,14] In patients with advanced operable disease, pregnancy is associated with a worse prognosis.[6]

PREGNANCY AFTER BREAST CANCER

After a diagnosis of breast cancer is made, subsequent pregnancy has not been shown to decrease overall survival.[6,10,13,14] However, the data on this issue are flawed and incomplete. The studies are uniformly retrospective and rely on physician recall, tumor registries, or hospital records to identify the population for analysis. Thus, the number of identified patients is lower than expected and selection bias is introduced.[10] Patients themselves may be responsible for some of this bias because women who perceive their cancer prognosis to be good are more likely to pursue pregnancy.[10,14] Cases and controls in these studies are not always matched with respect to age, stage, and nodal status, and so comparisons may not be valid. In addition, the status of recurrence may not be known. Logically, women would not attempt pregnancy if recurrent disease had been discovered, and these women may automatically enter the control group for comparisons.

The 5-year survival rate after pregnancy for patients diagnosed with stages I and II breast cancer is approximately 70 to 90 percent.[10] The time from cancer diagnosis to subsequent pregnancy affects the survival prognosis.[10,13] The risk of breast cancer recurrence is greatest within the first 2 years after diagnosis, and so conception should be delayed at least that long to allow early recurrence or metastases to become apparent.[14] The prognosis is worst if pregnancy occurs within 6 months of cancer diagnosis,[14] and it improves with time until after 4 years, survival approximates that with no subsequent pregnancy.[6,10] Multiple pregnancies after breast cancer diagnosis improve survival even more because healthy women are more likely to become pregnant and more time has elapsed since the diagnosis, indicating a better prognosis.[10]

Risk factors for the recurrence of breast cancer include the presence of lymph node metastases, tumor size over 3 cm, nuclear grade III, absence of ER, a high S-phase fraction (indicating proliferative activity), aneuploidy, and a high expression of cathespin D.[15] Appropriate counseling of patients at high risk for recurrence may aid them in decision making regarding plans for future pregnancy. These patients must know that they may not be alive or capable of caring for future offspring.

A woman young enough to be diagnosed with breast cancer during pregnancy should consider testing for genetic mutations that predispose to breast cancer

Genetic testing should be considered when breast cancer is diagnosed in youth.

(*BRCA1* and *BRCA2*). Because the results may have far-reaching implications (see Chap. 3), genetic counseling is required before testing is offered. The pros and cons of testing may then be discussed, and a careful decision can be made.

COMMONLY ASKED QUESTIONS

1. **Should a pregnancy in the first trimester be terminated when the diagnosis of breast cancer is made?** The decision to terminate pregnancy should be based on the stage of disease at diagnosis, the patient's ethical and religious beliefs, and the treatment deemed most likely to effect a cure of the cancer. An early-stage cancer may be treated by modified radical mastectomy and axillary node dissection alone. If lymph nodes are negative, no further treatment may be needed. However, advanced disease may require adjuvant therapy with cytotoxic drugs or radiation. Pregnancy termination may then be reasonable to prevent the deleterious effects on the fetus that these modalities are likely to cause in the first trimester. No available data indicate that pregnancy termination itself has a beneficial effect on prognosis other than allowing aggressive therapy to proceed without compromise.[6,12]

2. **Why doesn't a subsequent pregnancy adversely affect breast cancer prognosis?** The most likely reason is that the majority of breast cancers in young women are estrogen- and progesterone-receptor-negative. Therefore, the rising hormone levels of pregnancy are unlikely to affect the prognosis even if micrometastases or occult recurrence is present.[12] If, however, the receptor status of the cancer is positive, these hormones may cause growth. Theoretically, the very high hormone levels of pregnancy cause down regulation of receptors, and so the expected excessive progression may not occur.

3. **What is the likelihood of infertility after chemotherapy for the treatment of breast cancer?** The risk of ovarian failure after chemotherapy is dependent on the type of drug administered, the dose and duration of treatment, and the patient's age.[10] Alkylating agents are the drugs most likely to cause amenorrhea, and the likelihood increases proportionately with age. The multidrug regimen of cyclophosphamide, methotrexate, and 5-fluorouracil (CMF) is employed commonly in the treatment of breast cancer. Permanent amenorrhea is unlikely to occur after treatment with these drugs when the patient is under age 35.[10] However, the risk rises after age 40, and amenorrhea is more likely to be persistent. After the administration of doxorubicin (adriamycin), amenorrhea in women under age 35 is common but rarely is permanent (9 percent).[10] Tamoxifen has been associated with persistent amenorrhea in 66 percent of women over age 35.[10]

REFERENCES

1. Collins JC, Liao S, Wile AG. Surgical management of breast masses in pregnant women. *J Reprod Med* 1995; 40:785–788.
2. Sorosky JI, Scott-Conner CEH. Breast disease complicating pregnancy. *Obstet Gynecol Clin North Am* 1998; 25(2):353–363.
3. Yang WT, Suen M, Metreweli C, Chir MBB. Lactating adenoma of the breast: Antepartum and postpartum sonographic and color Doppler imaging appearances with histopathologic correlation. *J Ultrasound Med* 1997; 16:145–147.
4. Behrndt VS, Barbakorr D, Askin FB, Brem RF. Infarcted lactating adenoma presenting as a rapidly enlarging breast mass. *AJR* 1999; 173:933–935.
5. Scott-Conner CEH, Schorr SJ. The diagnosis and management of breast problems during pregnancy and lactation. *Am J Surg* 1995; 170:401–405.

6. Kuerer HM, Cunningham JD, Brower ST, Tartter PI. Breast carcinoma associated with pregnancy and lactation. *Surg Oncol* 1997; 6(2):93–98.

7. Merkel DE. Pregnancy and breast cancer. *Semin Surg Oncol* 1996; 12:370–375.

8. Nettleton J, Long J, Kuban D, et al. Breast cancer during pregnancy: Quantifying the risk of treatment delay. *Obstet Gynecol* 1996; 87:414–418.

9. Inbar MJ, Ron IG. Breast-conserving surgery and adjuvant chemotherapy in pregnancy. *Acta Obstet Gynecol Scand* 1996; 75:765–767.

10. Surbone A, Petrek JA. Childbearing issues in breast carcinoma survivors. *Cancer* 1997; 79:1271–1278.

11. Samuels TH, Liu F, Yaffe M, Haider M. Breast imaging: Gestational breast cancer. *Can Assoc Radiol J* 1998; 49:172–180.

12. DiFronzo LA, O'Connell TX. Breast cancer in pregnancy and lactation. *Surg Clin North Am* 1996; 76(2):267–278.

13. Surbone A, Petrek JA. Pregnancy after breast cancer: The relationship of pregnancy to breast cancer development and progression. *Crit Rev Oncol Hematol* 1998; 27:169–178.

14. Lethaby AE, O'Neill MA, Mason BH, et al. Overall survival from breast cancer in women pregnant or lactating at or after diagnosis. *Int J Cancer* 1996; 67:751–755.

15. Shivvers SA, Miller DS. Preinvasive and invasive breast and cervical cancer prior to or during pregnancy. *Clin Perinatol* 1997; 24(2):369–389.

16. Stefanidis K, Navrozoglou L, Mouzakioti E, et al. Breast cancer during pregnancy and lactation. *Eur J Gynaec Oncol* 1998; 19(5):487–488.

17. Mitre BK, Kanbour AI, Mauser N. Fine needle aspiration biopsy of breast carcinoma in pregnancy and lactation. *Acta Cytol* 1997; 41:1121–1130.

18. Mayr NA, Wen B, Saw CB. Radiation therapy during pregnancy. *Obstet Gynecol Clin North Am* 1998; 25(2):301–321.

19. Wobbes T. Effect of a breast saving procedure on lactation. *Eur J Surg* 1996; 162:419–420.

10

COMMON BREAST-FEEDING PROBLEMS

INTRODUCTION

Breast milk provides excellent nutrition for the baby as well as important antibodies to prevent infectious diseases.

For most women, the benefits of breast-feeding far outweigh any disadvantages. Breast milk provides excellent nutrition for the baby as well as important antibodies to prevent infectious diseases. It lowers the baby's risk of developing allergy-related problems such as eczema, asthma, and colic. Formula is expensive and requires preparation, whereas breast milk is always readily available and requires no time for cleaning up. In addition, many women describe a special emotional bonding with their infant that is facilitated by breast-feeding.

Despite these advantages, many women in the United States choose not to nurse their babies. Important social support from spouse, family, and friends may be lacking. Often women return to work soon after delivery and are not given the time and a place to pump or find it difficult to persevere. Obstetricians and general practitioners tend to place too little emphasis on the benefits of breast-feeding during prenatal care visits. Insufficient education is offered to pregnant women about how to initiate breast-feeding and how to anticipate and solve commonly encountered problems. The right of a woman to breast-feed in public has been recognized only recently.

Any discussion of the difficulties associated with the initiation and maintenance of the art of breast-feeding must begin with a review of pertinent anatomy and physiology regarding both the mother's breast and milk production and the infant's suckling mechanism. This chapter describes the most common breast-feeding pitfalls experienced in the first few postpartum weeks and some practical solutions.

ANATOMY AND PHYSIOLOGY OF THE BREAST

As was discussed in Chap. 1, the prolactin level starts to rise between 6 and 8 weeks of gestation in response to a rising estrogen level. Estrogen suppresses hypothalamic dopamine (the "pituitary inhibitory factor") and has a direct stimulatory effect on the pituitary to produce prolactin. This prolactin elevation, as well as prior exposure to other hormones (e.g., estrogen, progesterone, thyroid hormone, insulin, cortisol, and growth hormone), results in complete differentiation of the terminal alveolar cells into milk-producing units. Accompanying this differentiation is an increase in breast size that a woman may note as the first overt sign of pregnancy.

During pregnancy, active milk production is prevented by the antagonistic effect of progesterone on prolactin binding at its receptor. High estrogen levels also probably block prolactin action. Progesterone is produced by the placenta, and its inhibitory effect on lactation continues until placental expulsion occurs postpartum. True milk production begins once estrogen and progesterone levels decline 3 to 4 days postpartum. Until then, the alveoli are distended with colostrum, or "first milk," which is composed of sloughed central alveolar cells, leukocytes, and transudate. Rich in immunoglobulins, breast milk (including colostrum) confers protection from infections to a breast-feeding infant.

During pregnancy, active milk production is prevented by the antagonistic effect of progesterone on prolactin binding at its receptor.

Prolactin clearance is slower, usually taking about 7 days. In a non-breast-feeding patient, engorgement of the alveoli and ducts in the first few days postpartum flattens the cells and reduces their secretory activity. Prolactin levels wane, and milk production ultimately ceases after a week. The milk-producing apparatus regresses, and the breasts become smaller.

In patients who choose to breast-feed, several hormonal and nervous system events occur in concert to allow lactation to proceed. First, stimulation of the nipple and areola by suckling or breast pumping causes episodic peaks in prolactin secretion. The prolactin stimulates further milk production by the alveolar cells. Second, the afferent arc of a reflex pathway that involves nerve roots from thoracic levels 4, 5, and 6 is stimulated. This afferent arc is triggered by the tactile stimulation of receptors in the nipple and areola during suckling. However, hearing, seeing, smelling, or even thinking about the baby also can trigger the reflex. The afferent arc prompts the paraventricular and supraoptic nuclei in the hypothalamus to produce and release oxytocin for transport to the posterior pituitary. Oxytocin then enters the bloodstream and reaches the breast, where it stimulates contraction of the myoepithelial cells that surround the alveoli and ducts. Contraction of these cells causes transport of milk to the nipple and the underlying ampullae. This entire sequence of events is known as the "letdown" reflex. Although letdown can be initiated by numerous other triggers, continuation of lactation requires suckling or breast pumping. Not only does such stimulation promote prolactin release, suckling evacuates the milk already produced and prevents engorgement from decreasing alveolar cell secretion. Figure 10-1 (Plate 3) shows the pre- and postdelivery variations in hormone levels that are responsible for the initiation and maintenance of lactation.

Suckling causes the release of oxytocin (triggering the "letdown" reflex) and prolactin (promoting further milk production).

ANATOMY AND PHYSIOLOGY OF SUCKLING

Suckling and sucking are not synonymous. Suckling is the act of drawing the nipple and areola into the mouth and keeping it there by means of a slight negative pres-

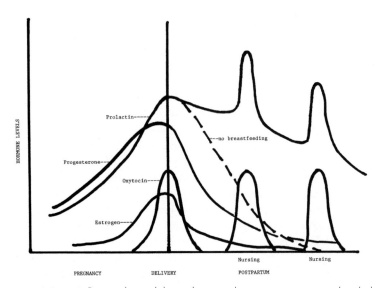

HORMONE LEVELS

Prolactin----

---no breastfeeding

Progesterone---

Oxytocin---

Estrogen----

Nursing   Nursing

PREGNANCY   DELIVERY   POSTPARTUM

FIGURE 10-1 (Plate 3) Pre- and postdelivery hormonal variations associated with the initiation and maintenance of lactation.

sure. Sucking involves the creation of a partial vacuum to draw fluid into the mouth, as in a straw or the nipple on a baby's bottle. When nursing, the infant empties the breast ducts of milk not by creating a vacuum but by opening and closing the jaws to eject milk from the ampullae beneath the nipple. As the milk is evacuated, more fills the ampullae as a result of the actions of oxytocin and prolactin, as was described above.

During the "latching-on" process the nipple and areola are drawn deeply into the baby's mouth and become flattened (Fig. 10-2). The nipple and areola are cupped by the baby's tongue, and the tongue rests on the infant's lower gum. The baby's lips are flanged outward. For latching on to occur optimally, one must take full advantage of the baby's rooting reflex. During rooting, the mouth opens, the tongue protrudes, and the face turns in response to light touch along the cheek or upper lip (Fig. 10-3). When the mouth opens widely, the mother, having flattened the nipple and areola between her thumb and fingers (Fig. 10-4), pulls the baby toward her breast. Trauma to the nipple and skin at the nipple-areola junction is common if too little of the areola is taken into the baby's mouth. Good latching on is demonstrated when the infant's nose and chin are touching the breast skin (Fig. 10-5).

As the infant's jaws open and close during suckling, milk is ejected from the ampullae beneath the nipple.

During breast-feeding, the infant's jaws open and close, expressing milk from the lactiferous sinuses (ampullae) into the infant's mouth. As this happens, peristaltic waves in the baby's tongue channel milk back to the oropharynx and initiate the swallowing reflex. Immediately after latching on, the infant typically displays short, fast bursts of suckling during which little milk flows. Then, as milk is ejected, the pattern becomes one of longer, slower jaw movements followed by swallowing and the generation of negative pressure. The negative pressure probably serves to keep the nipple and areola in the correct position for continued suckling.

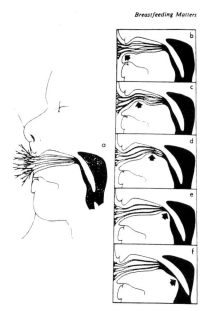

Breastfeeding Matters

FIGURE 10-2 Sagittal view of infant during the latching-on process. Note that the nipple and areola are drawn deeply into the baby's mouth and become flattened. [Reprinted from Woolridge MW. The anatomy of infant sucking. *Midwifery* 1986; 2(4):164–171, by permission of Churchill Livingstone.]

BREAST ASSESSMENT AND PRENATAL TEACHING

Physical evaluation of a patient during the first prenatal visit should include a thorough breast examination. In addition to inquiring about prior breast problems, the clinician should use this time to ask the patient about her plans for breast-feeding. Promotion of breast-feeding early in the pregnancy through discussion of its potential

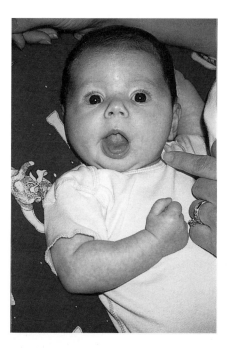

FIGURE 10-3 During the rooting reflex, the mouth opens, the tongue protrudes, and the face turns in response to light touch along the cheek or upper lip.

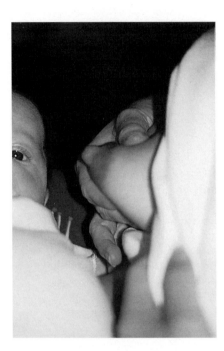

FIGURE 10-4 The mother flattens the nipple and areola between thumb and fingers to help the infant draw more areola into the mouth.

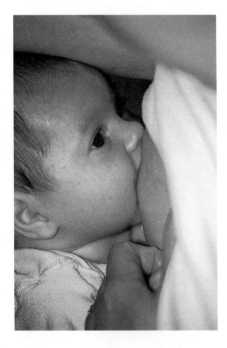

FIGURE 10-5 The infant's nose and chin must touch the breast to ensure correct latching on.

benefits is imperative to improve the low breast-feeding rate in this country. Clinicians should recommend that their patients and partners attend a breast-feeding class during the second or third trimester to help them prepare. Classes offer advice about ways to gain social support from partners, family, and friends; how to select appropriate clothing; how to initiate a dialogue with employers about the time and location for pumping; and what to expect during the first few weeks postpartum. Breast-feeding is not easy for all women and often requires a great deal of effort and patience. Only through preparation and encouragement can clinicians help patients continue nursing for an entire year, as is recommended by the American Academy of Pediatrics.

During the examination, the breasts should be inspected for size, symmetry, and the presence of surgical scars, skin changes, and nipple inversion. The patient should be reassured that only very rarely are breasts too small or too large to allow for normal lactation. She also should be counseled that preexisting asymmetry may become more noticeable as the breasts enlarge during pregnancy.

Surgical scars may signify past breast augmentation, reduction, or lump excision. Implants rarely impair lactation; however, many patients with implants are reluctant to initiate breast-feeding. Concern often centers on expected changes in cosmetic appearance after weaning or possible discomfort caused by distention of the already tense breast skin. Ptosis of the breast after weaning and discomfort resulting from engorgement commonly occur even in the absence of implants. Early supportive discussion may affect the patient's decision to try breast-feeding.

Patients who have undergone breast reduction surgery may or may not be capable of breast-feeding. A review of the operative records should help define realistic expectations. If the ducts beneath the nipple were severed to move the nipple to a more cephalad location, breast-feeding probably is not possible; however, ductal recanalization has been reported. Initial engorgement will be followed by regression of the milk-producing apparatus. If, however, the ductal connections to the nipple remain intact, breast-feeding may proceed unimpaired. Similarly, after excisional procedures (e.g., lumpectomy, breast biopsy, duct excision), integrity of the ductal system should not be affected.

Women with inverted nipples may or may not encounter difficulty breast-feeding. Even without intervention, the latching-on process is usually uneventful. However, some women will need to evert the nipple mechanically first, as is discussed below.

Physical examination also should include palpation of the breast and node-bearing areas for lumps. Palpation later in pregnancy, when the breasts are more dense and tender, will not be as likely to reveal the presence of a mass. In addition to palpation, the "pinch test" can be performed at the first or a subsequent prenatal visit. To perform the pinch test, the breast is cupped with the thumb superior and the fingers inferior to the areola (Fig. 10-6). Compression will cause the nipple to protract (move outward), retract (become flush with the areola), or invert (move deep to the areola). Normally, protraction of the nipple is seen. Retraction or inversion does not necessarily mean that the patient will have difficulty breast-feeding. However, such findings may prompt early referral to a lactation consultant.

Nipple retraction or inversion during the pinch test should prompt early referral to a lactation consultant.

ASSESSMENT OF THE MOTHER–BABY DYAD

Crucial to successful breast-feeding after release from the hospital is observation of the mother and baby together in the first 24 to 48 h. The mother should be taught at

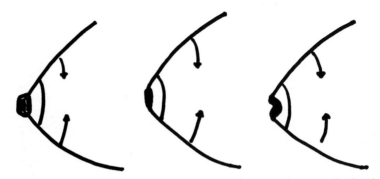

FIGURE 10-6 The pinch test is performed by cupping the breast between the thumb and fingers and compressing it just behind the areola (see Fig. 10-4). The nipple then will protract, retract, or invert, as shown here.

what point during the rooting reflex to bring the baby to the breast in order to allow as much areola as possible to enter the baby's mouth. The options for positioning the mother and baby should be demonstrated: the madonna hold, the football hold, and the side-lying position (Figs. 10-7, 10-8, and 10-9). Finally, the infant's suckling should be observed. To ensure adequate neonatal growth (after the first few days of life), the infant should nurse at least eight times in each 24-h period. Also, the infant should produce at least three stools and six voids per 24 h. While these parameters are widely accepted, they are not absolute. The mother should be taught to recognize the early cues of hunger (stirring, mouthing a fist, rooting) but should be encouraged to allow her sleeping baby to remain asleep for up to 5 h. The mother should sleep while the baby is sleeping and, as much as is possible, accept assistance when it is offered.

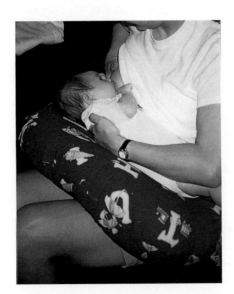

FIGURE 10-7 The madonna or cradle hold is the most frequently employed position for breast-feeding. The infant's head, shoulders, and hips should remain in the same plane to promote adequate latching on.

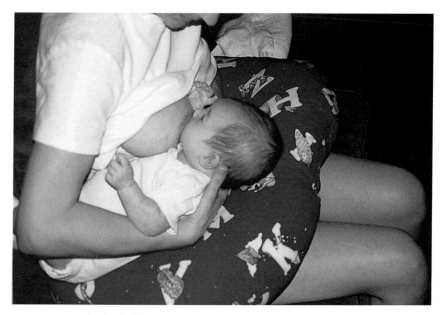

FIGURE 10-8 The football hold. This position offers an alternative to the cradle hold when the mother wishes to remain upright while breast-feeding.

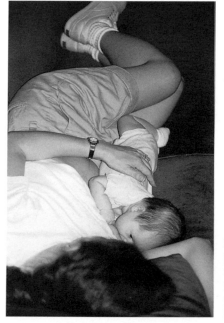

FIGURE 10-9 The side-lying position allows the mother to rest while breast-feeding. The infant may be positioned with the feet directed toward the head or foot of the bed.

COMMON PROBLEMS AND SOLUTIONS

NIPPLE OR BREAST PAIN

Normally, during the first few days postpartum, when production of "true milk" has not yet begun, the only discomfort felt by a new mother who is trying to breast-feed is the sensation of negative pressure on the ducts associated with latching on and the first few suckling bursts. As days pass and milk production ensues, a tingling sensation may be associated with letdown, and some women find this sensation uncomfortable. One solution to these usually minor problems is to start each feed with manual expression of milk, allowing letdown to begin without the trauma of latching on.

Breast engorgement is common in the first week of breast-feeding, when the production of true milk begins. Distention of the ducts and interlobular edema cause pain and swelling of the breast. The associated firmness may prevent effective latching on. Manual expression for a minute or two may help soften the breast and allow more areola to enter the baby's mouth during latching on. Application of ice to the breasts between feedings and the use of a supportive bra may offer some relief. Usually, the breast eventually becomes softer as the milk supply adjusts to the infant's demands.

The baby's mouth should be opened wide with the tongue protruding over the lower jaw at the time of latching on.

Nipple pain usually is caused by incorrect positioning, improper latching on, or a suckling problem. For example, cracked nipples (Fig. 10-10) may result from feeding in only one position and can improve simply by varying the way the baby is held. Fissures may develop at the base of the nipple if little or no areola enters the baby's mouth during latching on. Improvement in technique requires observation of the mother–baby dyad. Often the infant's head and shoulders are not aligned. Correct latching on is difficult with the baby's head turned to the side. The mother

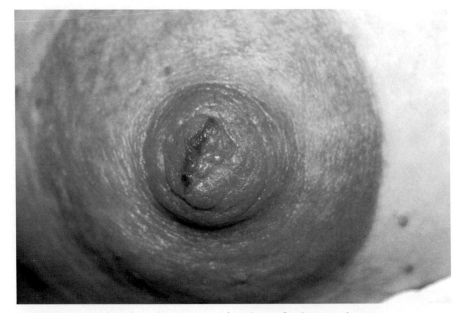

FIGURE 10-10 Cracked nipples may result from breast-feeding in only one position. (Courtesy of Kay Hoover.)

may be "bringing the breast to the baby" instead of "bringing the baby to the breast." The baby's mouth may not be opened wide, or the tongue may not be protruding at the time of latching on. These problems can be solved once they are recognized, and the assistance of a lactation consultant should be sought early on.

Trauma to the nipple also may be caused by the baby's tongue: either a short tongue or a short frenulum ("tongue-tied" infant). Most babies learn to feed normally over time even with a short tongue, but a short frenulum can easily be clipped in the clinician's office to facilitate breast-feeding.

Pure lanolin applied to the nipples after each feeding may help hasten the healing process and relieve discomfort. The bacteriostatic effect of breast milk has led some clinicians to recommend that breast milk be allowed to dry on the nipples after feeding. Others recommend local application of a mixture of antibacterial, antifungal, and steroid-containing ointments to treat traumatized nipples. Ice may help alleviate pain but does not solve the problem. Nipple shields are flexible silicone coverings for the nipple that are worn during breast-feeding to prevent nipple trauma (Fig. 10-11). While this is advocated by some clinicians as a means of allowing the nipple to heal while nursing continues, others voice numerous concerns: (1) Less nipple stimulation may lead to less prolactin secretion and less milk production, (2) the texture of the shield may result in "nipple confusion" and prevent the infant from wanting to return to nursing without the shield, and (3) the skin beneath the shield may become macerated if the shield remains in contact with the skin for long periods. Shells, as opposed to shields, are hard plastic domes with flexible silicone bases that have a hole in the center (Fig. 10-12). They are worn inside a bra, and the hole in the base allows the nipple to remain untouched by clothing. Another means to promote nipple healing and prevent pain is breast pumping. By avoiding the

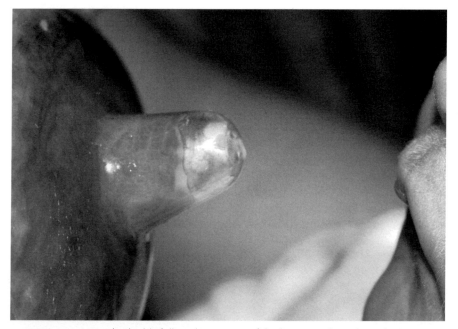

FIGURE 10-11 Nipple shields follow the contour of the breast and nipple and are intended to prevent nipple trauma during breast-feeding. (Courtesy of Kay Hoover.)

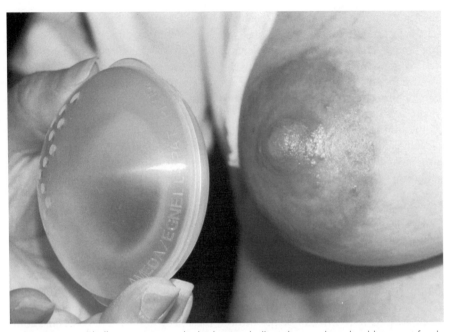

FIGURE 10-12 Shells are worn inside the bra and allow the nipple to heal between feedings without trauma from clothing. (Courtesy of Kay Hoover.)

trauma of latching on, the use of a pump for a short period may allow lactation to continue while giving the nipple time to heal.

Breast-feeding should not be a painful experience after the first week. Persistent or severe pain is abnormal and should not be ignored. Assistance from a lactation consultant may allow the problem to be corrected early enough that the mother does not abandon breast-feeding altogether.

PUERPERAL MASTITIS

Breast infection, or mastitis, most commonly occurs in the first few weeks postpartum. The acute onset of fever is accompanied by malaise and breast pain. Examination reveals a localized area of breast erythema, swelling, and tenderness. Bacteria (usually staphylococci) from the infant's mouth gain entry into the breast via a cracked or even a normal nipple. Stasis of milk then promotes bacterial growth. Treatment is with oral antibiotics (dicloxacillin 500 mg qid for 10 days) and continued breast-feeding. Massage and local heat also may improve the symptoms. Varying the positions for nursing to prevent ductal obstruction also may prevent milk stasis and recurrent mastitis. A lack of response to treatment suggests an underlying abscess, and in that case incision and drainage must be added to the antibiotic therapy.

INVERTED NIPPLES

Nipple inversion does not always cause difficulty with breast-feeding. However, if latching on is a problem, numerous techniques have been described to help draw out the nipple. One alternative is to wear a breast shell in the bra in an attempt to

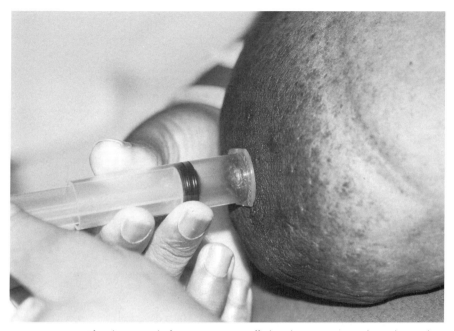

FIGURE 10-13 After the tip end of a syringe is cut off, the plunger is inserted into that end. The base of the syringe is placed over the inverted nipple, and gentle negative pressure generated by pulling back on the plunger helps draw the nipple out. This maneuver is followed immediately by bringing baby to the breast for latching on. (Courtesy of Kay Hoover.)

stretch the connective tissue that tethers the nipple inward. The pressure from the breast will push the nipple gently into the shell and allow it to protrude for latching on. Another option is to use the negative pressure generated by a breast pump or an inverted syringe to draw out the nipple (Fig. 10-13). The tip of a 12-mL syringe is cut off with a sharp knife, and the plunger is inserted into that end. With the base of the syringe over the nipple, gentle suction is created by pulling back on the plunger. Finally, one may try Hoffman's exercises to loosen the connective tissue beneath the nipple. To perform this technique, one finger from each hand is placed at positions 180 degrees away from each other at the base of the nipple. While gentle pressure is exerted, the fingers are pulled away from each other and away from the nipple. Even when performed several times per day, as recommended, this exercise is not uniformly helpful.

PLUGGED DUCT

Inadequate drainage of a duct leads to milk stasis. Occasionally, a plug of thickened milk may obstruct a duct completely. Evidence of the obstruction is seen on the nipple as a clear, white, or slightly yellow bleb (Fig. 10-14). The plug may cause localized pain in the nipple and a mass, or galactocele, may be palpable. Treatment consists of local warm compresses applied to the nipple (and the mass if present) followed by breast-feeding. Positioning so that the infant's chin is located over the involved lobule may help relieve the obstruction. The opening and closing of the baby's mandible massages the area and may help promote milk flow past the obstruction. If the plug persists, its removal in the clinician's office using a sterile hy-

A plugged duct is treated by the application of warm compresses, massage, and continued breast-feeding.

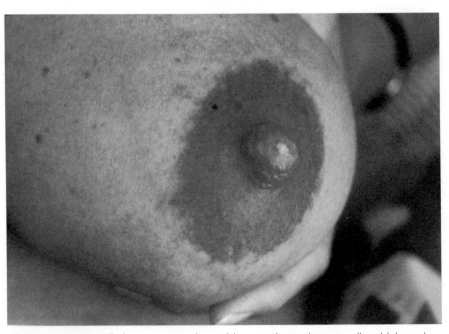

FIGURE 10-14 Ductal obstruction may be visible as a clear, white, or yellow bleb on the nipple. An associated lump caused by stasis of milk may be palpable.

podermic needle is indicated because persistent milk stasis is a common precursor to mastitis. If a mass persists after removal of the plug, needle aspiration of the mass should be performed to confirm the diagnosis of galactocele.

YEAST INFECTION

Nipple pain after the first week of breast-feeding and deep, burning, or shooting pain during or just after breast-feeding may be symptoms of breast candidiasis. Further support for this diagnosis is provided by the presence of oral or diaper-area thrush in the infant. On examination, the nipples are deep pink or red, or blisters may be present (Fig. 10-15). Treatment of both the mother and the baby is usually necessary. Topical nystatin, miconazole, or clotrimazole is effective when applied to the nipple after each feeding and to the baby's bottom after each diaper change. Oral thrush can be treated with oral nystatin suspension.

BLEEDING FROM THE NIPPLES

The most common cause of bleeding nipples is a crack or fissure resulting from traumatic latching on or improper positioning. Vascular engorgement and proliferation of fragile ductal epithelium during pregnancy also cause bloody secretions. Seldom is a bloody nipple discharge during pregnancy or lactation serious. However, blood emanating from a single untraumatized duct orifice may be due to an underlying intraductal papilloma or breast cancer. In this situation, referral to a general surgeon for evaluation is warranted.

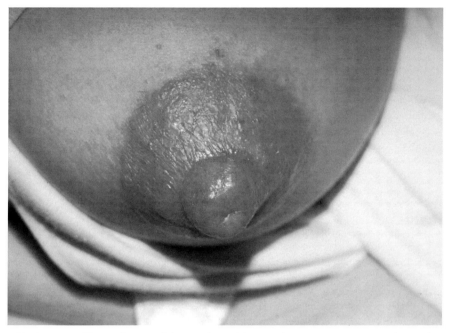

FIGURE 10-15 Yeast infection of the nipple and/or areola may appear as a red or pink sheen, or blisters may be seen.

SUMMARY

The advantages of breast-feeding include improving the infant's health, promoting emotional bonding, and minimizing cost and inconvenience. Many women are unaware of these benefits and decide against breast-feeding. The goal of clinicians should be to educate these women during pregnancy so that the decision is an informed one. Prenatal breast-feeding classes help prepare these patients and their families for the sometimes arduous task of breast-feeding. Timely referral of the patient to a lactation consultant when a problem such as nipple pain, plugged ducts, or engorgement occurs is crucial. With practice and sufficient guidance, breast-feeding is likely to be successful.

COMMONLY ASKED QUESTIONS

1. **How do I know that my baby is getting enough milk?** Many women are not aware of the demand–supply relationship associated with breast-feeding. The more often an infant nurses, the greater the prolactin release will be and the more milk will be produced. When a mother supplements the infant's intake with formula because of perceived inadequate milk production, she reduces the amount of time the infant is latched on. This decline in nipple stimulation results in less prolactin secretion and a decreased milk supply. By the end of the first postpartum week, the baby's output is a good indicator of how much milk he or she is receiving. Normally, the infant will produce at least six wet diapers and two to three stools per day. A weight gain of 4 to 8 oz per week, as documented during regular pediatric visits, also suggests adequate milk production.

Inadequate milk supply is uncommon. Even very small breasts are able to produce sufficient quantities. Failure of the "true milk" to come in after 3 to 4 days postpartum may be a result of continued progesterone production by a retained placental fragment. Rarely, hypopituitarism caused by intrapartum pituitary infarction, or Sheehan's syndrome, may be responsible.

2. **How long should I nurse on one breast before switching to the other?** A good rule of thumb is to allow the infant to finish feeding on one breast before offering the other one. When the baby's suckling slows down or he or she falls asleep, gently break the seal of the mouth on the breast by sliding a finger between the baby's gums all the way down to the nipple. Once the baby has been burped and wakes up, the other breast is offered. This sequence allows the baby to receive the "hindmilk," which is the high-fat portion of a feeding, from at least one breast. If the baby does not empty the second breast completely, manual expression or pumping can be used to prevent engorgement. Then the breast offered last during the current feeding is offered first during the next feeding.

3. **How can I prevent painful engorgement if I want to wean my baby before I go back to work?** Substitution of formula for one feeding the first day and an additional feeding each subsequent day will allow weaning to proceed without painful engorgement. When this regimen is used, the transition to another nutritional source can be completed in a week. Remember that the stimulus for prolactin release is nipple manipulation. If engorgement does occur, pumping or manual expression to reduce the pressure within the ducts will help relieve the pain. However, prolactin secretion will increase, and more milk will be produced.

When a breast-feeding mother must stop breast-feeding abruptly, painful engorgement can be expected. The prolactin level remains elevated for a few days, and milk production without evacuation results in distention of the lobules and ducts. The alveoli stop producing more milk, but several days pass before the engorgement subsides. Options for treatment include wearing a tight-fitting bra and wrapping the chest tightly to prevent further expansion. Application of ice reduces the sensation of pain. Frozen peas placed in a plastic bag conform better to the contour of the breast and may be more comfortable than ice cubes. Some lactation specialists recommend the application of cold, clean cabbage leaves to the skin beneath the ice packs as a means of "drawing out the milk," although no mechanism for this action has been proposed.

4. **Can I use oral contraceptive pills while I'm breast-feeding?** Progestin-only oral contraceptives (the minipill) are safe for use in breast-feeding women. Combination (estrogen plus progesterone) pills are more effective than the minipill but generally are withheld from breast-feeding patients because of concern that the estrogen component may cause a decline in milk production. This concern stems from the observation that high estrogen levels during pregnancy increase hypothalamic dopamine secretion, and dopamine inhibits prolactin secretion. Another reason to withhold combination pills is that small quantities of the medication can be found in the breast milk. Adverse effects that have been observed in neonates include jaundice and breast enlargement.

SUGGESTED READING

Hale T. *Medications and Mothers' Milk,* 9th ed. Amarillo, TX: Pharmasoft Publications; 2000.

Lawrence RA. *Breastfeeding: A Guide for the Medical Professional,* 5th ed. St. Louis: Mosby Year Book; 1999.

Mohrbacher N, Stock JS. *The Breastfeeding Answer Book.* Schaumburg, IL: La Leche League International; 1997.

Neifert M. Clinical aspects of lactation. Promoting breastfeeding success. *Clin Perinatol* 1999; 26(2):281–306.

Nelson WE, Behrman RE, Kliegman RM, et al, eds. *Nelson Textbook of Pediatrics,* 15th ed. Philadelphia: Saunders; 1996.

Newman J, Pitman T. *Guide to Breastfeeding.* Toronto: Harper Canada Publications; 2000.

Ramin SM, Cunningham FG. The breast in pregnancy and lactation. In: Cunningham FG, MacDonald PC, Gant NF, et al, eds. *Williams Obstetrics,* 20th ed., Supplement 6. East Norwalk, CT: Appleton & Lange; 1998.

Wilson-Clay B, Hoover K. *The Breastfeeding Atlas.* Manehaca, TX: Lactnews Press; 1999.

11 MALE BREAST CANCER

INTRODUCTION

Breast cancer usually is thought of as a disease of women. It occurs 100 times more often in females than in males, and the lifetime risk of a woman developing the disease is approximately 12 percent. Conversely, only 1400 cases of male breast cancer are diagnosed in the United States each year,[1,2] and it accounts for only 0.2 to 1 percent of all cancers in men.[3–5] Unfortunately, when it does occur, male breast cancer carries a high mortality rate, making early diagnosis and treatment crucial.

Only 1 percent of breast cancers occur in men, and male breast cancer accounts for only 0.2 to 1 percent of all cancers in men.

The literature on male breast cancer is relatively sparse, and most published reports are retrospective. Randomized clinical trials are not undertaken because the disease is rare. Conclusions about diagnosis and treatment therefore must be extrapolated from the experience with breast cancer in women. This chapter summarizes the unique features of male breast cancer and outlines a management strategy.

RISK FACTORS

Men with breast cancer typically present later in life than do women. The average age at diagnosis in men is 60 to 65 years, while most women with breast cancer are diagnosed in their early fifties.[4–6] The risk of developing breast cancer increases with age in both sexes. However, in men, a steady rise in incidence occurs throughout life, whereas in women, the rise is steeper in the premenopausal years.[2,5]

Risk factors for breast cancer include both genetic and environmental influences

(Table 11-1); however, most people diagnosed with the disease have no apparent risk factors. Several conditions associated with breast cancer in men suggest that a change in the normal ratio of estrogen to testosterone may be responsible. Klinefelter's syndrome, mumps orchitis, undescended testes, and testicular injury all result in impaired testicular testosterone production. The resultant relatively hyperestrogenic state may predispose a man to the development of breast cancer.[4,5] Ingestion of estrogen (e.g., for the treatment of prostate cancer) or occupational exposure to estrogen (e.g., in soap manufacturing or livestock processing) also may cause a hyperestrogenic state.[1]

Most risk factors for male breast cancer are associated with the presence of a relatively hyperestrogenic state.

Klinefelter's syndrome (47 XXY) is present in 3 percent of patients with male breast cancer, and 6 to 9 percent of patients with Klinefelter's syndrome develop breast cancer.[3,4,7] This condition is associated with gynecomastia, hypogonadism, and azoospermia. Gynecomastia, or excessive development of the male breast, is not in itself likely to be a risk factor for breast cancer.[1,2,5] Gynecomastia occurs in 30 to 50 percent of the general male population[3,5] and is present in up to 40 percent of patients with male breast cancer.[1,3,5] The high frequency of gynecomastia and the rarity of breast cancer in men make it unlikely that gynecomastia predisposes to breast cancer development.[3] Impaired testicular function is a more likely explanation for the increase in the risk of breast cancer associated with Klinefelter's syndrome.

Other risk factors related to alteration of the normal hormonal milieu include obesity and hepatic cirrhosis. Peripheral conversion of adrenal androstendione to estrone occurs in the fatty tissues of the body. Obesity therefore results in a higher estrogen state. Estrogen is metabolized in the liver, and so impaired liver function also may cause hyperestrogenism.[4]

The incidence of male breast cancer varies greatly, depending on the geographic location. The incidence is lowest in Japan and highest in Africa.[4,5] In Egypt, the incidence is 12 times greater than that in the United States.[4,5] In Zambia, 15 percent of all breast cancers have been reported to occur in men.[4,5] The high incidence in these countries may be due to hyperestrogenism caused by schistosomiasis-related liver damage.[4,5] Nonwhite race and heat-imposed reduction in testicular function are alternative explanations.[1,5] The incidence of male breast cancer also is higher in the Jewish population.[5]

Mutation of *BRCA2* on chromosome 13 has been linked to breast cancer–prone families in whom male breast cancer has occurred.[2,4] Other chromosomal abnormalities associated with male breast cancer include partial or

TABLE 11-1 RISK FACTORS FOR MALE BREAST CANCER

Decreased ratio of estrogen to testosterone
Klinefelter's syndrome, mumps orchitis, undescended testes, testicular injury
Obesity
Hepatic cirrhosis/liver disease

Genetic Factors
BRCA2
Complete or partial chromosome loss (e.g., chromosomes 17 and 18)

Increasing age

Environmental factors
Ionizing radiation (especially radiation therapy, fluoroscopy)
Electromagnetic radiation

complete loss of one chromosome 17, partial deletion of chromosome 18,[3] and other cytogenetic abnormalities.[4]

Exposure to electromagnetic radiation also has been proposed as a risk factor for male breast cancer.[4,5] Men who receive large doses of ionizing radiation, as occurs with repeated fluoroscopy or radiation therapy, are at increased risk as well.

PRESENTATION

Male breast cancer usually presents as a centrally located painless mass.

Male breast cancer usually presents as a centrally located painless mass.[2,4] Other associated symptoms may include nipple retraction, discharge, and breast tenderness. A left-sided predilection has been observed,[2,4,7] and palpable axillary adenopathy is present in 45 to 55 percent of these patients.[2,4] Because the male breast is smaller, involvement of the skin (ulceration, retraction), pectoralis fascia, or nipple is more common than it is in women.[4,5] Bilateral disease is less common in men, occurring in less than 5 percent of cases.[2,5] The mean diameter of the presenting mass is 3.0 to 3.5 cm.[4,5]

DIFFERENTIAL DIAGNOSIS

Because male breast cancer is rare, screening is not indicated. Breast self-examination is seldom mentioned to men during health maintenance visits. As a result, many men with breast cancer delay seeking medical attention for 6 to 9 months.[1,5]

The differential diagnosis includes cancer, gynecomastia, duct ectasia, fat necrosis, and nonmammary malignancy.

The differential diagnosis of a breast mass in a man includes cancer, gynecomastia, duct ectasia, fat necrosis, and nonmammary malignancy (chest wall sarcoma or cancer metastatic to the breast)[2] (Table 11-2). Approximately 85 percent of male breast masses are due to gynecomastia, the incidence of which increases with age.[5] Depending on whether the diagnosis is based on physical or histologic examination, gynecomastia is found in 12 to 40 percent of men with breast cancer.[2,3] Gynecomastia may be unilateral or bilateral and presents as a firm, tender area beneath the nipple.

Duct ectasia, or chronic inflammation of the subareolar ducts, may present as a small, firm retroareolar mass associated with nipple discharge. The diagnosis is uncommon unless gynecomastia is present. It is suspected if the multicolored discharge is guaiac-negative and imaging studies are otherwise unremarkable. Contrast mammography demonstrates dilated ducts without the presence of a mass. Treatment consists of the application of local heat and the administration of nonsteroidal anti-inflammatory agents.

TABLE 11-2 DIFFERENTIAL DIAGNOSIS OF BREAST MASSES IN MEN

Cancer
Gynecomastia
Duct ectasia
Fat necrosis
Nonmammary malignancy

Traumatic injury to the breast may result in fibrosis and calcification within a localized area. Skin retraction is common. Often the injury is unrecognized at the time when it occurs. Later, when a mass becomes palpable, the clinical findings are worrisome for cancer. Imaging studies may not be able to differentiate between fat necrosis and cancer, and biopsy often is required.

In a man with skin ulceration, flaking, or crusting near the nipple, the diagnosis of Paget's disease must be considered.[5] Imaging studies and biopsy are indicated.

DIAGNOSTIC TESTING

The mammographic findings of breast cancer are similar in men and women: a fairly well defined mass, spiculated margins, and microcalcifications.[4,5] With gynecomastia, no mass is present but a concentric, diffuse increase in radiographic density is seen.[5] Dense breast tissue can mask the presence of a distinct mass on mammography, and this problem is seen in women and in men with gynecomastia.[2] Mammography in men also can be problematic because of the small volume of breast tissue present.

Fine needle aspiration (FNA) cytology or open biopsy of any palpable mass in a male should be undertaken. FNA is quick, simple to perform, well tolerated, and helpful in guiding further management (see Chap. 4). For example, an FNA that is positive for cancer allows definitive surgical treatment to be planned without the need for two separate operations. However, a negative FNA usually should be followed by open biopsy.

Ultrasonography is less useful in men than in women because cysts, though uncommon, are more likely to be malignant.[4] However, ultrasonography may assist in the diagnosis of malignancy by detecting a hypoechoic mass with irregular margins.[5] Contrast mammography, or ductography, helps define the involved ducts when nipple discharge is present.[4]

STAGING

Clinical staging of male breast cancer follows the same algorithm as that for female breast cancer (see Chaps. 7 and 8) and includes physical examination, chest x-ray, and liver function tests.[1] Other imaging studies, such as bone scan and computed tomography (CT), should be performed if the symptoms suggest metastatic disease.

HISTOLOGY

Infiltrating ductal carcinoma is the most common histologic subtype of male breast cancer, occurring in 70 to 93 percent of cases.[1,2,5] Lobular carcinoma is rare because lobular development usually does not occur in men.[4,5] Ductal carcinoma in situ has been reported to account for 5 to 16 percent of male breast cancer cases.[1,4,5,8] Breast cancers in men are more often of a high histologic grade than are those in women, and hormone receptors are more commonly positive.[4] In men, estrogen receptors are positive in 65 to 92 percent of cases,[1,2,4]

Most male breast cancers are of the infiltrating ductal histologic subtype, and the majority are estrogen-receptor-positive.

whereas approximately 60 percent of breast cancers in women are positive.[5,7] DNA ploidy, epidermal growth factor (EGF), and HER-2 expression are not helpful predictors of the prognosis.[1,4] However, information about the S-phase fraction may be useful.[1,4]

TREATMENT

Modified radical mastectomy with axillary node dissection, with or without adjuvant radiation, chemotherapy, or hormonal treatment, is used for management of male breast cancer.

Because of the low incidence of the disease, no randomized clinical trials have been performed to determine the optimal mode of therapy for male breast cancer. Instead, treatment guidelines have been extrapolated from experience with breast cancer in women.[5] At the present time, modified radical mastectomy with axillary node dissection is the mainstay of therapy for patients with tumor confined to the breast.[1,4,5] In patients with chest wall invasion, radical surgery or preoperative therapy with cytotoxic agents or radiation may be indicated.[1,5]

Adjunctive radiation reduces local-regional recurrence but does not improve survival; therefore, its use is limited to patients at high risk for recurrence.[2,4,6] Radiation therapy for patients with large tumors or nodal disease should include the internal mammary and supraclavicular nodes because the centrally located cancers in men may more readily involve these nodes.[6] If radiation therapy is not employed postoperatively, it may be used as an adjunct to surgery for local recurrence.

Several retrospective cohort studies have been published that assess survival in patients who receive adjuvant systemic therapy. Tamoxifen has been shown to improve survival significantly in men with estrogen-receptor-positive stage II or operable stage III disease.[2,4] Multiagent chemotherapy with CMF (cyclophosphamide, methotrexate, and 5-fluorouracil) or FAC (5-fluorouracil, adriamycin, and cyclophosphamide) also may improve survival in these patients.[2,4] A reasonable management approach is to offer adjuvant chemotherapy to men at high risk for recurrent disease: locally advanced disease, nodal metastases, or negative estrogen-receptor status.[2,5]

Local recurrence of cancer in the breast usually is treated by surgical excision and systemic therapy (hormonal versus cytotoxic). If radiation was not used after the initial surgical management, excision of the recurrent tumor should be followed by radiation therapy.[1] If the recurrent tumor displays estrogen receptors, tamoxifen is administered; otherwise, cytotoxic therapy should begin.[1]

Metastatic disease occurs most frequently in the bone, lung, liver, and brain. Ablative hormonal therapy using orchidectomy, adrenalectomy, or hypophysectomy has had some success in the palliative treatment of recurrent or metastatic disease.[4] Numerous hormonal medications, primarily tamoxifen but also ketoconazole, cyproterone acetate, corticosteroids, androgens, progestins, aminoglutethimide, and buserelin, also have been tried with variable responses and constitute the first-line palliative treatment for metastatic disease.[2,4] Combination chemotherapy with CMF or FAC is considered to be second-line palliative therapy because the response rates are in the range of 40 to 50 percent.[2,4] Radiation therapy has been used to achieve local control of metastatic disease in the bone and brain.[5]

PROGNOSIS AND SURVIVAL

The strongest prognostic indicators for male breast cancer are stage and axillary node status.[2,4] In general, the prognosis for men with breast cancer is poorer than that for women with the disease. Men are typically older at diagnosis, their cancers are detected at a more advanced stage, and lymph nodes are more likely to be involved.[4,9] When matched for age and stage, however, survival is no different between the sexes.[2,4]

Nodal involvement at the time of diagnosis occurs in approximately 56 percent of cases and is more likely with larger tumors.[6] However, men are more likely to have positive nodes than are women, even with smaller primary tumors.[4,5] This finding may be related to the fact that cancers in men are closer to the skin. Dermal lymphatic invasion is more common in men than in women, and when studied in women, this lymphatic involvement is associated with a higher likelihood of metastases at diagnosis, rapid disease progression, and a poorer prognosis.[4] Histologically proved nodal spread is not always clinically apparent.[4,5] Axillary dissection therefore is a critical step in the determination of the prognosis and the formulation of plans for adjuvant therapy.

For men with breast cancer, the overall disease-specific 5-year survival (excluding deaths from other causes) is 43 to 74 percent.[6] When broken down on the basis of nodal status, the 5-year disease-specific survival for men with negative and positive nodes is 90 to 93 percent and 39 to 44 percent, respectively.[5] The crude survival rates are much lower because the diagnosis usually is made late in life, when other medical problems adversely affect longevity.

In women with breast cancer, tumor estrogen-receptor positivity increases with age and is associated with a better prognosis. In men, however, there is no age-related variation in receptor positivity and the response to hormonal therapy cannot be predicted consistently on the basis of receptor status.[1,4,7]

When matched for age and stage, men and women with breast cancer have similar survival.

SUMMARY

Male breast cancer is a rare disease that has many parallels with female breast cancer. Genetic and environmental risk factors have been described, and a state of relative estrogen excess has been implicated. In men, the disease presents as a painless central mass. Axillary examination does not always correlate with the histologic findings. Although it often is suspected clinically, the diagnosis must be confirmed histologically. Treatment consists of modified radical mastectomy and axillary node dissection with or without adjunctive radiation or systemic therapy. The prognosis depends on tumor size and nodal status.

REFERENCES

1. Winchester DI. Male breast cancer. *Semin Surg Oncol* 1996; 12:364–369.
2. Donegan WL, Redlich PN. Breast cancer in men. *Surg Clin North Am* 1996; 76(2):343–367.
3. Teixeira MR, Pandis N, Dietrich CU, et al. Chromosome banding analysis of gynecomastias and breast carcinomas in men. *Genes Chromosom Cancer* 1998; 23:16–20.

4. Ravandi-Kashani F, Hayes TG. Male breast cancer: A review of the literature. *Eur J Cancer* 1998; 34(9):1341–1347.
5. Jepson AS, Fentiman IS. Male breast cancer. *Int J Clin Pract* 1998; 52(8):571–576.
6. Cutuli B, Lacroze M, Dilhuydy JM, et al. Male breast cancer: Results of the treatments and prognostic factors in 397 cases. *Eur J Cancer* 1995; 31A(12):1960–1964.
7. Williams WL, Powers M, Wagman LD. Cancer of the male breast: A review. *J Natl Med Assoc* 1996; 88:439–443.
8. Cutuli B, Dilhuydy JM, DeLafontan B, et al. Ductal carcinoma in situ of the male breast: Analysis of 31 cases. *Eur J Cancer* 1997; 33(1):35–38.
9. Fullerton T, Lantz J, Sadler GR. Breast cancer among men: Raising awareness for primary prevention. *J Am Acad Nurse Pract* 1997; 9(5):211–216.

THE ROLE OF MAMMOGRAPHY IN THE DETECTION OF BREAST CANCER

INTRODUCTION

A woman's risk of developing breast cancer increases with age. Her lifetime risk of developing breast cancer is approximately 13 percent, or one in eight. Early detection of breast cancer allows a wide range of treatment options and leads to improved survival. Mammography plays a key role in the early detection of breast cancer and is the best screening tool available at this time.

OVERVIEW OF SCREENING STUDIES

Controversy still exists regarding the age at which screening mammography should begin. Analysis of screening trials in the United States, Holland, and Sweden has shown that regular screening mammograms unequivocally reduce mortality from breast cancer in women over age 50 by at least 31 percent.[1] Age 50 was chosen arbitrarily as the age to start mammographic screening in these trials because it is the approximate age when menses cease. However, because of the large number of women in the age group 40 to 49 years, the relative number of cancers occurring in that age group is similar to that occurring in the 50-to-59-year-old group.[2] Also, breast cancer is the leading cause of death in women 40 to 44 years of age, emphasizing the importance of screening in this age group.

Kopans and colleagues[3] showed that the positive predictive value of breast biopsies increased with the age of the patient but that there was not an abrupt change at age 50. The detection rate for breast cancer was 2.5 per 1000 for women 40 to 49 years of age, compared with 3.8 per 1000 for women in the age group from 50 to

79.[4] The recall rate after a screening mammogram in women age 40 to 49 years was not significantly different from the recall rate after age 50. In general, the recall rate after a first-time screening mammogram is approximately 10 percent.[5]

The breast cancer screening trials that attempted to evaluate women 40 to 50 years of age were flawed in many ways. The number of women included from this population group was statistically inadequate, the years of follow-up were too few, and the screening intervals were excessively long. Other problems included the use of a single mediolateral oblique (MLO) view for screening, poor technique, inadequate interpretation with higher thresholds for intervention, single instead of double reads, randomization problems (e.g., late-stage cancers were placed in the study group), control group women seeking mammography outside the trial, and participant noncompliance.[6,7]

Moskowitz[8] showed that the average lead time for breast cancers in women between ages 40 and 50 is 18 months. Mammography therefore must be performed annually in this population to reduce mortality from breast cancer. Screening performed at intervals greater than 12 months may result in a larger number of interval cancers, a higher stage at diagnosis, and no reduction in mortality. In addition, the use of a single MLO view for screening has been shown to reduce the rate of cancer detection.[9]

A meta-analysis of data from eight breast cancer screening trials showed a statistically significant > 18 percent reduction in breast cancer as a result of screening in women age 40 to 50.

Although there has been no single randomized trial to test the efficiency of screening women age 40 to 50, a meta-analysis of data from eight breast cancer screening trials showed a statistically significant > 18 percent reduction in breast cancer as a result of screening in this age group. The Breast Cancer Detection and Demonstration Project (BCDDP) showed that screening women in their forties is beneficial.[6] Survival rates in women age 40 to 49 were similar to those in women age 50 to 69. In 1995, the Surveillance, Epidemiology, and End Results (SEER) program showed an 8.1 percent decrease in breast cancer mortality among women age 40 to 49 between 1989 and 1992.[10] Perhaps yearly screening mammography will further decrease mortality from breast cancer in this age group as well as in older women.

CURRENT SCREENING GUIDELINES

Since 1997, the American College of Radiology (ACR) and the American Cancer Society (ACS) have recommended annual mammographic screening for women starting at age 40.[11] Guidelines from other physician organizations vary, with some organizations recommending a baseline at age 35. In addition, mammography may benefit women younger than age 40 who are at increased risk for breast cancer. If a woman has a family history of premenopausal breast cancer in a mother or sister, mammographic screening should begin at age 30, closer to the age when the affected person was diagnosed.[12]

FDA CERTIFICATION IN MAMMOGRAPHY

The quality of mammography has improved dramatically since the clinical trials of the Health Insurance Plan of New York (HIP) in the 1960s and the BCDDP in the 1970s. Advances in mammographic technology have been accompanied by strict U.S. Food and Drug Administration (FDA)-imposed quality control rules and regulations. FDA certification of mammography facilities is required under the Mammography Quality Standards Act (MQSA) of October 1994 and has resulted in standardization of quality between facilities. The certification process includes a survey of the facility and its personnel, quantification of the radiation dose to the patient, and quality assessment of mammographic images, equipment, and film processing. Each facility is inspected annually by the FDA and must adhere to the guidelines for equipment, personnel, mammograms, and reports.

Reports must use ACR Breast Imaging Reporting and Data System (BI-RADS) terminology:[13]

0 Incomplete, needs additional imaging or comparison to prior studies
1 Negative, routine follow-up
2 Benign finding but also negative for cancer, routine follow-up
3 Probably benign, 98 percent probability of benign but short interval follow-up recommended
4 Suspicious, biopsy should be considered
5 Highly suggestive of malignancy, biopsy required

As of April 30, 1999, mammography facilities must inform patients in writing of the results of their mammograms. In addition, patients who are self-referred must receive a copy of the report as well as a letter in lay language stating the results of the mammogram. Each facility is responsible for the tracking and follow-up of all patients who have a positive or suspicious mammographic finding. To satisfy these requirements, the facility must have a computerized database for follow-up and tracking of patients. The mammography facility also must ascertain that all recommendations are followed by directly communicating with the referring facility or physician. Although very time-consuming for the facility, these measures were added to ensure that patients with positive findings would not be lost to follow-up.

RADIATION DOSE TO THE BREAST

The current understanding of radiation-induced carcinogenesis stems from extrapolation of the effects seen in radiation therapy patients and nuclear bombing survivors. The mean glandular dose of radiation to the breast for each mammographic exposure is approximately 0.2 rad, well below the dose associated with the risk for radiation-induced cancer. A woman's breast tissue is less sensitive to radiation after she has completed a full-term pregnancy and after age 40. However, some difference in susceptibility to radiation may depend on an individual's genetic makeup. The hypothetical risk of breast cancer death from radiation exposure from mammographic screening beginning at age 45 was calculated to be 5 in 1 million women. These 5 deaths would be in addition to the 750 deaths resulting from the 15,000 naturally occurring breast cancers that would have gone undetected without screening. Therefore, the risk of developing breast cancer from mammography is negligible.[2]

The mean glandular dose of radiation to the breast for each mammographic exposure is approximately 0.2 rad.

MAMMOGRAPHIC TECHNIQUE

The goal of mammography is to produce high-resolution images of the breast while minimizing radiation exposure to the patient. Mammographic equipment is specifically designed to use low-energy x-rays to achieve excellent contrast between fat, glandular tissue, masses, and calcifications.

Two views of each breast are required for routine screening mammography of an asymptomatic patient: the craniocaudal (CC) view and the MLO view (Fig. 12-1). For future films to be compared easily, the nipple must be in profile. The MLO view contains the most breast tissue and should include the pectoral muscle down to the level of the nipple.

Mammogram labeling is standardized, and a marker is placed on the lateral aspect of each image. The location of a lesion within the breast then can be determined by noting its position relative to the nipple on the two views. To describe the location of a lesion, the breast can be divided into quadrants or the lesion's location can be described relative to the numbers on a clock face. Markers may be placed on nipples, prominent skin lesions, or scars to aid in the evaluation of mammographic findings. Often, a nipple or skin lesion may give the appearance of a mass on a mammogram (Fig. 12-2).

To obtain the CC and MLO views, the breast must be positioned between two compression plates, one of which contains the film (Fig. 12-3). Compression reduces radiation exposure and spreads the breast tissue into a uniform thickness, allowing small masses to be better visualized. Unfortunately, breast compression can be very uncomfortable for some women. The technologist must be skilled in positioning the patient to obtain optimal compression with minimal discomfort. For premenopausal women, the experience may be improved if mammography is scheduled to occur during the proliferative phase of the menstrual cycle, when the breasts may be less tender.

Eklund and colleagues[14] developed a technique for screening mammography in women with breast implants. These patients require four views of each breast to maximize the amount of breast tissue that is imaged. The two standard compression views include as much of the posterior breast tissue as possible. Additional CC and MLO views are taken of the anterior breast tissue by pulling the tissue forward over the implant while pushing the implant back toward the chest

Compression reduces radiation exposure and spreads the breast tissue into a uniform thickness, allowing small masses to be better visualized.

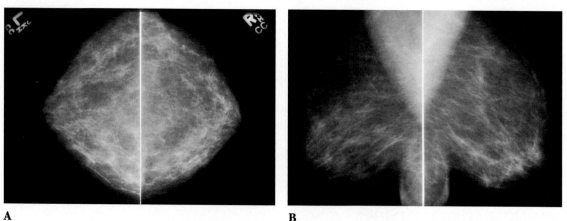

A   **B**

FIGURE 12-1 The standard mammographic images are the craniocaudal *(A)* and mediolateral oblique *(B)* views of both breasts compared side by side for symmetry. Note the inclusion of the pectoral muscle down to the level of the nipple on the MLO view.

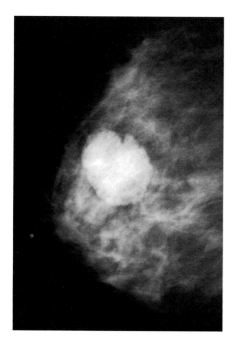

FIGURE 12-2 This large seborrheic kerato-sis projects as a mass on the mammogram.

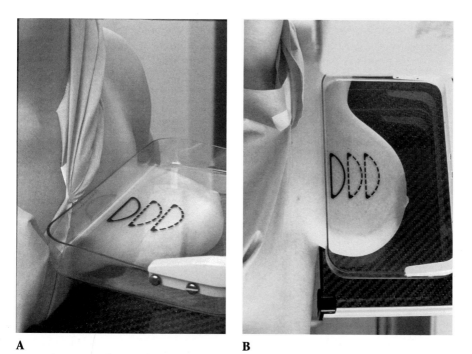

A   **B**

FIGURE 12-3 *A.* The craniocaudal view is obtained by positioning the breast between a compression plate and an image detector that is aligned horizontally. ***B.*** The mediolateral view requires that the plates be angled vertically along the plane of the pectoral muscle.

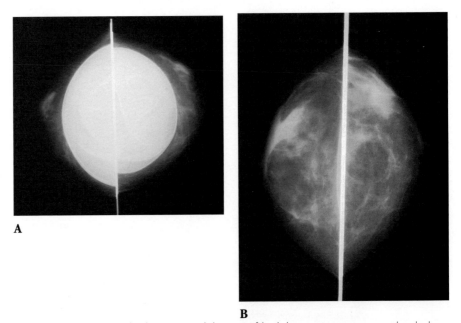

FIGURE 12-4 *(A)* Standard craniocaudal views of both breasts in a patient with subglandular implants. Note that only a small amount of breast tissue is imaged around the implant. *(B)* With the implant displacement views, improved compression and imaging of the tissue behind the nipple area are obtained.

wall (Fig. 12-4). This technique is easier to perform in patients with subpectoral implants. Patients with capsular contractures or hardening of implants are more difficult to image. Although the additional views increase the amount of breast tissue visualized on the mammogram, not all the breast tissue can be imaged. Clinical breast examination in these patients is extremely important. Because of the additional time required to perform mammography on patients with implants and the possible need for repeated views, these patients should be imaged at a permanent facility instead of a mobile screening setting (e.g., a traveling van.)

SYMPTOMATIC PATIENTS

Patients who have symptoms of a lump or breast pain require special care. Their testing should take place in a standard facility, and a radiologist should be present to evaluate the films before the patient's departure. If a mass is palpable, a skin marker must be placed over the mass on both views. The presence of the skin marker on the mammogram indicates that the mass was included on the film.

In addition to the standard CC and MLO views, other images may be needed to assess an area of abnormality completely. The spot compression view utilizes focal compression to spread the tissues and separate an area of suspicion from overlapping parenchyma. The magnification view allows improved delineation of mass borders as well as the shape and number of calcifications. Additional views, such as a straight lateral view or a laterally exaggerated CC view, can be tailored to the mammographic finding or the patient's symptoms. These additional images aid in distinguishing a discrete lesion from overlapping breast tissue.

Ultrasound is a useful adjunct for the evaluation of patients with a palpable mass (see below). In fact, for the initial evaluation of a mass in a pregnant or young (< 25 years old) woman, ultrasound is the procedure of choice. Also, in a symptomatic patient with implants, additional evaluation with ultrasound may be helpful in determining whether a palpable mass is in the breast tissue or is related to the implant. Both ultrasound and magnetic resonance imaging (MRI) of the breast can be used to evaluate implant rupture.

NORMAL MAMMOGRAMS

Breasts are composed of a combination of fatty tissue and glandular parenchyma. Mammographically, breasts that are primarily fatty have a low-density, almost transparent appearance. Conversely, dense, glandular breasts appear nearly opaque white. The BI-RADS classification divides mammographic patterns into four groups: almost entirely fatty breast tissue, scattered fibroglandular elements, heterogeneously dense, and extremely dense. A woman's age and hormonal status play a role in determining the mammographic appearance of her breasts. Young women usually have very dense breasts, making visualization of abnormalities difficult (Fig. 12-5). With aging, the glandular tissue is replaced with fat and the breasts appear less dense (Fig. 12-6). Approximately 24 percent of women who begin hormone replacement therapy display a mammographic increase in breast density (Fig. 12-7). The detection of cysts and fibroadenomas also increases with the use of estrogen replacement therapy[15] and may contribute to an increase in the false-positive rate of mammography.

Screening mammograms are compared side by side for symmetry as well as for more specific findings, such as masses and calcifications. To improve the detection of abnormalities, mammograms should be viewed on a special light scope with no

Screening mammograms are compared side by side for assessment of symmetry and the presence of masses or calcifications. Comparison with prior films ensures that subtle changes will be detected.

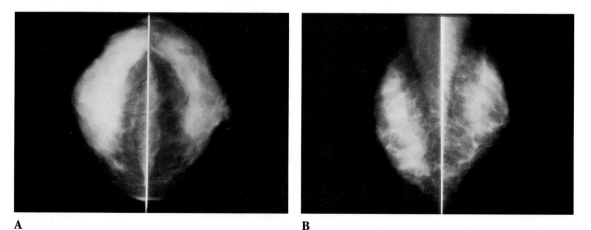

A   **B**

FIGURE 12-5 Craniocaudal *(A)* and mediolateral oblique *(B)* views demonstrating the normal mammographic appearance of the dense breasts of a 30-year-old woman.

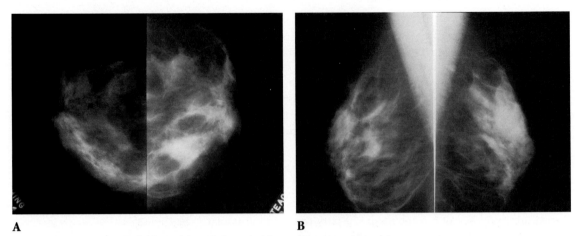

A   **B**

FIGURE 12-6 Craniocaudal *(A)* and mediolateral oblique *(B)* views of an older patient showing fatty replacement of glandular breast tissue. Asymmetry may develop as the breasts change with age.

ambient light in the room. In addition, current mammograms must be compared with prior studies to ensure that subtle changes are detected.

The false-negative rate of mammography is approximately 10 percent. False negatives can be attributed to dense breast tissue that obscures the abnormality, small size of the lesion, a lesion seen only on one view, subtle or atypical findings, inadequate mammographic technique, and interpretation error.[16] A negative or benign mammogram interpretation should not delay the biopsy of a clinically suspicious mass.

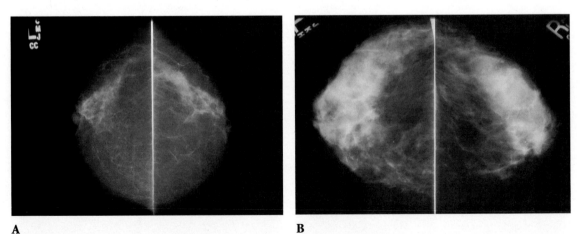

A   **B**

FIGURE 12-7 Craniocaudal views before hormone replacement therapy *(A)* and 2 years after the initiation of hormone replacement therapy *(B)* demonstrate an increase in mammographic density.

MAMMOGRAPHIC SIGNS OF MALIGNANCY

Mammographic signs of breast cancer include the presence of a mass and/or clustered microcalcifications. Although any mass seen on mammography is suspicious, the presence of irregular or microlobulated borders is especially foreboding. A nonpalpable, poorly marginated, spiculated mass found on a mammogram carries a 74 percent positive predictive value for breast cancer (Fig. 12-8). If the mass is palpable and spiculated in appearance, the positive predictive value increases to approximately 99 percent. Masses are seen more commonly in invasive breast cancers than in intraductal cancers. Other disease processes that can present with a spiculated mass are complex sclerosing lesions, postsurgical scars, fat necrosis, and benign granular-cell tumors. A well-circumscribed mass that is round or oval has only a 2 percent chance of being cancer.[17]

A nonpalpable, poorly marginated, spiculated mass found on a mammogram carries a 74 percent positive predictive value for breast cancer.

Calcifications are a common mammographic finding. Microcalcifications are less than 500 μ in diameter and, when "clustered" in a group of at least five, often represent cancer. The suspicion for cancer increases when the calcifications vary in size, shape, and density. The most suspicious shapes are linear branching forms and granular shapes, which may be arranged in a ductal segment and directed toward the nipple (Fig. 12-9). The microcalcifications associated with breast cancer may reflect calcification of necrotic tumor cells or secretion of calcium by tumor cells.

When microcalcifications are not associated with a mass, they have a positive predictive value for cancer of approximately 20 percent and are a common finding

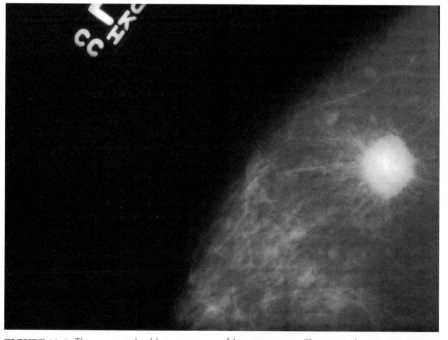

FIGURE 12-8 This mass is highly suggestive of breast cancer. The central mass is very dense, has irregular borders, and shows the typical spiculations extending out from the edges of the mass. These spiculations may represent extension of the cancer or fibrosis from a desmoplastic reaction to the cancer.

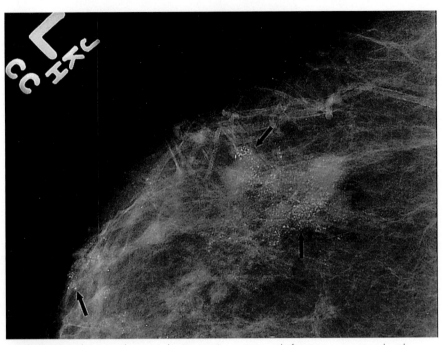

FIGURE 12-9 The tiny white specks *(arrows)* are microcalcifications associated with breast cancer. This patient had an invasive ductal cancer as well as an extensive intraductal component. Note the microcalcifications extending to the nipple area.

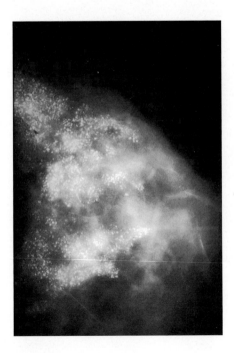

FIGURE 12-10 Mammogram demonstrating the ground-glass calcification pattern seen with comedocarcinoma. This extensive cancer was not palpable.

in ductal carcinoma in situ (DCIS). Comedocarcinoma is the most common type of DCIS, and the associated microcalcifications may represent necrosis accompanying rapid growth. The comedo type of DCIS may be multicentric, and the extent of involvement correlates with the extent of the microcalcifications (Fig. 12-10). This is not true for a noncomedo DCIS, in which the calcifications on the mammogram probably underestimate the extent of the DCIS.[18] Only 1 to 2 percent of cases of DCIS are associated with lymph node metastases. DCIS accounts for 22 to 45 percent of all breast cancers diagnosed mammographically.[19]

Twenty percent of patients with breast cancers display subtle, indirect signs of malignancy on mammography. These signs include asymmetry, architectural distortion, a unilateral focus of prominent ducts, and a developing neodensity. Comparison to prior mammograms is especially important in evaluating these findings. Although a dilated asymmetric duct pattern is rarely indicative of cancer, this finding is of increased significance when the dilated duct represents an interval change, contains microcalcifications, or is in a nonsubareolar location.[20] Nipple retraction and skin thickening are late manifestations of breast cancer that are better appreciated clinically.

BREAST ULTRASOUND

INTRODUCTION

Breast ultrasound is an excellent adjunct to mammography; however, ultrasound is not useful for breast cancer screening because it cannot detect the small clustered microcalcifications that may be an early sign of breast cancer. Its use in breast imaging has evolved from the simple determination of whether a mass is cystic or solid to the characterization of a mass as probably benign or malignant. The development of the handheld linear array transducer with multiple movable focal zones from 5 to 12 MHz and the availability of real-time imaging have enhanced the usefulness of ultrasound in breast diagnosis.[21] However, differentiation of benign from malignant solid lesions is still not completely reliable with current ultrasound technology.

The use of ultrasound in breast imaging has evolved from the simple determination of whether a mass is cystic or solid to the characterization of a mass as probably benign or malignant.

INDICATIONS

The primary utility of breast ultrasonography lies in the assessment of a palpable mass. For young (< 25 years old) or pregnant women, ultrasound is the initial imaging study of choice to evaluate a palpable lump. Ultrasound also can be used to characterize a nonpalpable mammographically detected mass. In this case, the mammographic finding must be correlated with the ultrasound finding to ensure that the correct area of the breast is evaluated. In postoperative patients, ultrasound can differentiate between scar formation and fluid collections. In a high-risk patient with dense breast tissue, ultrasound examination may be used as an adjunct to mammographic screening.[22] It may be useful in evaluating patients with nipple discharge or complications of breast implants. Ultrasound also may be employed to guide fine needle aspirations, needle drainage procedures, core biopsies, and needle-localization procedures.

For young (< 25 years old) or pregnant women, ultrasound is the initial imaging study of choice to evaluate a palpable lump.

TECHNIQUE

The patient is scanned in the supine position with the arm raised above the head and the body rotated slightly so that the breast tissue is distributed more evenly over the chest wall. This position allows better visualization of the tissues between the skin and the rib cage and reduces motion of the breast. The use of a linear array transducer with dynamic focusing and frequencies of 7.5 MHz or higher is ideal. The breast should be scanned in both the transverse and the longitudinal planes. Examination in a radial plane may be needed to evaluate ducts of the extension of a mass along a duct. The ultrasonographer should be familiar with the appearance of normal breast tissue: Fatty tissue appears hypoechoic, and fibroglandular tissue is echogenic.[23]

EVALUATION

Ultrasound can be used to determine the location, size, shape, and border characteristics of a mass. In addition, the internal composition of a mass can be seen as echogenic, hypoechoic, or anechoic. A simple cyst appears as an anechoic mass with a round or oval shape with smooth walls, sharp anterior and posterior borders, and good through transmission of sound with posterior acoustic enhancement (Fig. 12-11). A simple cyst does not need to be aspirated unless it is symptomatic or interferes with future breast examinations.[24] Typical ultrasonographic features of a malignant mass include larger longitudinal than transverse dimensions, angular margins, spiculated borders, a hypoechogenic texture, and distal shadowing behind the mass (Fig. 12-12).

DUCTOGRAMS

Spontaneous unilateral nipple discharge that is bloody, serous, or watery should be evaluated cytologically, and a mammographic examination of the breasts should be performed. If the discharge emanates from only one or two ducts, contrast mammography, or ductography, may identify and localize the area of abnormality, facilitating surgical excision. First, the involved duct orifice is dilated slowly to allow the insertion of a small, blunt-tip needle or a 24-gauge angiocatheter (Fig. 12-13). Then a small amount of iodinated contrast material, usually less than 0.5 mL, is injected carefully into the duct. Appropriate mammographic images then are examined for evidence of a ductal filling defect, irregularity, dilatation, or complete obstruction; these signs often are associated with carcinoma (Fig. 12-14). The size and location of the lesion, as well as its distance from the nipple, should be noted.[26,27]

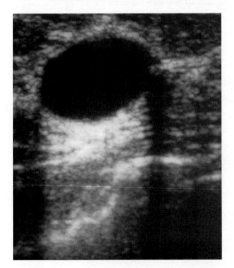

FIGURE 12-11 The typical ultrasound appearance of a simple cyst. Note the well-defined borders, the lack of echoes within the mass, and the posterior acoustic enhancement.

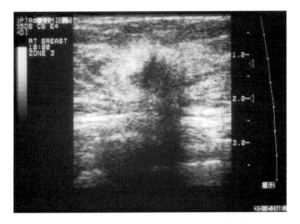

FIGURE 12-12 The ultrasound appearance of breast cancer. Note the fingerlike projections extending from the mass, the hypoechogenic texture, and the distal shadowing behind the mass.

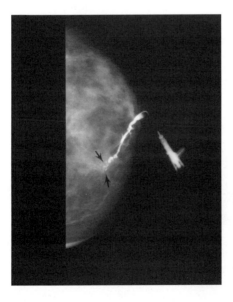

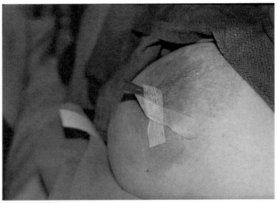

A   **B**

FIGURE 12-13 Dilation of the draining duct allows the insertion of a 24-gauge angiocatheter *(A)* through which contrast can be injected *(B).*

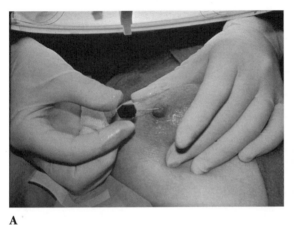

FIGURE 12-14 Ductogram performed to evaluate a bloody nipple discharge. The abrupt cutoff of contrast within the duct occurs at the site of a cancer.

ROLE OF MRI IN BREAST IMAGING

MRI is slowly evolving as a useful tool in the evaluation of breast problems. MRI of the breast employs a dedicated coil with tissue-specific sequences tailored to produce images in the transverse, longitudinal, and coronal planes. It has become the study of choice to diagnose rupture of a silicone implant. With intracapsular rupture, in which the silicone remains contained within the fibrous capsule surrounding the implant, the collapsed shell of the implant is seen as serpiginous folds, or the "linguine sign" (Fig. 12-15).[28]

The introduction of gadolinium-diethylene triamine pentaacetic acid (Gd-DTPA) contrast has improved the utility of breast MRI. Some masses can be distinguished as malignant on the basis of certain tissue enhancement characteristics with contrast. However, normal breast tissue and benign lesions also may enhance with contrast; therefore, the diagnostic utility of MRI alone remains limited.

MRI can detect chest wall invasion as well as multicentric and multifocal lesions (Fig. 12-16). It can be used to evaluate the effect of chemotherapy on a breast cancer and can distinguish between scar tissue and recurrent disease. MRI may be a useful adjunct in the evaluation of patients with dense breast tissue who are at increased

With intracapsular rupture, in which the silicone remains contained within the fibrous capsule surrounding the implant, the collapsed shell of the implant is seen as serpiginous folds, or the "linguine sign."

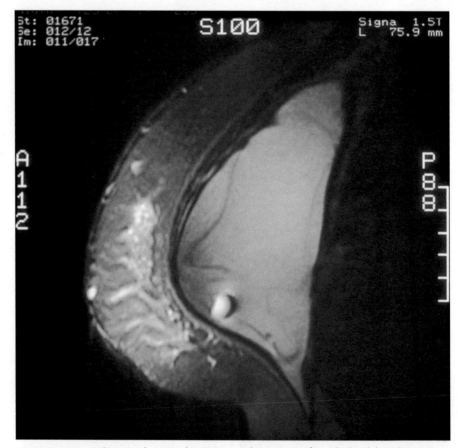

FIGURE 12-15 MRI scan showing the intracapsular rupture of a subglandular silicone implant. The dark wavy lines represent the collapsed shell of the implant. The silicone remains contained within the fibrous capsule surrounding the implant.

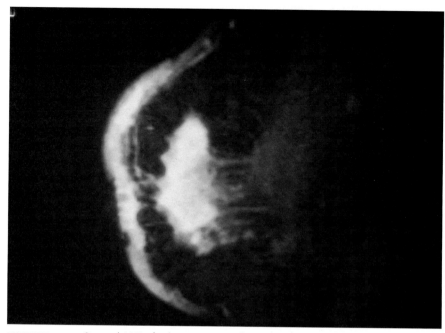

FIGURE 12-16 Sagittal MRI of a breast using a fat-suppressed sequence makes the fat appear black, while the tumor mass and skin are white. Note the stringlike extension of the tumor to the pectoral muscle.

risk for breast cancer and in whom a mammogram is not definitive. A special coil is under development to facilitate the biopsy of lesions found on MRI.[29]

ROLE OF NUCLEAR MEDICINE IN BREAST IMAGING

Technetium-99m-sestamibi is a radioactive isotope that plays a complementary role in the diagnosis of breast cancer. Ten minutes after its intravenous injection, lateral and anterior scans of the breast are taken. The isotope concentrates in malignant tissue and involved lymph nodes appear on the scan as a dark area of increased up-take. This type of imaging has a high positive predictive value for breast cancer and is particularly useful in patients with dense breast tissue in whom mammographic interpretation is limited. However, it is not useful in the evaluation of microcalcifications or the detection of masses less than 2 cm in diameter. At the present time, this procedure remains an adjunct for evaluating difficult cases and high-risk patients.[30–32]

NEEDLE BIOPSY PROCEDURES

FINE NEEDLE ASPIRATION

To perform fine needle aspiration (FNA) of a breast mass, a 20- to 25-gauge needle is introduced into the mass to sample its contents. Negative pressure generated by an attached syringe allows removal of fluid if the mass is cystic or of cellular material if the mass is solid. The contents thus withdrawn can be evaluated cytologically. Initially, this procedure was possible only if the patient's mass was palpable. Now, stereotactic and ultrasound guidance techniques allow sampling of nonpalpable lesions as well. The procedure has minimal associated morbidity, and with a cytopathology technician present for processing, the results are available quickly. The fairly high false-negative rate associated with FNA is affected by the skill of the clinician performing the aspiration and cytopathologist interpreting the smears. An FNA diagnosis of malignancy may help guide patient management, but a negative result is not as helpful because it does not definitively exclude the possibility of cancer. Also, DCIS cannot be distinguished from an invasive cancer by FNA cytology.[33]

CORE NEEDLE BIOPSY

As opposed to FNA, in which a cytologic sample is obtained, core needle biopsy removes strips of tissue that can be evaluated histologically.

As opposed to FNA, in which a cytologic sample is obtained, core needle biopsy removes strips of tissue that can be evaluated histologically. The spring-driven biopsy gun can accept anything from an 18-gauge needle to an 11-gauge needle (Fig. 12-17). Commonly, a 14-gauge needle removes strips of tissue large enough for the pathologist to interpret. Not only can benign tissue be distinguished from malignant tissue, but in situ versus invasive cancer and type of cancer can be discerned. The accuracy of the procedure is at least 96 percent when a 14-gauge needle is used. The technique initially was developed for use with stereotactic guidance, but ultrasound guidance has become practical as well.[34,35] The complication of hematoma formation can be avoided by ensuring that the patient has not taken anticoagulants, including aspirin, for at least 5 days before the procedure. The other problem associated with core biopsy is inadequate sampling as a result of obtaining insufficient tissue from the mass or missing the mass altogether.[36]

Stereotactic guidance allows precise placement of a needle to within 1 mm of a lesion, assuming that the patient does not move during the procedure. Stereotactic core breast biopsy can be performed with the patient in one of two positions: (1) lying prone with the breast positioned through a hole in the table and the lesion targeted from below (Fig. 12-18), or (2) sitting up, with the lesion targeted from above. Both masses and clustered microcalcifications can be targeted easily for biopsy.

With the patient lying prone, the compression device and the x-ray tube are located beneath the table. Only a small region of the breast is imaged, and the lesion to be biopsied is centered within the window of the compression plate. Once the scout view has been taken, two stereo pair images are taken 30 degrees apart from each other, 15 degrees away from midline. Using digital imaging, the images are processed within seconds. Next, the center of the lesion is marked on both of the stereo pairs and the computer calculates the X, Y, and Z axes of the lesion. These dimensions are transferred to the computerized gun at the biopsy table.

The breast within the window of the compression plate is cleansed with betadine. Lidocaine 1% is injected to anesthetize the skin, and 1% lidocaine with 1:100,000 epinephrine is used for deeper local anesthesia. After a 14-gauge needle is attached to the spring-driven gun, an initial core biopsy specimen is taken from the center of the lesion (Fig. 12-19). Additional tissue samples are taken 2 to 3 mm from the center. When a mass is biopsied, at least five core samples are removed. When microcalcifications are targeted, up to 10 additional passes with the biopsy needle may be necessary to sample the area adequately. A specimen radiograph of the core samples will ensure that the calcifications in question are present within the sample.[37]

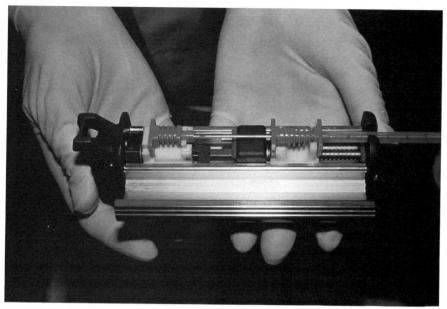

FIGURE 12-17 A. A spring-driven core biopsy gun.

A vacuum-assisted biopsy device that uses an 11- or 14-gauge needle may improve the sampling of microcalcifications because the needle is not removed from the breast once it has been inserted. The opening of the needle's cutting device is rotated in a clockwise direction to sample the area around the needle. When an 11-gauge needle is used to remove an entire lesion, a small metallic clip can be inserted

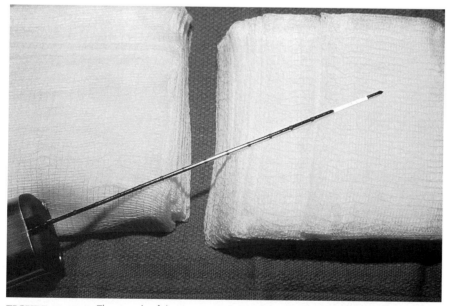

FIGURE 12-17 B. The trough of the cutting portion of the needle is visible near the tip of the needle.

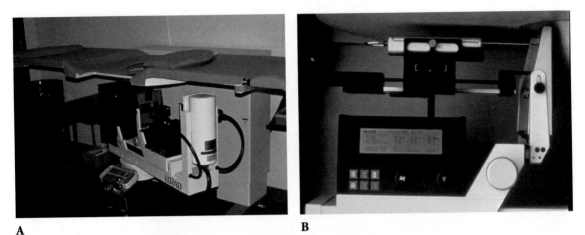

A   **B**

FIGURE 12-18 *A.* The patient lies prone on the core biopsy table. *B.* Her breast is positioned between the compression plate and the image detector located under the table.

Histologic evaluation of a core biopsy specimen can differentiate carcinoma in situ from invasive cancer. However, if atypical ductal hyperplasia or DCIS is found, excisional biopsy is still needed to exclude an invasive cancer.

into the breast at the end of the procedure to mark the location of the biopsy. Then, if cancer is diagnosed, the biopsy site can be reexcised. With these larger samples, bleeding is a more common complication. A clinically evident hematoma forms in approximately 4 percent of cases in which the vacuum-assisted device is used. Other complications include infection and inadequate sampling. A histologic result discordant from the mammographic diagnosis occasionally occurs.[38,39]

Core needle biopsy offers the advantage over FNA of enabling the pathologist to differentiate carcinoma in situ from invasive cancer. However, if atypical ductal hyperplasia or DCIS is found, excisional biopsy is still needed to exclude an invasive cancer.[40] The mammographic appearance of a lesion should always be compared with the histologic report. In a multi-institutional study of 6152 biopsied lesions,

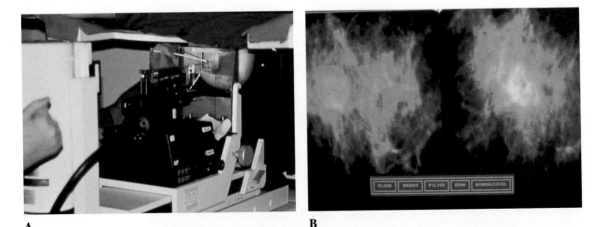

A   **B**

FIGURE 12-19 *A.* After the skin is cleansed and local anesthesia is administered, a 2-mm nick in the skin is made with a scalpel. The core biopsy needle is introduced into the skin incision, and the biopsy gun is fired. *B.* The samples are taken from predetermined locations; the three-dimensional coordinates are programmed into the computerized gun by the clinician after a review of the stereopair images.

the false-negative rate ranged from 0.3 to 0.6 percent with a cancer miss rate of 1.2 to 1.5 percent.[41] Core needle biopsy decreases the cost of cancer diagnosis by approximately 50 percent compared with excisional biopsy.[42]

ULTRASOUND-GUIDED NEEDLE BIOPSY

Core needle biopsy of the breast using ultrasound guidance is an alternative to stereotactic breast biopsy when a mass is visible on ultrasound (Fig. 12-20). The procedure is performed in the supine position rather than prone, as on the stereotactic biopsy table. Using ultrasound, the needle's path is monitored from its insertion into the skin (Fig. 12-21) to its entry into the mass. The needle can be introduced perpendicular to the mass or from a lateral or oblique position. Because microcalcifications often are difficult to visualize on ultrasound, stereotactic guidance may be the more appropriate technique to use in that setting.[43]

NEEDLE-LOCALIZATION PROCEDURES FOR EXCISIONAL BIOPSY

Before a nonpalpable breast lesion can be excised, it first must be localized by using mammographic or ultrasound guidance. A hollow needle is placed into the mass, through which a wire with a terminal hook or barb is inserted. The wire is left in place to guide the surgeon accurately to the lesion and help minimize the volume of breast tissue excised.

On the morning of surgery, the patient is brought to the mammography suite for placement of the needle and hook wire. The patient is positioned in the mammography machine with the windowed alphanumeric compression plate on the skin surface from which the needle will be inserted. A scout film is taken with the breast

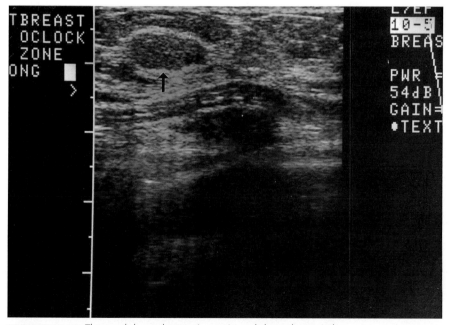

FIGURE 12-20 This oval-shaped mass *(arrow)* is solid on ultrasound.

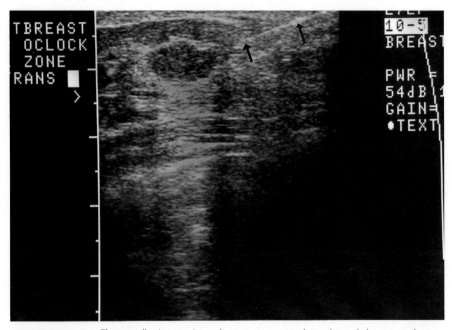

FIGURE 12-21 *A.* The needle *(arrows)* can be seen approaching this solid mass in the prefire image.

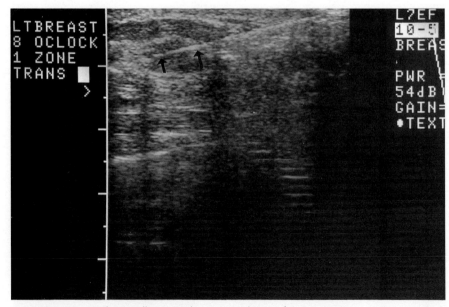

FIGURE 12-21 *B.* The needle enters the mass in the postfire image.

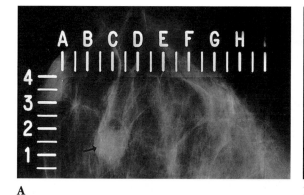

A

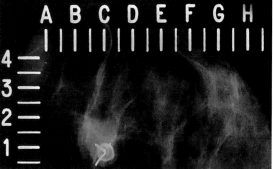

B

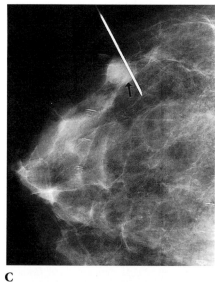

C

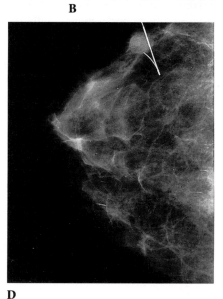

D

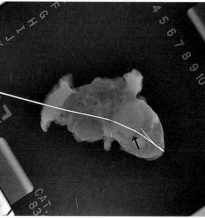

E

FIGURE 12-22 A. The patient is placed in the mammography machine with the breast positioned so that the shortest distance to the lesion is at the opening of the windowed part of the alphanumeric compression plate. **B.** The needle is then positioned into the mass. **C.** If the positioning is satisfactory, the breast is taken out of compression, and an orthogonal view at 90 degrees is done to determine the depth of the lesion relative to the needle. **D.** If the position of the needle is satisfactory, the wire is deployed and the needle is removed. One final film is taken to show the position of the lesion to the barb of the wire *(arrow).* **E.** A radiograph of the specimen should always be performed to demonstrate that the lesion has been excised.

in compression, and the compression plate is left in place to guide needle placement. Depending on the location of the lesion and the preference of the surgeon, the needle is inserted from the skin surface that provides the shortest distance to the lesion while the needle remains parallel to the chest wall. If the patient has no known allergies, her skin is cleansed with betadine and anesthetized with 1% lidocaine. The needle and wire are inserted, and a mammogram is taken. If the position of the needle is satisfactory, the patient's breast is removed from compression and an orthogonal view is taken. If accurate placement is confirmed, the needle is removed and the wire is left in place. One final film is taken with the wire in position, and the lesion is marked on the film. The distance from the barb to the skin surface is measured. The films accompany the patient to the operating room. After excision, a radiograph of the specimen and the attached wire is performed to ensure that the entire lesion has been removed and that the wire is intact (Fig. 12-22).

COMMONLY ASKED QUESTIONS

1. **My doctor found a lump in my breast last week, but my mammogram was normal. Should I have any further evaluation?** A discrete mass in the breast must be evaluated histologically to ensure that it is benign. Because mammography carries a false-negative rate of 10 to 15 percent, a normal mammogram does not rule out the possibility of malignancy. Ultrasonography should be performed to determine whether the lump is a simple cyst, in which case no further evaluation may be necessary, or a solid mass. If it is solid, it should be sampled (fine needle aspiration or core biopsy) or excised. If there is little clinical suspicion, fine needle aspiration may suffice. Occasionally, a fairly localized area of denser breast tissue may prompt the workup described here. If the clinical impression is benign, mammography is negative, and ultrasonography does not demonstrate a mass, follow-up with serial physical examinations may be all that is necessary.

2. **Won't the repeated radiation exposure from mammography over time put me at increased risk for breast cancer?** The radiation dose for routine mammographic imaging is only 0.4 rad per breast (0.2 rad per view). The hypothetical risk of breast cancer from repeated exposure to such small doses of radiation is far outweighed by the potential benefit of early cancer detection.

3. **I found my first mammogram to be extremely painful, and I was sore for weeks afterward. Why do they have to compress my breasts so flat?** The breasts are not uniform in thickness and must be flattened between the two compression plates to minimize radiation exposure and maximize visualization. To avoid unnecessary discomfort, premenopausal women should undergo mammography during the follicular phase of the menstrual cycle and postmenopausal women taking hormone replacement therapy may wish to discontinue their medication for a few weeks before the scheduled appointment. A skilled technician usually can manage to obtain adequate views with minimal patient discomfort.

4. **I was told I need to have a "core biopsy" of some calcifications in my breast. What can I expect that procedure to be like?** When you arrive for the core biopsy, you probably will be asked to lie facedown on a table that has a hole cut out of one end. Your breast will dangle through the hole and will be positioned between two compression plates underneath the table. A mammogram will be repeated in this position to locate the abnormal area. A computer will calculate exactly where the biopsy needle should go. With your breast still lying between the plates, your skin will be cleansed and anesthetized. A small incision will be made in your skin with a scalpel so that the needle is not dulled by the skin. The spring on the needle gun is released, and the needle samples tissue from the area targeted by the computer. The number of passes made with the needle depends on the size and shape of the abnormality, but expect at least 5 to 10. Most women say that the procedure is not very

painful, and some do not feel anything after the local anesthetic is injected. After the procedure, you will keep pressure on the incision site for about 10 min. A bandage then will be placed. Application of ice when you get home may help prevent bruising.

REFERENCES

1. Hall FM. Screening mammography (editorial). *AJR* 1986; 147:195–197.
2. Feig SA. Screening guidelines and controversies. In: Bassett LW, Jackson V, Johan R, Bralow L, eds. *Diagnosis of Diseases of the Breast.* Philadelphia: Saunders; 1997:329–343.
3. Kopans DB, Moore RH, McCarthy KA, et al. Positive predictive value of breast biopsy performed as a result of mammography: There is no abrupt change at age 50 years. *Radiology* 1996; 200:357–360.
4. Kopans DB, Moore RH, McCarthy KA, et al. Biasing the interpretation of mammography screening data by age grouping: Nothing changes abruptly at age 50. *Breast J* 1998; 4:139–145.
5. Moskowitz M. Retrospective reviews of breast cancer screening: What do we really learn from them? *Radiology* 1996; 199:615–620.
6. Feig SA. Determination of mammographic screening intervals with surrogate measures for women aged 40–49 years. *Radiology* 1994; 193:311–314.
7. Miller AB, Baines CJ, To T, Wall C. Canadian National Breast Screening Study: I. Breast cancer detection and death rates among women aged 40–49 years. *Can Med Assoc J* 1992; 147(10):1459–1476.
8. Moskowitz M. Breast cancer: Age-specific growth rates and screening strategies. *Radiology* 1986; 161:37–41.
9. Moskowitz M. Impact of a priori medical decisions on screening for breast cancer. *Radiology* 1989; 171:605–608.
10. Cardenosa G, Eklund GW. Screening mammography in women 40–49 years old. *AJR* 1995; 164:1104–1106.
11. Feig SA, D'Orsi CJ, Hendrick RE, et al. American College of Radiology Guidelines for Breast Cancer Screening. *AJR* 1998; 171:29–33.
12. Moskowitz M. Breast cancer screening: All's well that ends well, or much ado about nothing? *AJR* 1988; 151:659–665.
13. American College of Radiology (ACR). *Illustrated Breast Imaging Reporting and Data System (BI-RADS TM),* 3d ed. Reston, VA: American College of Radiology; 1998.
14. Eklund GW, Busby RC, Miller SH, Job JS. Improved imaging of the augmented breast. *AJR* 1988; 151:469–473.
15. Stomper PC, Van Voorhis BJ, Ravnikar VA, Meyer JE. Mammographic changes associated with postmenopausal hormone replacement therapy: A longitudinal study. *Radiology* 1990; 174:487–490.
16. Huynh PT, Jarolimek AM, Daye S. The false-negative mammogram. *Radiographics* 1998; 18:1137–1154.
17. Moskowitz M. Breast imaging. In: Donegan WL, Spratt JS, eds. *Cancer of the Breast,* 3d ed. Philadelphia: Saunders; 1988:167–205.
18. Rebner M, Raju U. Noninvasive breast cancer. *Radiology* 1994; 190:623–631.
19. Cardenosa G. *Breast Imaging Companion.* Philadelphia: Lippincott-Raven; 1997:204–205.
20. Huynh PT, Parellada JA, Shaw de Paredes E, et al. Dilated duct pattern at mammography. *Radiology* 1997; 204:137–141.
21. Heywang-Kobrunner SH, Schreer I, Dershaw DD. Sonography. In: Heywang-Kobrunner SH, Schreer I, Dershaw DD. *Diagnostic Breast Imaging.* New York: Thieme; 1997:81–91.
22. Kolb TM, Lichy J, Newhouse JH. Occult cancer in women with dense breasts: Detection with screening US—diagnostic yield and tumor characteristics. *Radiology* 1998; 207:191–199.

23. Cardenosa G. Breast ultrasound. In: Cardenosa G. *Breast Imaging Companion.* Philadelphia: Lippincott-Raven; 1997:128–151.
24. Venta LA, Dudiak CM, Salomon CG, Flisak ME. Sonographic evaluation of the breast. *Radiographics* 1994; 14:29–50.
25. Stavros AT, Thickman D, Rapp CL, et al. Solid breast nodules: Use of sonography to distinguish between benign and malignant lesions. *Radiology* 1995; 196:123–134.
26. Cardenosa G, Doudna C, Eklund GW. Ductography of the breast: Technique and findings. *AJR* 1994; 162:1081–1087.
27. Baker KS, Davey DD, Stelling CB. Ductal abnormalities detected with galactography: Frequency of adequate excisional biopsy. *AJR* 1994; 162:821–824.
28. Gorczyca DP, Sinha S, Ahn CY, et al. Silicone breast implants in vivo: MR imaging. *Radiology* 1992; 185:407–410.
29. Hulka CA, Kopans DB. Magnetic resonance imaging. In: Kopans DB. *Breast Imaging,* 2d ed. Philadelphia: Lippincott-Raven; 1998:617–636.
30. Clifford EJ, Lugo-Zamudio C. Scintimammography in the diagnosis of breast cancer. *Am J Surg* 1996; 172:483–486.
31. Villanueva-Meyer J, Leonard MH, Briscoe E, et al. Mammoscintigraphy with technetium-99m-sestamibi in suspected breast cancer. *J Nucl Med* 1996; 37:926–930.
32. Chen EM, Khalkhali I, Cutrone JA, et al. Tc-99m sestamibi exam finds niche in breast dx. *Diagn Imaging,* August 1997, pp. 61–65.
33. Kopans DB. *Breast Imaging,* 2d ed. Philadelphia: Lippincott-Raven; 1998:644.
34. Parker SH, Lovin JD, Jobe WE, et al. Stereotactic breast biopsy with a biopsy gun. *Radiology* 1990; 176:741–747.
35. Parker SH, Lovin JD, Jobe WE, et al. Nonpalpable breast lesions: Stereotactic automated large-core biopsies. *Radiology* 1991; 180:403–407.
36. Sullivan DC. Needle core biopsy of mammographic lesions. *AJR* 1994; 162:601–608.
37. Parker SH, Jobe WE. *Percutaneous Breast Biopsy.* New York: Raven Press; 1993.
38. Parker SH. Interventional breast procedures and the evolution of minimally invasive breast biopsy. *Semin Breast Dis* 1998; 1:64–70.
39. Liberman L. Advantages and disadvantages of minimally invasive breast biopsy procedures. *Semin Breast Dis* 1998; 1:84–94.
40. Liberman L, Dershaw DD, Rosen PP, et al. Stereotaxic core biopsy of breast carcinoma: Accuracy at predicting invasion. *Radiology* 1995; 194:379–381.
41. Parker SH, Burbank F, Jackman RJ, et al. Percutaneous large-core breast biopsy: A multi-institutional study. *Radiology* 1994; 193:359–364.
42. Liberman L, Fahs MC, Dershaw DD, et al. Impact of stereotaxic core breast biopsy on cost of diagnosis. *Radiology* 1995; 195:633–637.
43. Harvey JA, Moran RE. US-guided core needle biopsy of the breast: Technique and pitfalls. *Radiographics* 1998; 18:867–877.

MAMMOGRAPHIC APPEARANCE OF COMMON ABNORMALITIES

INTRODUCTION

Mammography is the single most useful screening test for breast cancer; however, other imaging modalities are important adjuncts for the evaluation of symptomatic patients. For example, ultrasound is the initial imaging study of choice for patients who are pregnant or lactating and for women under age 25 (Fig. 13-1). In these patients, the density of breast tissue may obscure the visualization of a mass on mammography.

BREAST CANCER

The mammographic findings with the highest positive predictive value for breast cancer are clustered microcalcifications and a spiculated mass; however, other signs also are common. For example, invasive ductal carcinoma may appear as a well-circumscribed mass (Fig. 13-2). In fact, the medullary, papillary, and mucinous subtypes of this cancer often present in this way.[1]

Medullary carcinoma is more common in younger women and accounts for approximately 3 percent of breast cancers. Despite a rapid growth rate, the prognosis usually is favorable. Typically, a patient will present with a well-defined mass that was noticed only recently (Fig. 13-3). Papillary carcinoma usually is diagnosed later in life, most often in the seventh decade. This cancer has a slower growth rate and may be accompanied by nipple discharge and cyst formation (Fig. 13-4). Mucinous carcinomas account for approximately 2 percent of breast cancers. They also have a slower growth rate and a favorable prognosis (Fig. 13-5).

The mammographic findings with the highest positive predictive value for breast cancer are clustered microcalcifications and a spiculated mass.

149

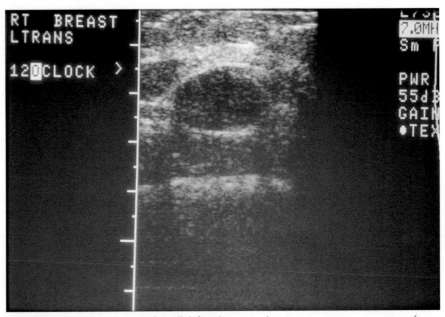

FIGURE 13-1 The oval-shaped, well-defined mass in this young patient represents a fibroadenoma.

Lobular carcinoma is the most difficult type of cancer to diagnose mammographically. Commonly, it presents as a palpable mass that is not seen on mammography because the tumor cells infiltrate the breast tissue in a single file (Fig. 13-6). Ultrasound may be helpful in evaluating the palpable abnormality (Fig. 13-7). Occasionally, shrinkage and hardening of the involved breast occur (Fig. 13-8). Lobular carcinoma is associated with an increased risk of bilateral disease.

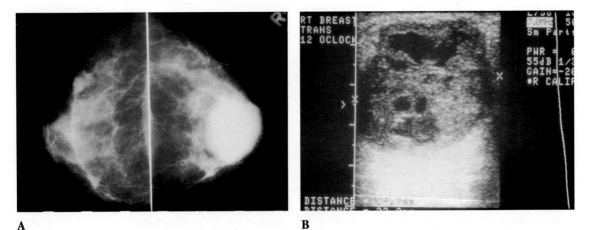

A   B

FIGURE 13-2 **A.** The mass in the retroareolar region of the right breast is an invasive ductal cancer. **B.** The cystic areas within the mass on ultrasound represent tumor necrosis.

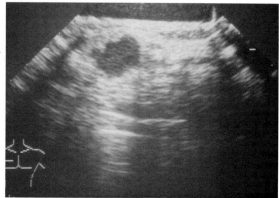

B

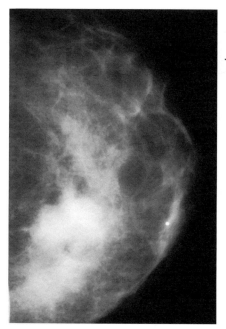

A

FIGURE 13-3 *A.* The palpable medullary carcinoma in the lateral right breast is partially obscured by the overlying glandular tissue. *B.* The mass is solid on ultrasound.

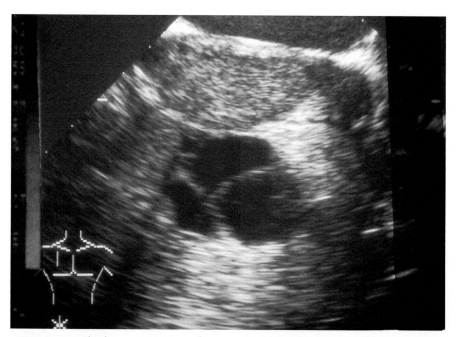

FIGURE 13-4 This large invasive papillary carcinoma showed both solid and cystic components on ultrasound.

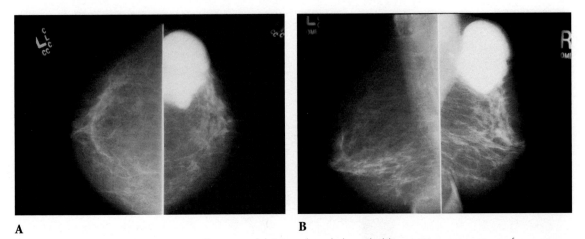

A   **B**

FIGURE 13-5 Craniocaudal *(A)* and mediolateral oblique *(B)* mammograms of a muci-nous carcinoma demonstrating a well-circumscribed dense mass in the upper outer quad-rant of the right breast.

With inflammatory breast cancer, the pattern of spread is via the dermal lym-phatics. As a result, this cancer presents clinically with swelling and erythema of the breast and a peau d'orange appearance to the skin. The mammogram shows an overall increase in density of the breast tissue, limiting the perception of a discrete mass (Fig. 13-9). Skin thickening may be visible around the areola.

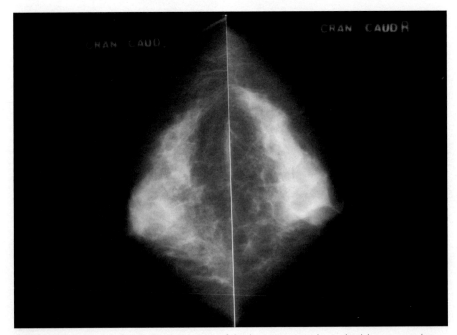

FIGURE 13-6 Except for slight asymmetry of the breast tissue, the palpable mass in the right breast representing an invasive lobular carcinoma is not evident on the mammogram.

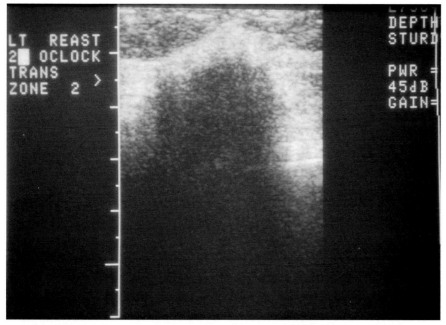

FIGURE 13-7 The characteristic appearance of invasive lobular carcinoma is demonstrated in this ultrasound by the presence of an echogenic mass with fingerlike projections and marked attenuation of sound.

Paget's disease of the breast presents clinically as reddening, scaling, and bleeding of the nipple that prompts biopsy. Mammography may show an underlying mass or suspicious microcalcifications.

Breast cancer may be multifocal or multicentric (Fig. 13-10). Bilateral breast cancers also can occur. Evaluation of all mammographic findings must be undertaken before the patient's treatment is planned.

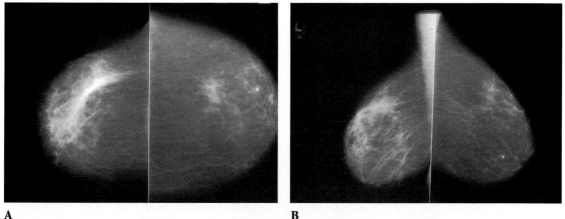

A **B**

FIGURE 13-8 Craniocaudal *(A)* and mediolateral oblique *(B)* mammograms demonstrating the asymmetry in size and density of the breast associated with an invasive lobular cancer.

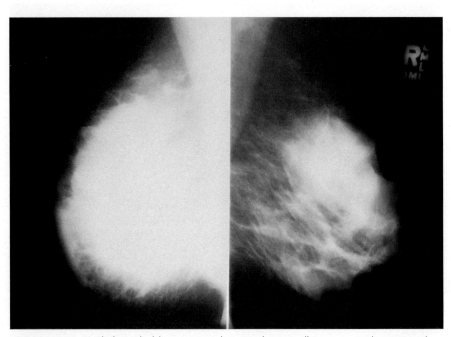

FIGURE 13-9 Mediolateral oblique views showing the overall increase in the size and density of the breast in a patient with inflammatory breast cancer.

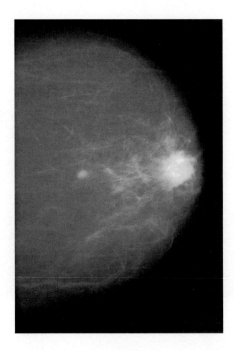

FIGURE 13-10 Both the large and the small masses in this breast are invasive ductal cancers.

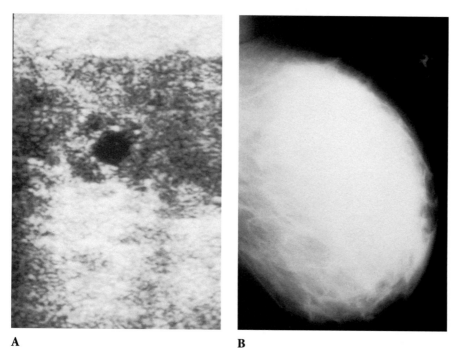

A   **B**

FIGURE 13-11 This 27-year-old pregnant patient presented with a palpable breast mass. **A.** Ultrasound shows a solid mass with thickening of the overlying skin. **B.** The mammogram shows dense tissue. Biopsy revealed invasive ductal carcinoma.

Breast cancer is an infrequent occurrence during pregnancy. Pregnant patients have very dense breasts, making breast ultrasound a more useful initial imaging study than mammography. If ultrasound shows a worrisome solid mass, mammography of the symptomatic breast is warranted to look for malignant calcifications (Fig. 13-11). Pregnancy should not delay imaging or biopsy of a suspicious finding. Hematoma formation, milk fistula, and infection are complications of breast biopsy that occur more commonly in a pregnant woman.[2] Therefore, needle biopsy may be a reasonable alternative to excisional biopsy to reduce the likelihood of such complications.

Pregnancy should not delay imaging or biopsy of a suspicious finding.

FIBROADENOMA

Fibroadenomas are the solid masses that occur most frequently in the breast and occur most frequently in adolescent girls. These benign fibroepithelial tumors are estrogen-dependent, and so they typically enlarge during pregnancy and involute after menopause. The mean age of occurrence is 30 years, but they can be found in all age groups.[3]

Mammographically, a fibroadenoma appears as a well-circumscribed rounded to oval mass (Fig. 13-12). Lobulation of the margins often is seen. Fibroadenomas are multiple in approximately 15 percent of cases (Fig. 13-13). Since fibroadenomas contain functional tissue, secretory changes can occur (Fig. 13-14).

During involution, characteristic coarse popcorn-type macrocalcifications occur

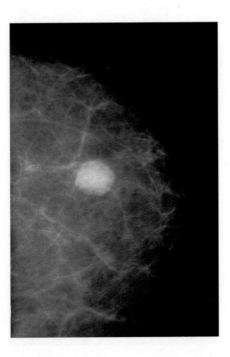

FIGURE 13-12 The rounded mass on this craniocaudal view represents a fibroadenoma.

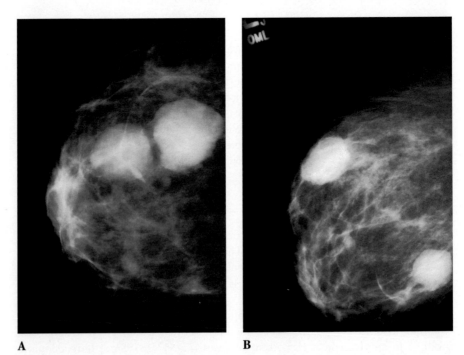

A   B

FIGURE 13-13 Craniocaudal *(A)* and mediolateral oblique *(B)* mammograms showing well-circumscribed masses in the upper outer and lower outer quadrants of the left breast. Both masses are fibroadenomas.

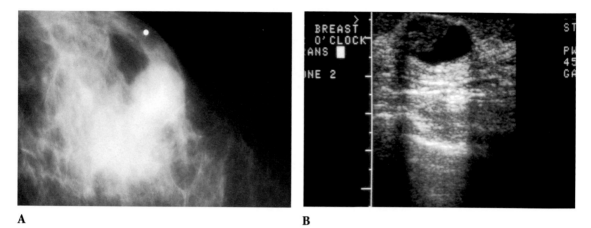

FIGURE 13-14 **A.** The partially obscured mass in the upper right breast is a fibroadenoma with secretory changes. **B.** Note the solid and cystic area on the ultrasound of the mass.

within the fibroadenoma (Fig. 13-15). These calcifications develop over time and begin in a peripheral location along the margins of the mass. The location and appearance of the calcifications aid in the diagnosis (Fig. 13-16). Occasionally, microcalcifications within the epithelial spaces of a fibroadenoma appear similar to malignant microcalcifications, making biopsy necessary (Fig. 13-17).

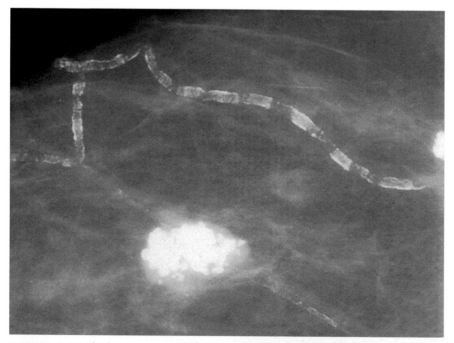

FIGURE 13-15 The large coarse calcification is characteristic of a degenerating fibroadenoma.

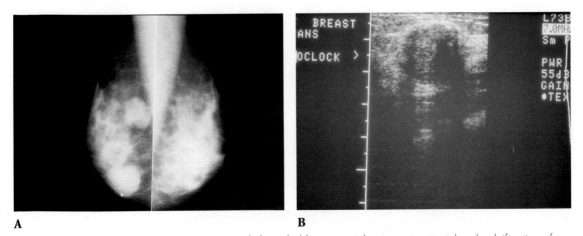

A   B

FIGURE 13-16 *A.* Mediolateral oblique view demonstrating peripheral calcification of a fibroadenoma in the inferior left breast. *B.* The calcification causes the shadowing noted on ultrasound.

Giant fibroadenomas (also called juvenile fibroadenomas) (Fig. 13-18), tubular adenomas, and lactating adenomas are subtypes of common fibroadenomas. They all appear similar on mammographic imaging[4]; however, tubular adenomas contain more ductal elements on histopathologic examination (Fig. 13-19). Lactating adenomas, in contrast, contain ductal elements but lack a significant fibrous component. Lactating adenomas occur most commonly during pregnancy (Fig. 13-20). Giant fibroadenomas

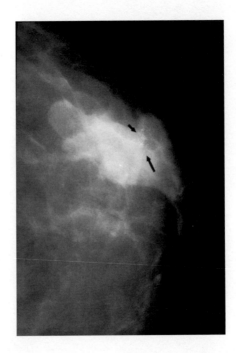

FIGURE 13-17 The arrows point to microcalcifications in a fibroadenoma.

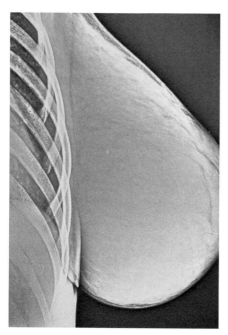

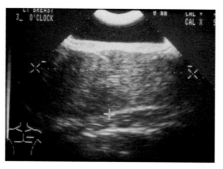

A

B

FIGURE 13-18 *A.* The tubular structure overlying the anterior aspect of the breast on this xeromammogram represents an engorged skin vein. *B.* The large breast mass is a giant fibroadenoma that measured almost 10 cm in diameter on the ultrasound examination.

often are over 5 cm in size at the time of presentation and enlarge rapidly. They account for approximately 4 percent of fibroadenomas and usually occur in women under 20 years of age. The size of the mass may cause asymmetry of the breasts as well as venous distention and ulceration of the overlying skin.

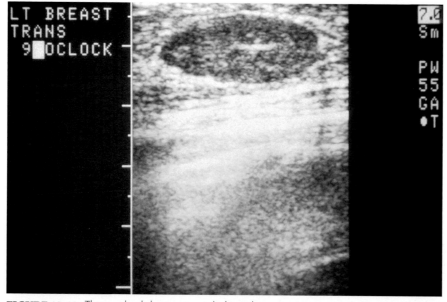

FIGURE 13-19 This oval solid mass is a tubular adenoma.

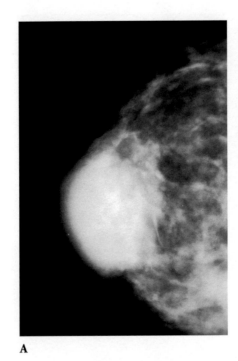

A

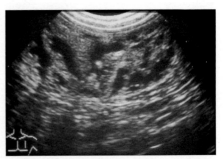

B

FIGURE 13-20 *A.* The mass in the retroareolar region of the left breast is a lactating adenoma. *B.* The cystic spaces on the ultrasound represent secretory changes.

CYSTOSARCOMA PHYLLODES

Cystosarcoma phyllodes (phyllodes tumor) is a rapidly growing fibroepithelial tumor that is benign in approximately 85 percent of cases.

Cystosarcoma phyllodes (phyllodes tumor) is a rapidly growing fibroepithelial tumor that is benign in approximately 85 percent of cases. The mean age at occurrence is 45 years. Incomplete excision may result in local recurrence. The malignant variety rarely metastasizes, but hematogenous spread can occur. A phyllodes tumor presents as a palpable mass with imaging features similar to those of a fibroadenoma. Calcifications are uncommon (Fig. 13-21).

AGGRESSIVE FIBROMATOSIS

Aggressive fibromatosis refers to a rare spindle-cell tumor that occasionally involves the breast. The clinical features and imaging characteristics of these lesions mimic those of breast cancer. They have been reported after breast trauma, after breast augmentation, and in association with pregnancy (Fig. 13-22). Wide excision of the lesion is needed to avoid recurrence.[3]

HAMARTOMA

A hamartoma, or fibroadenolipoma, is a benign encapsulated mass that is composed of fat, fibrous tissue, and glandular elements (Fig. 13-23). Hamartomas may not be distinctly palpable because of their fat content but may cause asymmetry and thickening of the breast tissue. Also, since hamartomas are composed of normal tis-

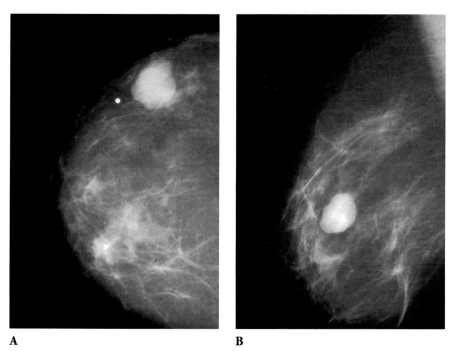

<table>
<tr><td>**A**</td><td>**B**</td></tr>
</table>

FIGURE 13-21 The well-circumscribed mass in the upper outer quadrant of the left breast on craniocaudal (CC) *(A)* and mediolateral oblique (MLO) *(B)* views appears very similar to a fibroadenoma; however, the histologic diagnosis is a benign phyllodes tumor.

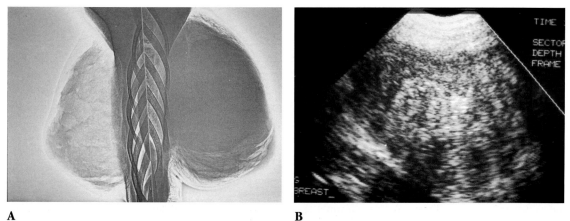

A **B**

FIGURE 13-22 *A.* The large mass that occupies the entire right breast in this 16-year-old patient has an appearance similar to that of a giant fibroadenoma. *B.* This mass was solid on ultrasound. Surgery revealed aggressive fibromatosis that was fixed to the chest wall.

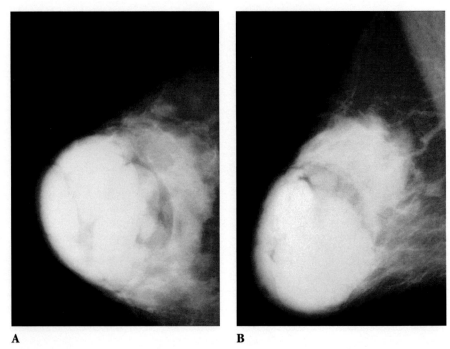

A   **B**

FIGURE 13-23 The large mass in the anterior left breast on the craniocaudal **(A)** and mediolateral oblique **(B)** views contains both fatty and glandular components. This appearance is characteristic of a hamartoma.

sue, ultrasound may not show a definable mass.[5] Because of the characteristic mammographic appearance, biopsy is not indicated. Surgical excision may be indicated to improve cosmesis.

LIPOMA

A lipoma is a benign mass of fatty tissue surrounded by a thin fibrous capsule (Fig. 13-24). Lipomas usually are soft and well-circumscribed on palpation of the breast. The mammographic appearance is very characteristic, and biopsy is not necessary. Again, surgery to improve the cosmetic appearance may be indicated. Generally, masses that contain fat are benign.

FAT NECROSIS AND OIL CYSTS

The fibrosis and calcification that occur in the later stages of healing can make fat necrosis difficult to distinguish from breast cancer, both clinically and radiographically.

Traumatic oil cysts and fat necrosis are two other breast masses that contain fat. They arise after traumatic or surgical injury to the fatty tissue of the breast (Fig. 13-25). Fat necrosis also can be seen with Weber-Christian disease, in which nodular panniculitis is associated with fever and other constitutional symptoms.[6] In contrast to a lipoma, fat necrosis often presents as an indurated mass with indistinct borders (Fig. 13-26). The fibrosis and calcification that occur in the later stages of healing can make fat necrosis difficult to distinguish from breast cancer both clinically and radiographically. Biopsy often is needed.

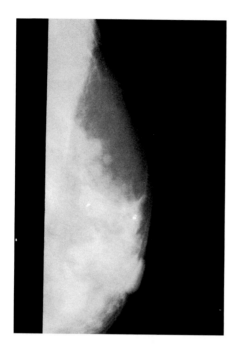

FIGURE 13-24 The fatty mass in the lateral right breast on this exaggerated craniocaudal view is a lipoma. It is surrounded by a thin opaque band that represents the lipoma's capsule.

HEMATOMA AND BREAST TRAUMA

Trauma to the breast from the shoulder restraint portion of an automobile seat belt causes a characteristic bandlike area of increased opacity on a mammogram. The opacity represents a contusion or hematoma at the site of the injury (Fig. 13-27). The location of the finding varies, depending on whether the patient was the driver

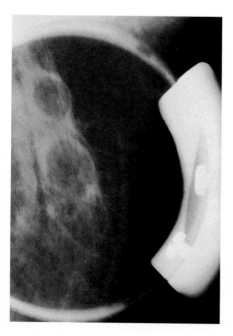

FIGURE 13-25 The central fat within these small, palpable masses represents areas of fat necrosis from a previous biopsy.

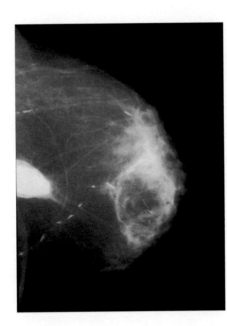

FIGURE 13-26 The hard, palpable mass in the anterior aspect of the right breast on this craniocaudal view contains fat. Biopsy revealed fat necrosis. A port from a catheter is visible.

or a passenger. Usually the driver sustains an injury to the upper inner quadrant of the left breast and/or the lower inner quadrant of the right breast.[7] These areas may later calcify and form palpable oil cysts.

Trauma to the breast from a fall can cause a sizable hematoma to form, especially if the patient is taking anticoagulant medication (Fig. 13-28). The resultant mass may be difficult to differentiate from breast cancer. Hemorrhage into an existing cancer mass also must be considered.

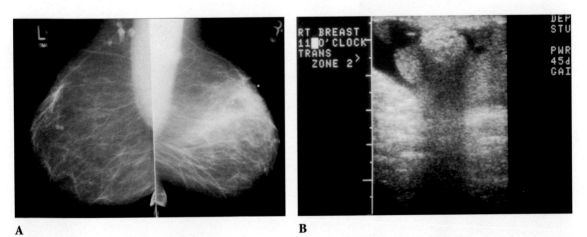

A   **B**

FIGURE 13-27 *A.* The band of increased opacity on the mediolateral oblique view is characteristic of a seat belt injury to the breast. *B.* The ultrasound findings are consistent with a hematoma.

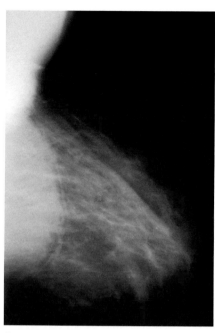

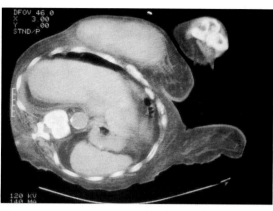

B

FIGURE 13-28 *A.* The mass in the posterior aspect of the right breast is a hematoma. *B.* It is seen as an opaque mass in the posterior aspect of the right breast on computed tomography of the chest.

A

FIBROCYSTIC CHANGES

Fibrocystic changes are characterized by breast lumps on clinical examination that may or may not be associated with breast pain. Specific findings seldom are seen on mammography or ultrasound examination of the breast. However, distinct histopathologic changes such as cysts, fibrosis, intraductal papillomatosis, and sclerosing adenosis may be found.

BREAST CYSTS

Breast cysts are fluid-filled masses that develop in the terminal lobular units along the milk ducts. When continuity with the ductal system is maintained, a cyst may be associated with nipple discharge. An imbalance between secretion and resorption of fluid in the breast lobules may result from changes in estrogen levels. Cysts commonly occur between ages 30 and 50 years. Cysts are a common cause of breast pain, and a cyst may present as a rapidly enlarging mass.

The typical mammographic appearance is that of a well-circumscribed rounded to oval mass. The borders of the mass may be obscured if the glandular tissue is dense (Fig. 13-29). Cysts may contain calcium, which can be shown to layer out on a lateral mammogram (Fig. 13-30).

Ultrasound shows an anechoic mass with a well-delineated wall and good through transmission of sound (Fig. 13-31). Occasionally, echoes may be present within the cyst because of the high fat or protein content of the fluid. When this oc-

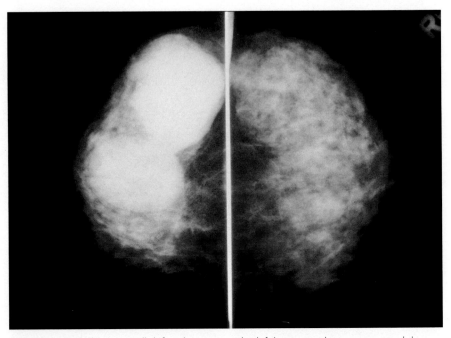

FIGURE 13-29 The two well-defined masses in the left breast on these craniocaudal views are cysts.

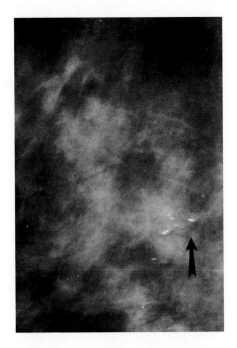

FIGURE 13-30 The sedimented calcium *(arrow)* has a "teacup" appearance in these tiny milk cysts.

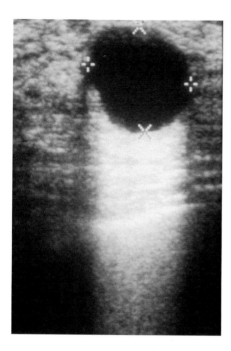

FIGURE 13-31 Ultrasound of this cyst demonstrates the absence of internal echoes, well-defined walls, and posterior acoustic enhancement.

curs, distinction from a solid mass is difficult and aspiration is recommended. Cysts also should be aspirated when their presence interferes with clincial breast examination or when they produce pain.

GALACTOCELE

A galactocele is a milk cyst that develops during lactation. The mammographic appearance varies, depending on the fat content and fluidity of the inspissated milk as well as the density of the surrounding breast tissue.[8] The mass may be indistinguishable from other breast lesions by ultrasound, and fine needle aspiration or biopsy is needed for diagnosis (Fig. 13-32).

MASTITIS AND BREAST ABSCESS

Mastitis is an inflammatory process involving the breast that most commonly occurs during the puerperal period in breast-feeding women. Occasionally, nonpuerperal infection may follow nipple piercing, mammaplasty, or breast biopsy procedures. Mammographically, the skin may be thickened and the breast tissue appears more dense. Although rare in young patients, inflammatory carcinoma should be considered in the differential diagnosis of breast inflammation, particularly when the patient does not respond to antibiotics (Fig. 13-33). A poor response to antibiotics also may occur when the inflammatory process has progressed to abscess formation (Fig. 13-34). The differential diagnosis of breast inflammation also includes lymphoma and edema of the breast from congestive heart failure or superior vena cava obstruction.

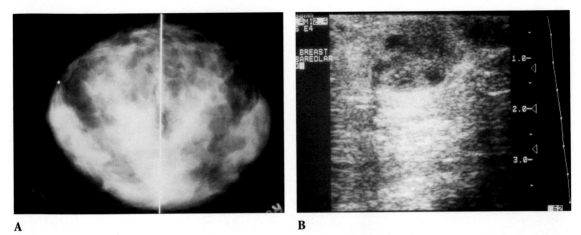

A **B**

FIGURE 13-32 *A.* The palpable mass in the retroareolar area of the left breast on these craniocaudal views is marked by a ball bearing. *B.* The mass is solid on ultrasound. A galactocele was diagnosed by excisional biopsy.

MONDOR'S DISEASE

Mondor's disease is thrombophlebitis that occurs in a superficial vein in the breast. Symptoms of pain and tenderness are accompanied by the presence of a cordlike thickening of the involved vein. Mondor's disease may resemble mastitis or cancer with erythema of the overlying skin. Occasionally, the involved vein is visible on a mammogram or ultrasound as a tubular structure.[9]

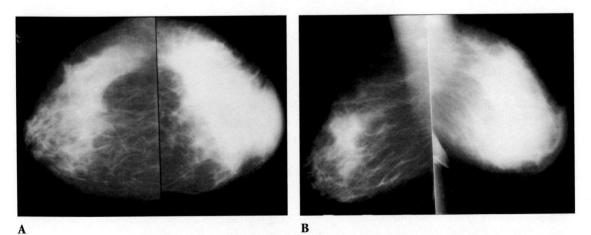

A **B**

FIGURE 13-33 The clinical presentation of this 27-year-old patient suggested mastitis. The craniocaudal *(A)* and mediolateral *(B)* mammograms show increased stromal density of the right breast, representing inflammatory breast cancer.

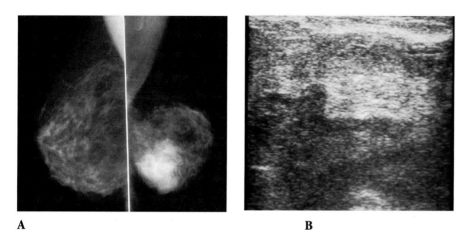

A   **B**

FIGURE 13-34 The mass in the inferior right breast on the mediolateral oblique view *(A)* in this diabetic patient is an abscess. Culture grew *Staphylococcus aureus*. **B.** The mass is poorly defined on ultrasound.

DUCT ECTASIA

Duct ectasia is a nonspecific dilation of the ducts beneath the nipple. The patient presents with nipple discharge or a palpable mass caused by secretions retained within the ducts. The mammogram or ductogram shows dilated ducts in the retroareolar region (Fig. 13-35). As the process continues, the secretory material in the ducts undergoes saponification and calcification, producing characteristic

Duct ectasia is a nonspecific dilation of the ducts beneath the nipple. The patient presents with nipple discharge or a palpable mass caused by secretions retained within the ducts.

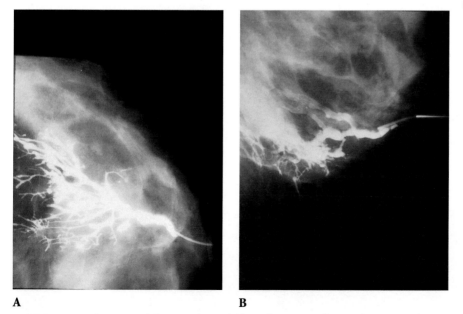

A   **B**

FIGURE 13-35 Craniocaudal *(A)* and straight lateral *(B)* views from a ductogram show dilated ducts in this patient with duct ectasia.

needlelike calcifications in the ducts that appear to be directed toward the nipple (Fig. 13-36). This process is termed plasma cell mastitis, and the calcifications are called secretory calcifications.

BENIGN PAPILLARY LES3IONS

Benign papillary lesions of the breast include a solitary intraductal papilloma, multiple papillomas, and papillomatosis. A solitary intraductal papilloma is central in location, arising within a duct close to the nipple. The average age at presentation is 48 years.[10] The patient presents with a spontaneous bloody or serous nipple discharge that usually emanates from a single duct.[11] Mammograms are usually negative, but on occasion a mass or a dilated duct may be seen behind the nipple (Fig. 13-37). The characteristic finding on ultrasound is an intracystic mass (Fig. 13-38). Ductography is very useful, particularly in cases with nipple discharge in which the mammographic findings are negative or nonspecific (Fig. 13-39). The ductogram helps locate the lesion and evaluate its extent (Fig. 13-40). Such mapping is helpful to the surgeon in planning duct excision.

Multiple papillomas usually arise peripherally in the terminal lobular units. They more commonly present with a palpable mass or a mammographic finding (Fig. 13-41A). Again, ultrasound is helpful in demonstrating an intracystic mass (Fig. 13-41B). In the series of Cardenosa and Eklund,[11] a subtype of multiple papillomas was described to be central in location. The risk of breast cancer associated with multiple papillomas is greater than the risk associated with a solitary papilloma.

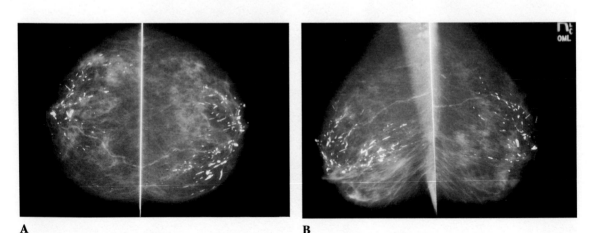

A **B**

FIGURE 13-36 Craniocaudal *(A)* and mediolateral oblique *(B)* views of both breasts show characteristic secretory calcifications. Note the orientation of the calcifications toward the nipple.

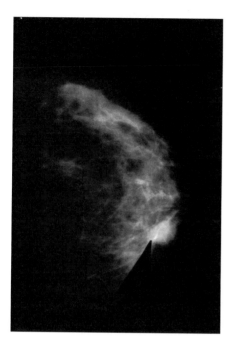

FIGURE 13-37 The mass (arrow) in the retroareolar region is a papilloma.

Papillomatosis occurs in the peripheral ducts and is characterized by epithelial hyperplasia. As part of the spectrum of fibrocystic changes, papillomatosis is usually an incidental finding during biopsy of another lesion. Occasionally, it can present as a cluster of microcalcifications or a mass on a mammogram. In a patient with nipple discharge, the ductogram may show minimal irregularity of the ductal lumen.

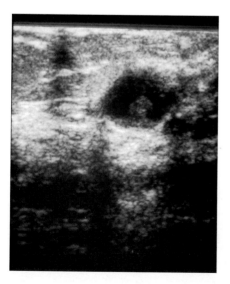

FIGURE 13-38 The small solid mass protruding into the cystic space is an intraductal papilloma.

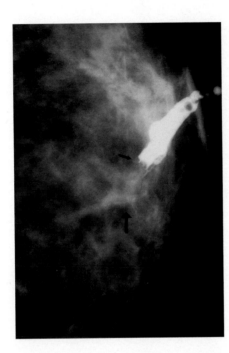

FIGURE 13-39 This patient presented with serous nipple discharge. Contrast in the duct shows an abrupt cutoff at the location of the papilloma. The appearance cannot be distinguished from that of cancer.

FOCAL FIBROSIS

Focal fibrosis may be part of the spectrum of fibrocystic changes or may represent involutional change. It usually presents as a poorly marginated mass on mammographic imaging and has solid features on ultrasound (Fig. 13-42). Occasionally, it is discovered incidentally during the evaluation of other symptoms (Fig. 13-43).

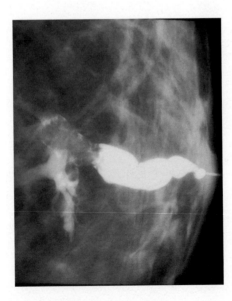

FIGURE 13-40 Bloody nipple discharge prompted this ductogram. Contrast fills the draining duct. The mass outlined in the posterior duct is an intraductal papilloma.

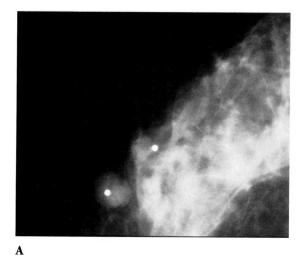

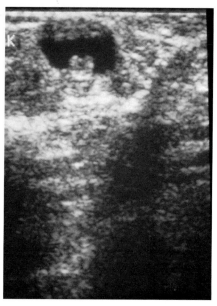

FIGURE 13-41 This patient presented with two palpable masses in the lateral left breast. ***A.*** A cranio-caudal view cropped to the area shows the masses marked with ball bearings. ***B.*** Ultrasound showed characteristic intracystic masses.

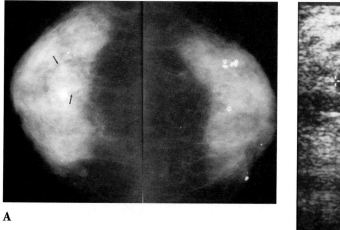

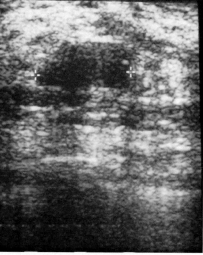

FIGURE 13-42 The partially obscured mass *(arrows)* in the left breast on these craniocaudal views *(A)* is solid on ultrasound *(B).* Excisional biopsy revealed focal fibrosis.

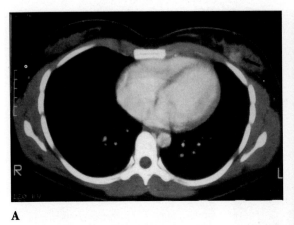

FIGURE 13-43 The finding of a mass in the left breast on computed tomography *(A)* prompted the mammogram *(B).* Focal fibrosis was found on excisional biopsy.

A

B

DIABETIC MASTOPATHY

Benign fibrous tumors of the breast have been described in young patients with long-standing insulin-dependent diabetes.[12,13] The patient presents with a firm, palpable mass that can be several centimeters in diameter. Bilateral masses may be found. Because of the dense glandular breast tissue in a young patient, the mass often is not visible mammographically, and ultrasound is needed for evaluation. The mass is echogenic on ultrasound, and marked distal shadowing is present (Fig. 13-44). Although the clinical appearance in a young diabetic patient is classic, the similarity to cancer on ultrasound necessitates biopsy in many patients. Ultrasound guidance of the core biopsy needle can be performed to assure that the mass is sampled adequately.

EPIDERMAL INCLUSION CYSTS

Epidermal inclusion cysts are retention cysts in the skin that may arise from obstruction of hair follicles. Inclusion cysts are the most common type of cyst arising in the skin of the breast. Mammographically, a well-defined mass is noted, and it may change in size over time. If it is palpable, a tangential view of the mass shows its proximity to and continuity with the skin (Fig. 13-45). If the mass is inflamed, excision may be needed. A marker should be placed on any skin lesion before mammography is performed to prevent misinterpretation.

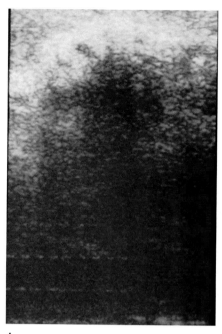

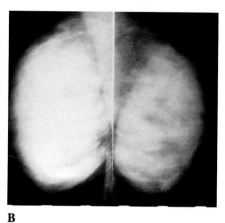

B

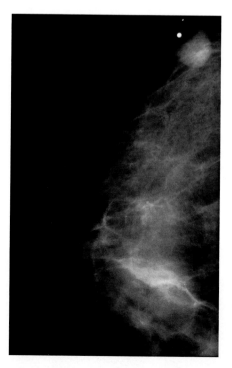

A

FIGURE 13-44 This young diabetic patient presented with a palpable mass in the left breast. **A.** Ultrasound of the mass shows it to be solid with marked attenuation of sound. **B.** Mediolateral oblique views of both breasts show asymmetry with no discrete findings. Core needle biopsy of the mass revealed fibrosis.

FIGURE 13-45 The small mass marked by the ball bearings is an inclusion cyst in the skin.

Steatocystoma multiplex is a rare autosomal dominant condition in which multiple inclusion cysts are present in the skin. This entity appears on the mammogram as multiple fat-containing cysts[13] (Fig. 13-46).

SKIN CALCIFICATIONS

Calcium deposition in the skin may occur within sebaceous cysts, areas of trauma, tattoos, or keloids (Fig. 13-47). These calcifications may project within the breast tissue on the mammogram and may be difficult to differentiate from malignancy. Mammographically, the calcifications can be targeted in a localization grid, and a tangential view then confirms their location in the skin[14] (Fig. 13-48).

FOREIGN BODIES

Foreign bodies may be seen within the breast as a result of past trauma or surgery. Occasionally, bullet fragments or shrapnel may be visible on a mammogram. In one patient, a sewing needle was found in the breast (Fig. 13-49). Calcified suture material, metallic sutures, or surgical clips may be present (Fig. 13-50). Also, the retained sheath from a Hickman catheter can on occasion be seen within the breast (Fig. 13-51).

BREAST IMPLANTS

In 1992, the U.S. Food and Drug Administration (FDA) banned the routine use of silicone breast implants.[15] As women who still have silicone implants reach the appropriate age for breast cancer screening, special positioning techniques are being

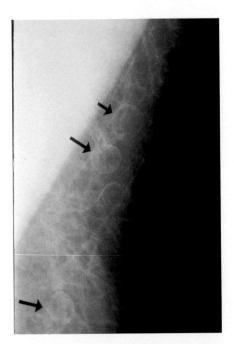

FIGURE 13-46 The fat-containing inclusion cysts of steatocystoma multiplex project as small oil cysts in the skin (arrows). Clinically, these cysts appear as skin papules.

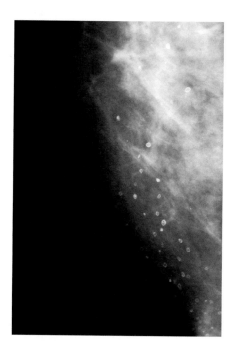

FIGURE 13-47 These rounded calcifications with lucent centers are typical of the calcifications that occur in keloids.

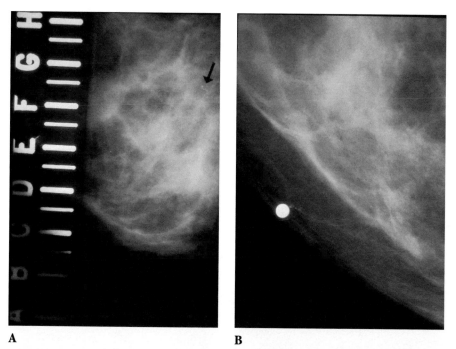

A

B

FIGURE 13-48 *A.* The arrows point to the calcifications targeted in the localization grid. A skin marker is placed on the calcifications with the patient in the grid. *B.* A tangential view in the region of the marker shows that the calcifications are within the skin.

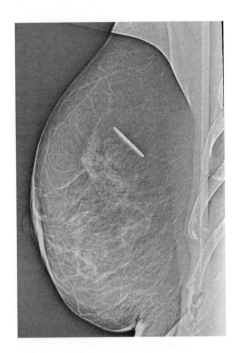

FIGURE 13-49 This xeromammogram demonstrates a sewing needle in the upper breast. The patient was not aware of the needle's presence but reported helping her mother with sewing as a child.

used to improve mammographic visualization of breast tissue around the implants. With the technique of Eklund and associates,[16] four views of each breast are taken. The type of implant and its position in the breast usually are apparent from the mammogram (Fig. 13-52). Silicone implants are densely opaque, whereas the folds

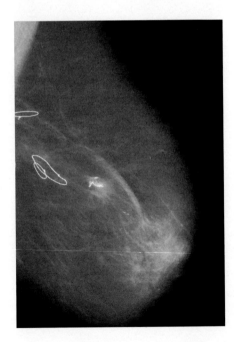

FIGURE 13-50 The calcified sutures are from a prior benign biopsy..

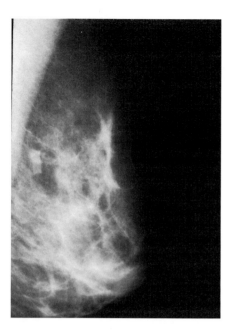

FIGURE 13-51 The tubular structure in the posterior right breast represents a retained cuff from the sheath of a previously placed Hickman catheter.

or valve of a saline implant may be visible through the shell of the implant (Fig. 13-53). The double chamber of some implants also can be noted (Fig. 13-54). Occasionally, the presence of implants is noted on chest x-ray because the calcifications that form along the capsule of the implants are visible (Fig. 13-55).

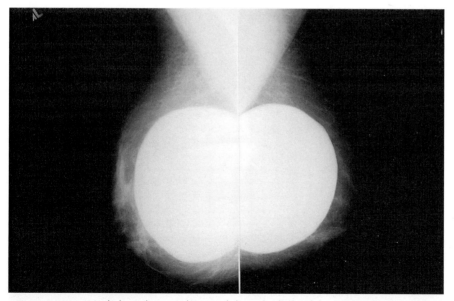

FIGURE 13-52 Mediolateral views showing bilateral subglandular implants positioned anterior to the pectoral muscle. The opaque implant obscures visualization of the underlying tissue.

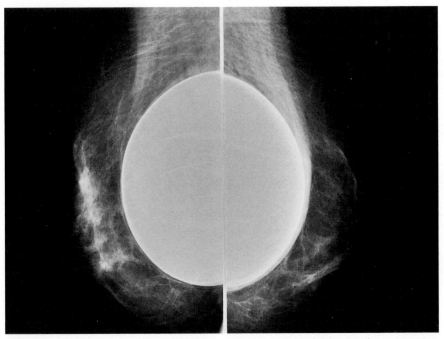

FIGURE 13-53 Horizontal folds are visible in these retropectoral saline implants.

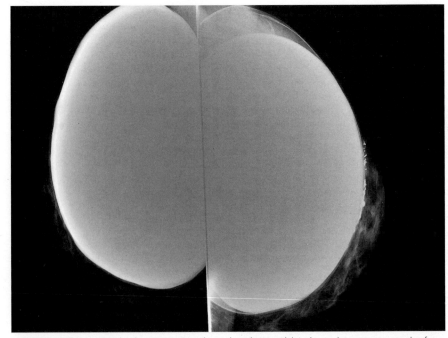

FIGURE 13-54 Note the lucent outer saline chamber visible along the superior and inferior margins of the double-lumen implant on the right.

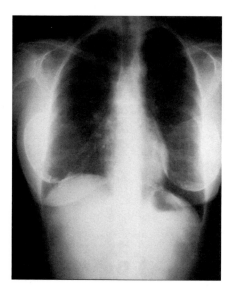

FIGURE 13-55 The rounded calcified masses overlying the lower chest are calcified breast implants.

Evaluation of breast symptoms in patients with implants is sometimes problematic. Palpable lumps may represent a mass or may be related to leakage of silicone. Mammography can determine whether silicone is present outside a ruptured implant or after the removal of a ruptured implant (Fig. 13-56). Retained capsules after

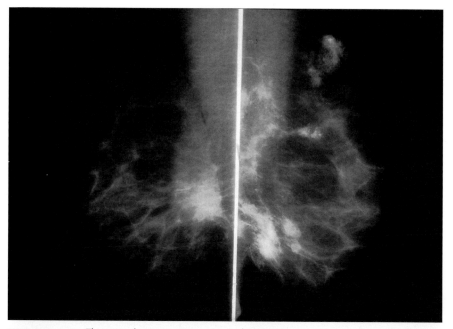

FIGURE 13-56 The irregular, opaque areas on these mammograms represent residual silicone in the breast after the removal of ruptured implants.

implant removal can appear as masses on mammography (Fig. 13-57). Ultrasound is a particularly helpful adjunct in evaluating patients with implants (Fig. 13-58).

Breast cancer can present as a palpable mass or as a nonpalpable lesion detected only by screening (Fig. 13-59). Although there is no correlation between silicone implants and breast cancer, the presence of implants can delay the diagnosis. Since it is difficult to image all of the breast tissue in these patients, clinical examination is very important. Clustered pleomorphic microcalcifications or spiculated masses are highly suspicious for breast cancer (Fig. 13-60). Occasionally, the cancer will appear on the mammogram only as an indentation along the margin of the implant that disturbs its contour (Fig. 13-61).

Rupture of silicone implants can be intracapsular or extracapsular. With intracapsular rupture, the implant's shell collapses within the inner silicone gel but both are contained within the fibrous capsule that forms around the implant. Therefore, the silicone does not extrude into the surrounding breast tissue. Intracapsular rupture cannot be diagnosed by mammography since the silicone is contained by the fibrous capsule. With extracapsular rupture, the silicone gel extrudes into the breast tissue and can be seen on mammography as extension of silicone from the implant (Fig. 13-62). Frequently, the silicone extends along the plane of the pectoral muscle toward the axilla (Fig. 13-63). Mammography also can detect rupture of a saline implant by demonstrating deflation of the implant.

Ultrasound is useful in evaluating implant rupture. Extraluminal silicone within the breast tissue appears as a "snowstorm" pattern on ultrasound (Fig. 13-64). Implants that are ruptured may show increased interior echogenicity (Fig. 13-65). Also, wavy lines within the implant represent shell collapse (Fig. 13-66).

Intracapsular rupture cannot be diagnosed mammographically since the silicone is contained by the fibrous capsule. With extracapsular rupture, the silicone gel extrudes into the breast tissue and can be seen mammographically.

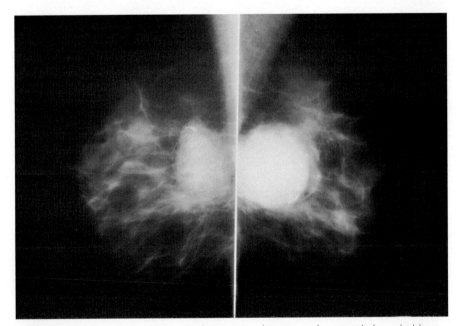

FIGURE 13-57 The masses present in the posterior breasts on these mediolateral oblique views represent the fibrous capsules left after implant removal.

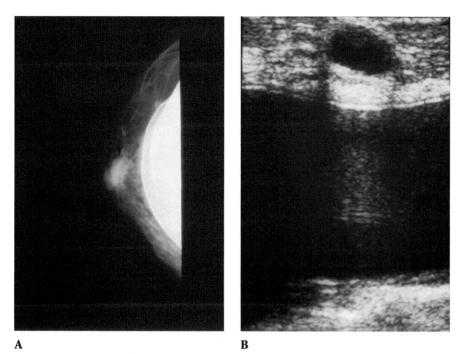

A   **B**

FIGURE 13-58 The small mass in the retroareolar region on the mammogram *(A)* was a cyst on ultrasound *(B).* The cyst is anterior to the normal-appearing sonolucent silicone implant.

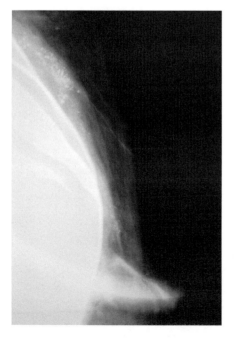

FIGURE 13-59 The fine granular microcalcifications anterior to the superior margin of this saline implant represent invasive ductal carcinoma. The patient had metastatic liver disease at the time of the diagnosis.

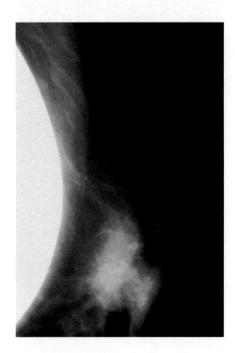

FIGURE 13-60 The spiculated mass in the retroareolar region anterior to this subpectoral silicone implant is an invasive ductal carcinoma.

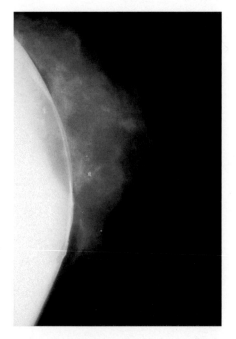

FIGURE 13-61 Fading of the anterior contour of this implant is caused by the mass effect of the patient's breast cancer.

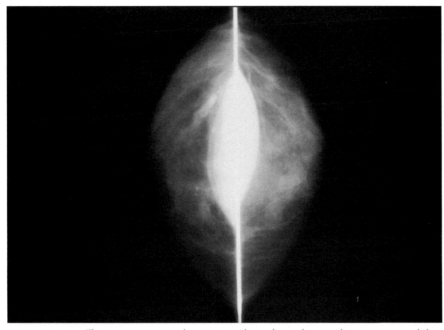

FIGURE 13-62 The opaque material anterior to the right implant on these craniocaudal views represents silicone extruding from an extracapsular rupture.

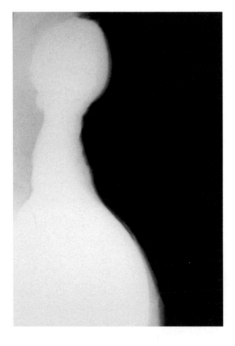

FIGURE 13-63 Note the clublike appearance of the silicone as it extends into the axilla after extracapsular rupture.

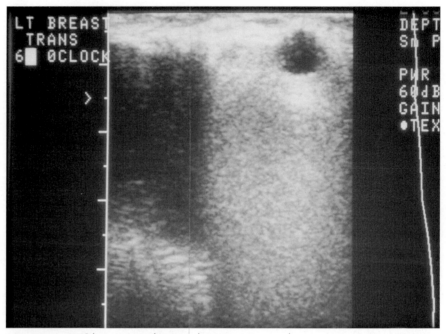

FIGURE 13-64 Silicone extending into the tissue is very echogenic.

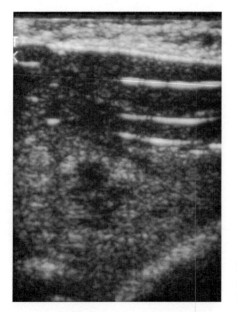

FIGURE 13-65 This silicone implant is not sonolucent. The increased echogenicity is indicative of implant rupture.

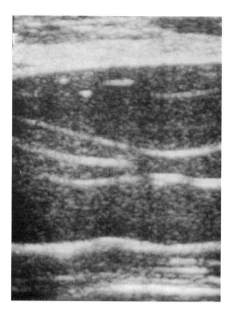

FIGURE 13-66 Serpiginous lines within the implant represent the collapsed shell floating in the silicone gel.

Magnetic resonance imaging (MRI) of the breast is the most definitive procedure for evaluating intracapsular rupture of a silicone implant. Although various findings may be seen, the characteristic abnormality is called the "linguine sign," in which a series of dark wavy lines within the implant represent the collapsed shell of the implant floating within the gel (Fig. 13-67).

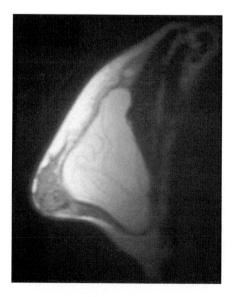

FIGURE 13-67 The dark wavy lines within the silicone implant indicate intracapsular rupture.

COMMONLY ASKED QUESTIONS

1. **I'm now 20 weeks pregnant, and I found a lump in my breast. My doctor wants me to have a mammogram, but isn't the radiation going to hurt my baby?** The first step in the evaluation of a breast lump during pregnancy is usually ultrasonography or fine needle aspiration. Either procedure can determine whether the lump is cystic, in which case no further evaluation may be necessary. Ultrasonography also may be able to distinguish a true mass from parenchymal asymmetry. Because the breasts are more dense during pregnancy, mammography often yields images that are very opaque and difficult to interpret. However, if a mass is solid or clinically suspicious for cancer, mammography is recommended. The radiation dose to the patient is only 0.2 rad, per view, and with shielding, the dose to the fetus is very low.

2. **I have a soft lump in my breast that is thought to be a lipoma. Should it be removed?** Lipomas are benign fatty tumors that usually cause no symptoms other than the presence of a lump. On examination, they are soft, well defined, and nontender. Mammographically, lipomas have a characteristic appearance because they are composed of fat. Unless the size or location of the lipoma causes a cosmetic problem, excision is not required.

3. **Should I still undergo screening mammography even though my implants take up almost all of my breasts?** Mammographic screening for breast cancer is recommended for all women beginning at age 40 even in the presence of implants. In fact, because implants can obscure clinical examination, annual screening between ages 40 and 50 (instead of every other year) is warranted. Mammography is technically more difficult with implants, especially if they are located superficial to the pectoralis major muscles. Four mammographic views per breast are taken in patients with implants: the two standard views and then two views in which the breast tissue is pulled over the implant while the implant is pushed toward the chest wall (the Eklund technique).

REFERENCES

1. Kopans DB. *Breast Imaging.* Philadelphia: Lippincott-Raven; 1998.
2. Harris JR, Hellman S, Henderson IC, Kinne DW. *Breast Diseases.* Philadelphia: Lippincott, 1991.
3. Rosen PP. *Rosen's Breast Pathology.* Philadelphia: Lippincott-Raven; 1997.
4. Powell DE, Stelling CB. *The Diagnosis and Detection of Breast Disease.* St. Louis: Mosby; 1994.
5. Adler DD, Jeffries DO, Helvie MA. Sonographic features of breast hamartomas. *J Ultrasound Med* 1990; 9:85–90.
6. Bernstein JR. Nonsuppurative nodular panniculitis (Weber-Christian disease): An unusual cause of mammary calcifications. *JAMA* 1977; 238:1942–1943.
7. DiPiro PJ, Meyer JE, Frenna TH, Denison CM. Seat belt injuries of the breast: Findings on mammography and sonography. *AJR* 1995; 164:317–320.
8. Gomez A, Mata JM, Donoso L, Rams A. Galactocele: Three distinctive radiographic appearances. *Radiology* 1986; 158:43–44.
9. Conant EF, Wilkes AN, Mendelson EB, Feig SA. Superficial thrombophlebitis of the breast (Mondor's disease): Mammographic findings. *AJR* 1993; 160:1201–1203.
10. Haagensen CD. *Diseases of the Breast,* 3d ed. Philadelphia: Saunders; 1986.
11. Cardenosa G, Eklund GW. Benign papillary neoplasms of the breast: Mammographic findings. *Radiology* 1991; 181:751–755.
12. Logan WW, Hoffman NY. Diabetic fibrous breast disease. *Radiology* 1989; 172:667–670.
13. Cardenosa G. *Breast Imaging Companion.* Philadelphia: Lippincott-Raven; 1997.

14. Berkowitz JE, Gatewood OD, Donovan GB, Gayler BW. Dermal breast calcifications: Localization with template-guided placement of skin marker. *Radiology* 1987; 163:282.
15. Reynolds HE. Evaluation of the augmented breast. *Radiol Clin North Am* 1995; 33(6):1131–1145.
16. Eklund GW, Busby RC, Miller SH, Job JS. Improved imaging of the augmented breast. *AJR* 1988; 151:469–473.

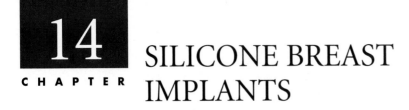

SILICONE BREAST IMPLANTS

HISTORY OF BREAST AUGMENTATION

Breast augmentation has been popular since the late 1800s, and it currently is the most frequently requested cosmetic surgical procedure. Early attempts to enlarge the breast involved transplantation of autologous fatty tissue. However, those operations did not employ microsurgical techniques and resulted in fat necrosis and less than optimal results.

Another procedure performed before breast implants became available was the injection of paraffin into the breast. This practice was common in Asia, where the materials injected were neither controlled nor of pharmaceutical quality. Paraffin was selected because it remains liquid at body temperature. The paraffin was mixed with various oils or petroleum jelly to facilitate injection. The performance of this procedure continued until shortly after World War II. Acceptable cosmetic results were short-lived, resulting in the loss of popularity of the technique. Unfortunate recipients of these injections developed diffuse granulomas throughout the injected sites (Fig. 14-1), with or without draining sinus tracts.

Injection of medical-grade silicone fluid was used for breast augmentation during the 1950s and 1960s. Currently, silicone fluid injection is not approved by the U.S. Food and Drug Administration (FDA), and patients who wish to undergo the procedure must travel to Mexico or Asia. As with paraffin injection, granulomas often form and the firm masses and associated fibrosis result in a less than optimal cosmetic appearance. Subcutaneous mastectomy to remove granulomas is commonly required. In addition, silicone fluid has been injected either intentionally or inadvertently into skeletal muscle. Liquid silicone may track along anatomic planes

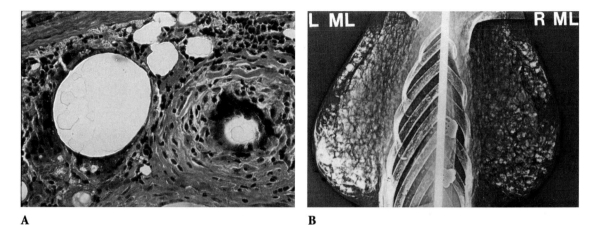

A   **B**

FIGURE 14-1 **A.** After paraffin injection, the foreign material elicits a brisk granulomatous response that almost uniformly results in an unacceptably firm breast with an uneven cobblestone texture. Some women who underwent paraffin injection also developed draining sinuses. Most of these women were treated with subcutaneous mastectomy and reconstruction. Resected tissue is remarkable for dense fibrosis in spheres and surrounding empty spaces. Any remaining paraffin is removed in the deparaffinization step of tissue processing, leaving only the resulting granulomas and dystrophic calcification, as seen here. **B.** Film screen mammogram demonstrating diffuse distribution of silicone after injection into the breast.

of least resistance when pressure is applied, resulting in the formation of soft tissue depots of silicone in sites outside the breast. Histologically, silicone granulomas display varying degrees of concentric fibrosis with central multinucleate giant cells surrounding refractile, water-clear foreign material. The foreign material is seen histologically and has a tendency to remain in the rims of the vacuoles or strands in the resected tissue. Some of the silicone is removed during tissue processing (Fig. 14-2).

Early attempts to implant breast prostheses surgically involved the use of synthetic materials with the consistency of sponges. However, the tissue ingrowth and shrinkage associated with the prostheses eventually necessitated their removal.

In 1963, silicone gel breast prostheses were introduced. The silicone gel is enclosed in a shell composed of silicone elastomer (Fig. 14-3). The rubbery elastomer is a more highly cross-linked silicone polymer preparation than the silicone gel or liquid. Over time, a specialized scar known as an implant-related capsule develops around the implant's elastomer shell. As surgeons gained experience with implants, they noted that contractures of the implant-related capsule would cause an undesirable change in the contour of the augmented breast. Implant manufacturers were prompted to consider ways in which the elastomer shell could be altered to improve the long-term cosmetic outcome. Between 1968 and 1984, surface texture was added to the original smooth silicone elastomer shell in an effort to reduce the formation of capsular contractures. Theoretically, the texture would facilitate anchoring of the implant in the breast and interrupt the ability of the myofibroblasts to contract concentrically. Most textures are applied as the shell is cast; polyurethane foam, however, is glued onto the silicone elastomer shell. In some cases, fragments of the elastomer texture become incorporated into the host tissue.

Over time, a specialized scar known as an implant-related capsule develops around the implant's elastomer shell.

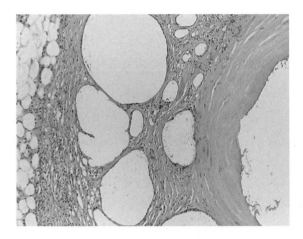

FIGURE 14-2 Compared with the paraffin granuloma in Fig. 14-1, the silicone granuloma shown here has unique-appearing macrophages whose multiple vacuoles vary in size. Some vacuoles contain rims of refractile foreign material. Multinucleate giant cells surround larger droplets of silicone, and stranding of the water clear foreign material may be observed in the cytoplasm of these aggregates.

Before the Medical Device Amendments of 1976, the FDA did not assure the safety and effectiveness of medical devices. Breast implants were in use before the law was passed, and so they were allowed to remain on the market after the amendments passed. Manufacturers were given until 1991 to gather scientific evidence about the safety and effectiveness of the gel-filled devices. Because insufficient supporting data were presented, the FDA withdrew gel-filled implants from the market. Gel-filled implants are currently available only in FDA-approved clinical studies.

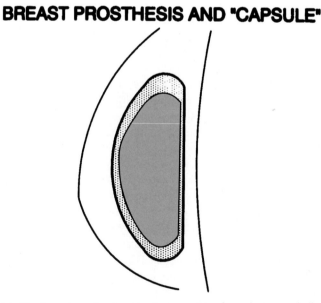

FIGURE 14-3 The breast prosthesis or implant consists of an elastomer shell of silicone rubber filled with silicone gel or saline. Once it is implanted within the soft tissue of the breast, a specialized scar, or implant-related capsule, forms around the implant in an attempt to reduce friction.

Participation in these studies requires that each patient agree to be followed for a specified period after implantation.

Saline-filled implants are currently available for both augmentation and reconstruction. The manufacturers were notified in 1993 to gather safety and effectiveness data, and since 1994, companies that market saline-filled implants have been required to enroll patients in clinical trials to gather these data. The results of these clinical trials are confidential unless the manufacturers choose to make them public.

BREAST IMPLANT–RELATED CAPSULES

After the placement of a prosthesis, the tissue surrounding the foreign body creates a specialized scar or capsule. This capsule is variable in thickness and frequently contracts. Contracture may occur days, weeks, months, or even years after the placement of the implant. When the capsule contracts, the space holding the implant is constrained, often resulting in folds of the elastomer shell (Fig. 14-4). Folding may be detected on physical examination when the points of the folds are palpable. Furthermore, the contracted capsule visibly stands out from the surrounding breast tissue and is palpably firm (Fig. 14-5). Capsular contracture is graded clinically from I to IV, with grade IV being the most severe (Table 14-1).

Histopathologic study of breast implant–related capsules has led to insight into the host response to breast prostheses, including the mechanism behind capsular contracture. Capsules form to reduce the friction that results from mechanical disruption and cavitation of connective tissue, especially in response to a foreign

When the capsule contracts, the space holding the implant is constrained, often resulting in folds of the elastomer shell.

CAPSULAR CONTRACTURE

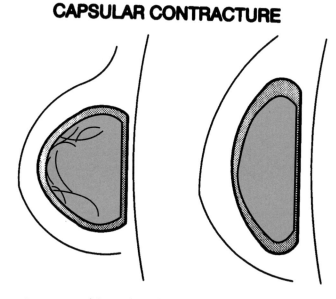

FIGURE 14-4 Contracture of the implant-related capsule causes the profile of the implanted breast to change from the cosmetically desired contour to a rounder, more projected profile. As the space allowed for the implant becomes constricted, the elastomer shell folds on itself. The silicone elastomer is not strong when folded and will develop fold flaws and eventual rupture at the site of the folds.

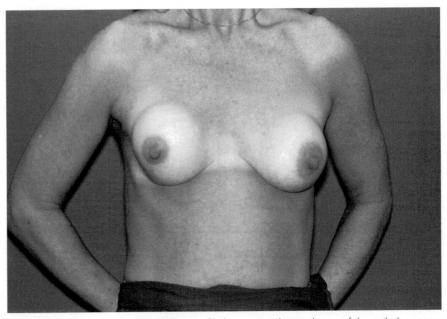

FIGURE 14-5 Note asymmetry between the breasts, with angulation of the right breast in the anterior axillary line causing lateral projection of the nipple.

body.[1–3] This characteristic host response has been used to therapeutic advantage in preparing the forearm to accept a tendon graft.[4]

Histologically, the early capsule resembles granulation tissue (Fig. 14-6), the body's attempt to close a defect caused by tissue cavitation. When the granulation tissue is unable to bridge the cavity (as occurs when the implanted foreign material prevents tissue approximation), synovium develops to reduce surface friction. The finding that the lining of breast implant–related capsules demonstrates synovial differentiation is important. Rather than functioning as a barrier to the movement of foreign material, the synovium actually moves particulate matter away from the capsular space and toward deeper tissues. Its cellular components, stromal structure, and absence of a basement membrane facilitate this action.[5,6] The movement of particulate matter away from the capsule may explain why contracted capsules may or may not be thicker than noncontracted capsules.[7] Furthermore, particles in the form of silicone gel droplets or elastomer shell fragments are not required for clinically evident capsular contracture to oc-

TABLE 14-1 CLASSIFICATION OF IMPLANT-RELATED CAPSULAR CONTRACTURE

Grade I	Breast feels as soft as unoperated breast
Grade II	Breast is less soft, and implant can be palpated but is not visible
Grade III	Breast is firmer; implant is visible or causes distortion and can be palpated easily
Grade IV	Breast is hard, tender, painful, and cold; distortion of breast is present

SOURCE: Bostwick J. Breast reconstruction. In: McCarthy JG, ed. *Plastic Surgery: The Trunk and Lower Extremity*, Vol 6. Philadelphia: Saunders; 1990:3897–3928.

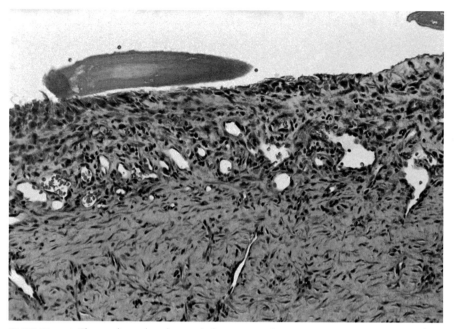

FIGURE 14-6 The implant-related capsule begins as a host response to tissue injury. When granulation tissue is unable to bridge the gap caused by the implant, the body creates a surface lined by synovium around the implant to reduce friction. The surface of the implant determines the histologic appearance of this specialized scar, or implant-related capsule.

cur. Numerous authors have documented capsular contracture in patients with saline implants, although its occurrence is less common than it is with gel-filled implants.[8,9]

Capsule formation and contracture have been delayed, but not prevented, by the creation of textured implant elastomer. Histologic examination of capsules with such textures has shown that the texture may become partially or completely incorporated into the capsule.[10,11] When this occurs, the texture is covered by host tissue to create a plane of reduced friction. Incorporation of foreign material into the capsule therefore adds tissue to the capsular surface, sometimes reducing the space for the implant. If the elastomer shell folds to fit the smaller available space (Fig. 14-7), the shell is predisposed to rupture. Worton and associates[12] noted that when folds occurred in elastomer shells, "fold flaws" or perforations occurred at the tips of the folds. Therefore, capsular contracture resulting in the wrinkling of an intact elastomer shell may precede and indeed predispose to rupture of the implant.

The mechanism behind capsular contracture with smooth saline implants is less clear. Scanning electron microscopy of explanted elastomer shells reveals pits and blebs on the surface from shearing of the elastomer or phagocytosis in situ by macrophages. In addition, some explants are surrounded by an opacifying "film"[13] that may correspond to the protein observed in the capsular space and on the capsule surface.[14]

If the elastomer shell folds to fit the smaller available space, the shell is predisposed to rupture.

TYPES OF IMPLANTS

The original breast implants were manufactured with smooth elastomer shells (Fig. 14-8). Subsequently, the silicone elastomer shell thickness and external texture were

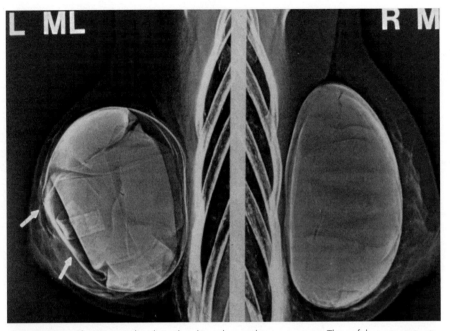

FIGURE 14-7 This patient developed unilateral capsular contracture. The soft breast retains its normal profile, while the contracted breast's implant-related capsule is associated with an increase in projection. Note the folds of the elastomer shell and the points at the end of the folds. These points may be palpable on examination and predispose the implant to rupture.

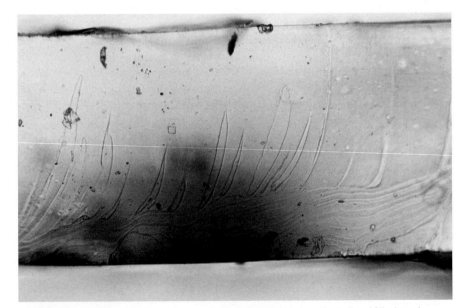

FIGURE 14-8 Most manufacturers initially introduced the smooth shell gel-filled implants shown here. The elastomer shell may vary in thickness and composition in an effort to reduce the phenomenon called gel bleed, or passage of silicone liquid through an intact shell.

varied in an attempt to modify capsular contracture. A smooth shell saline-filled implant has a predictably simple and relatively hypocellular implant-related capsule (Fig. 14-9). Implants have a single or a double lumen, and either shell may hold saline or gel. Occasionally, two implants are placed, one stacked on the other, to create the desired contour.

The McGhan Company, one of the companies that still manufactures implants, introduced a texture (Fig. 14-10) that is available on both saline and gel-filled implants (Fig. 14-11). This cuboidal texture creates mirror-image villous projections in the implant-related capsule (Fig. 14-12) that contain microscopic pieces of elastomer broken from the surface of the implant (Fig. 14-13). This foreign material is embedded in the implant-related capsule and will remain unless the entire capsule is removed during explantation. The foreign body chronic inflammatory response to the elastomer shell fragments consists of lymphocytes, macrophages, and occasionally plasma cells. Inflammatory cells are known to secrete cytokines that can produce systemic symptoms when they circulate in sufficient quantities. Whether this foreign material accounts for any of the symptoms reported by breast implant recipients (fever, malaise, rash, aches, and pains) is unclear. Research must be carried out to establish whether a cause-and-effect relationship exists.

The Mentor Company, which also still manufactures implants, introduced a texture that is available on both saline and gel-filled implants (Fig. 14-14, Plate 4; and Fig. 14-15). This texture does not have sharp edges and is associated with less breakage of elastomer particles. Therefore, the implant-related capsule has quite a different appearance and synovial differentiation is readily seen (Fig. 14-16). The cells lining synovial membranes in any site are macrophages interspersed with fibroblasts.

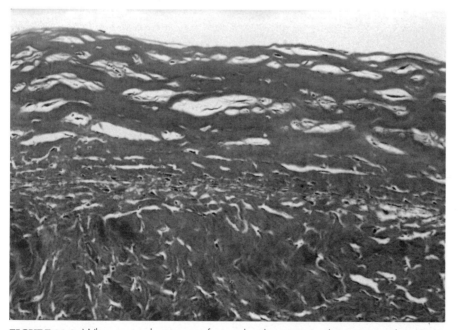

FIGURE 14-9 When an implant is manufactured without texture, the corresponding implant-related capsule is smooth. If no silicone gel or fluid is present, the capsule is fairly hypocellular.

FIGURE 14-10 Cubical indentations in the elastomer shell of a Biocell implant.

The macrophages are oriented with processes directed toward the capsule lumen. Neither macrophages nor fibroblasts produce basement membrane material, and so the implant-related capsule does not present a barrier to the migration of the macrophages.

Dow Corning is no longer making implants but manufactured more implants in its history than any other company to date. Dow created a uniquely textured shell

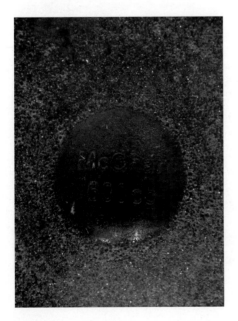

FIGURE 14-11 This McGhan Biocell textured saline-filled tissue expander can be placed temporarily at the time of mastectomy to allow soft tissue to be stretched gently to accommodate the final prosthesis.

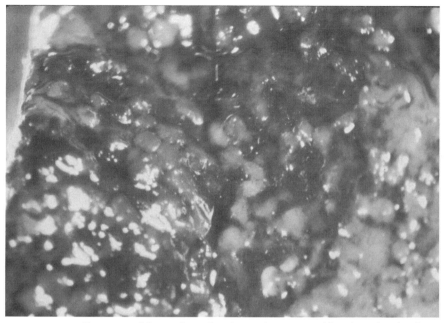

FIGURE 14-12 The tissue of the implant-related capsule grows to fill in the cubical indentations of the texture, resulting in a cobblestone appearance to the capsule on gross inspection.

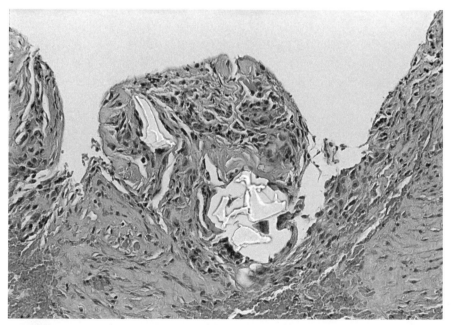

FIGURE 14-13 Histologic examination of the implant-related capsule surrounding a Biocell implant demonstrates the villous projections that are noted grossly. These projections consist of well-vascularized fibrous tissue with occasional embedded irregular sheets of water clear foreign material surrounded by multinucleate giant cells. These are fragments of elastomer shell texture incorporated into the capsule.

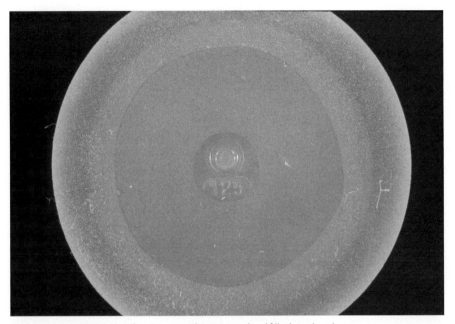

FIGURE 14-14 (Plate 4)   This Mentor Siltex textured gel-filled implant has an opaque appearance. A relatively large patch covers the majority of the back of the implant. In the center of the back is a circle containing a central raised gel fill point with the size marked in an oval.

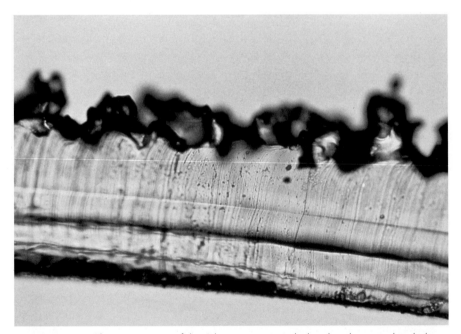

FIGURE 14-15   Close inspection of the Siltex texture reveals that the elastomer has bulbous ends.

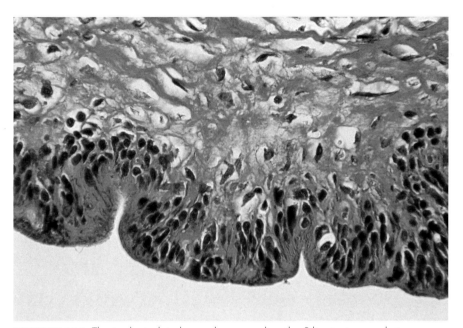

FIGURE 14-16 The implant-related capsule surrounding the Siltex texture rarely incorporates fragments of elastomer shell. The histology of this capsule is structurally and functionally identical to that of synovium.

on its Micro Structured Implant (MSI) (Fig. 14-17) that consisted of sturdy pillars of silicone elastomer (Fig. 14-18). Interestingly, the mirror-image indentations in the implant-related capsule contained no elastomer shell fragments (Fig. 14-19). However, innumerable vacuolated macrophages could be seen containing refractile water clear droplets of foreign material consistent with silicone fluid. These vacuolated macrophages can be observed even when the implant appears intact. The silicone fluid "sweats" or "bleeds" from or through the elastomer shell.

The silicone fluid can escape fom the intact elastomer shell.

Surgitek, which no longer manufactures implants, is one of several companies that used polyurethane foam to add texture to smooth elastomer shells (Fig. 14-20). The foam (Fig. 14-21) was glued on with silicone-based adhesive. The purpose of the texture was to promote tissue ingrowth in an attempt to reduce friction in the implant-related space and by interrupting concentric contraction by myofibroblasts. In the implant-related capsule, tissue ingrowth into the foam actually lifted the foam from the elastomer shell in many cases. Because of the incorporation of the polyurethane foam into the capsule, it is important to perform capsulectomy at the time of removal of these implants.[15] If capsulectomy is not performed, foam remains in the tissue, accompanied by a brisk chronic inflammatory response (Fig. 14-22). The subsequent contracted mass can create concern about cancer on follow-up mammograms, and another operation to remove the capsule must later be performed. Occasionally, women with foam-covered implants undergo biopsy of enlarged axillary lymph nodes. Careful inspection of the nodes reveals not only silicone oil or gel droplets but also triangular fragments of polyurethane foam (Fig. 14-23).

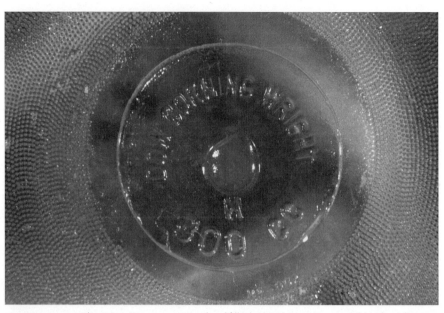

FIGURE 14-17 The Dow Corning textured gel-filled MSI (Micro Structured Implant) has a back patch with a central fill point. The size is noted in cubic centimeters, and the texture appears to be in orderly rows when viewed on end.

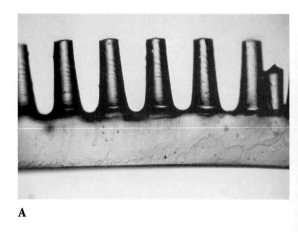

A

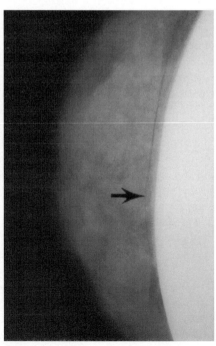

B

FIGURE 14-18 *A.* MSI texture imparts an orderly columnar arrangement to the elastomer texture. *B.* This particular texture is associated with accumulation of fluid in the capsular space, creating a characteristic appearance on mammography or MRI of the breast.

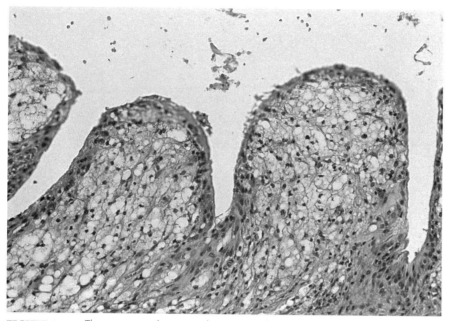

FIGURE 14-19 The corresponding capsule opposite the MSI texture demonstrates villous projections. In this case, the stroma is packed with back-to-back histiocytes with vacuoles of foreign material consistent with silicone. This texture is not incorporated into the patient's tissue; however, silicone liquid is evident in spite of a grossly intact elastomer shell.

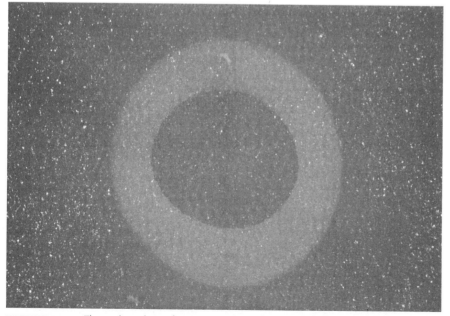

FIGURE 14-20 This polyurethane foam-covered, gel-filled Surgitek implant has an even more opaque white ring.

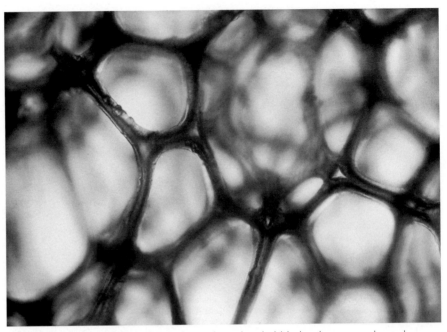

FIGURE 14-21 Polyurethane is a polymer that when bubbled with gas, produces the foam most familiar to people as furniture cushions. A thin layer of polyurethane foam is glued to the elastomer shell, usually with a silicone adhesive.

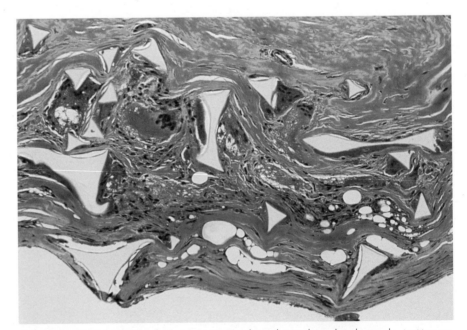

FIGURE 14-22 Polyurethane foam is incorporated into the implant-related capsule, inciting an intense fibrotic reaction. Histologically, multinucleate giant cells surround fragments of foam and are accompanied by lymphocytes and histiocytes with variable-size vacuoles containing silicone. Although the elastomer shell may appear intact to inspection upon removal, silicone and polyurethane are invariably present in the capsular tissue.

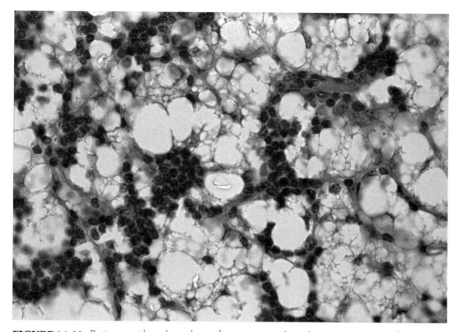

FIGURE 14-23 Patients with polyurethane foam–covered implants may note axillary adenopathy. Biopsy may show minute triangular fragments and other irregular pieces of firm foreign material within the vacuoles of histiocytes. Other histiocytes have rims of refractile foreign material consistent with silicone.

Several manufacturers, including Dow Corning, used Dacron patches on the backs of implants to anchor them to the chest (Fig. 14-24). Like polyurethane foam, Dacron fibers were intended to encourage tissue ingrowth and become incorporated into the implant-related capsule (Fig. 14-25). Histologically, the fibers are accompanied by a brisk chronic inflammatory response (Fig. 14-26).

Implants, especially those with Dacron patches, may be associated with confluent calcification of the implant-related capsule. This radiopaque calcification presents an imaging challenge at the time of mammography (Fig. 14-27) as well as an impressive gross appearance (Fig. 14-28). Capsules with "eggshell" calcification to this degree are correspondingly firm to palpation, and some of these patients complain of pain.

Implants, especially those with Dacron patches, may be associated with confluent calcification of the implant-related capsule.

The implant-related capsule is not a barrier to the migration of silicone. In some cases, the pectoralis or serratus muscles are infiltrated with macrophages containing vacuoles of silicone (Fig. 14-29), and this may be seen in the absence of elastomer shell rupture. Less commonly, silicone may be observed in the lumen of venules in the subcapsular soft tissue (Fig. 14-30). Once silicone enters the vascular system, it theoretically may be found in a variety of distant locations. No one knows whether this movement of silicone has clinical significance. Patients with chronic disease (e.g., renal failure, diabetes) often are presented with small doses of silicone in the vascular system through dialysis tubing and the silicone lubrication in syringes. If these patients complained of fatigue, muscle aches, or skin rash, their symptoms probably would be attributed to their disease, not to silicone exposure.

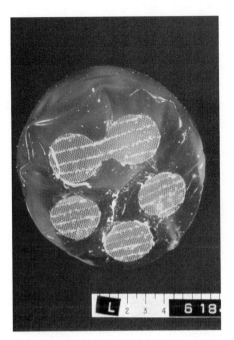

FIGURE 14-24 This Dow Corning gel-filled implant has a fixation patch on its back. Fixation patches were designed to prevent rotation of the implant within the capsule. The patches are affixed to the surface of the elastomer shell and are composed of a Dacron mesh. The mesh is intended to encourage tissue ingrowth. The pattern of the fixation patches can help identify the implant's manufacturer. For example, five round patches with two connected in a dumbbell fashion indicate that Dow Corning was the manufacturer.

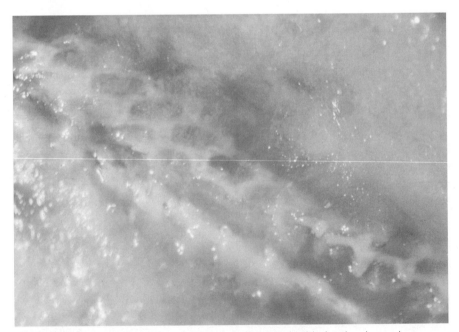

FIGURE 14-25 Threads of the Dacron patch become embedded within the implant-related capsule. Some of these fibers become physically separated from the implant. Therefore, removal of the capsule at the time of explantation is important to ensure that no foreign material remains within the body.

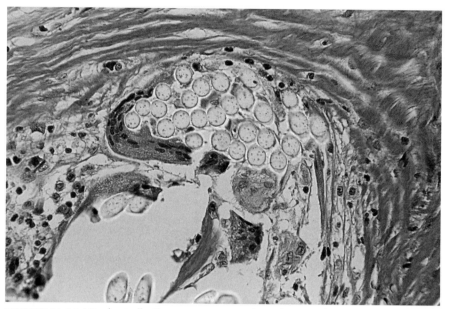

FIGURE 14-26 Histologically, Dacron incorporated into the capsule resembles a multifilament suture. These fibers are associated with a dense fibrosis and an intense histiocytic multinucleate giant-cell response.

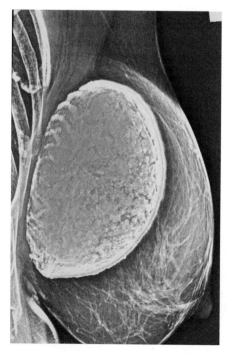

FIGURE 14-27 This retroglandular implant is associated with extensive calcification of the implant-related capsule.

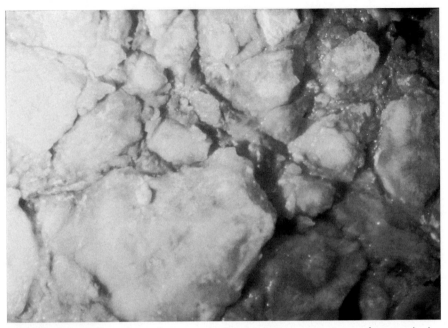

FIGURE 14-28 Surface dystrophic mineralization can vary in appearance from cracked eggshells when the entire capsule is involved (as shown here) to a fine, translucent stiff area on an otherwise pliable capsule. The mineralization process is more confluent in association with implant rupture and implants with Dacron patches.

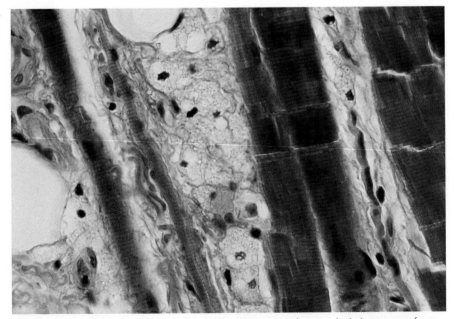

FIGURE 14-29 After successful closed capsulotomy, a procedure in which the surgeon forcefully "presses" on a contracted capsule in order to release it, silicone from a ruptured implant may travel via tissue planes to rest in other areas of the chest wall. Here skeletal muscle of the chest is infiltrated by macrophages containing fine vacuoles of refractile foreign material.

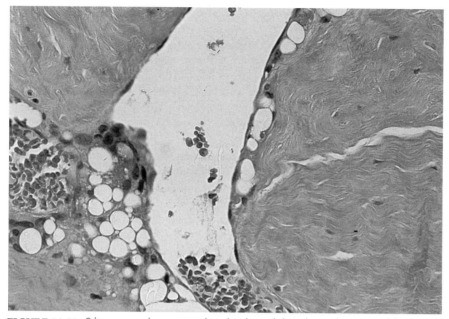

FIGURE 14-30 Silicone reaches regional nodes through lymphatic drainage of the breast. Any silicone that is not deposited in the nodes may enter the venous circulation through the thoracic duct. On rare occasions, silicone is observed in vascular spaces deep to the implant-related capsule, as is shown here. Seldom are other tissues included with an implant-related capsule for histologic evaluation; however, the possibility that silicone will reach other tissue sites via the vasculature is not excluded.

INDICATIONS FOR BREAST AUGMENTATION

Breast augmentation is widely available by request. Very few insurance plans cover the cost of the procedure, and so patients who desire augmentation pay out of pocket. Several psychological studies have compared women seeking augmentation mammaplasty to control groups. A recurring theme is that women who request augmentation are highly self-conscious, especially about their unclothed bodies, and place emphasis on dress and external appearance.[16] In one study, nearly two-thirds of the control group of women thought their breasts were small or very small, while presumably all the women requesting augmentation thought the same.[17] Certainly, media depictions of what is "normal" add to any woman's perception that her body is somehow abnormal or unattractive.

Obstetrician-gynecologists have a unique opportunity to reassure women during a breast examination that their breasts are normal. Furthermore, an opportunity for patient education presents itself, since many women are not aware that breasts continue to change in size and shape long after menarche. Therefore, patients may choose to undergo breast augmentation before breast development is complete.

Women who choose breast reconstruction after surgical removal of the breast because of cancer have very different motivational and psychological profiles. They choose reconstruction to reduce the sense of deformity brought on by their cancer diagnosis and treatment. Not surprisingly, they demonstrate greater satisfaction with the results of reconstruction than do women undergoing augmentation.

PHYSICAL EXAMINATION OF THE BREAST AFTER AUGMENTATION

Women who undergo breast augmentation have the same, if not a greater, risk of developing breast masses as women without augmentation. Implant-related masses may be granulomas from silicone located in soft tissues adjacent to the implant-related capsule (Figs. 14-31 and 14-32). Distant silicone granulomas related to the passage of silicone via tissue planes, retained implant-related capsules, and foreign material after implant removal are other implant-related masses.[15]

Breast implants may be inserted through inframammary, periareolar, or axillary incisions.

Breast implants may be inserted through inframammary, periareolar, or axillary incisions (Fig. 14-33). The majority of breast tissue usually is located anterior to the implant, but the implant may be placed either superficially or deep to the pectoralis major muscle (Fig. 14-34). Compression of the normal tissue as a result of the prosthesis may challenge the clinical examination of the glandular breast tissue. As always, examination of the axillae is important, keeping in mind that implants sometimes are associated with axillary adenopathy.

Occasionally, the treatment of capsular contracture includes forcible rupture of the capsule by the application of external pressure to the breast in a procedure called closed capsulotomy. After closed capsulotomy, extrusion of silicone along tissue planes may result in the later formation of granulomas. Common locations of tissue granulomas related to implants are adjoining and deep to the implant capsule as well as along fascial planes to the axilla or abdominal wall. Rarely, masses can be found as far away as the back, elbow, or groin.

When a mass is detected after breast augmentation, it should be evaluated in the same way as a mass occurring in a woman without implants. Short of tissue diagnosis, there is no way to distinguish a silicone granuloma from a breast neoplasm. Fine

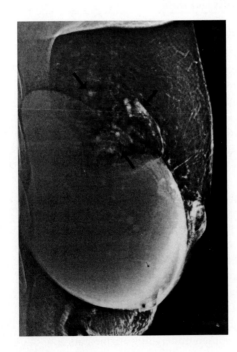

FIGURE 14-31 Silicone from the ruptured implant has entered the soft tissue of the chest and axilla. Silicone gel in soft tissues creates an exuberant foreign body response, and the resulting fibrosis may be palpable as a mass or granuloma.

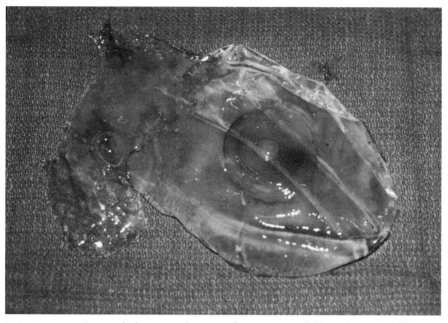

FIGURE 14-32 Ruptured silicone implants usually are removed. The surgeon should re-move the implant with the implant-related capsule intact to be certain that the foreign mate-rial is completely excised. If the silicone gel has traversed the capsule, further surgery may be needed to remove the foreign material.

INCISION SITES FOR AUGMENTATION MAMMAPLASTY

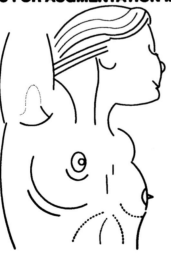

FIGURE 14-33 The incisions for the placement of breast prostheses may be inframam-mary, subareolar, or axillary in location. Skillful surgeons create such subtle scars that they may be overlooked easily on physical examination. Patients should be queried about prior cosmetic surgery, since some may be reluctant to volunteer that history.

PROSTHESIS PLACEMENT

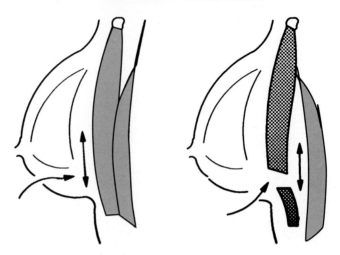

FIGURE 14-34 The prosthesis usually is placed in a retroglandular position anterior to the pectoralis major muscle or in a submuscular location behind the pectoralis major and serratus anterior muscles. The retroglandular location provides ease of placement and removal of the implant, but submuscular placement is associated with a lower incidence or delayed onset of capsular contracture.

needle aspiration is a suitable technique to evaluate possible silicone granulomas. If they are given adequate historical information, pathologists will recognize the foreign material in histiocytes obtained on needle aspiration.

RECOMMENDATIONS FOR MAMMOGRAPHY AFTER BREAST AUGMENTATION

Patients should be referred for mammography after augmentation according to risk factor and age guidelines for women without augmentation.

Patients should be referred for mammography after augmentation according to risk factor and age guidelines for women without augmentation. Although both patients and physicians may be concerned that the compression required for mammography may rupture breast implants, no evidence supports this fear. However, if an implant is ruptured before mammography, the compression may be sufficient to squeeze silicone from the broken elastomer shell into the implant-related capsule. The technique for mammography in the presence of implants attempts to displace the opaque implant away from the compression plates.

Magnetic resonance imaging (MRI) is more expensive than mammography and usually is not recommended for breast cancer screening. However, it is used frequently to evaluate the integrity of breast implants and does not require compression. Ultrasound may be used to assess soft tissues of the chest and axillae for the presence of silicone granulomas and silicone-related adenopathy.

SOURCES OF INFORMATION FOR PATIENTS CONSIDERING BREAST AUGMENTATION OR BREAST RECONSTRUCTION

Patients considering augmentation procedures may ask for sources of information in addition to those supplied by the plastic surgeon. The FDA breast information hot line for consumers and health professionals can be reached by dialing 1-888-463-6322. A Web site with similar information can be found at http:\\www.fda.gov\cdrh\breastimplants\indexbip.html. A visit to that site gives the patient access to a publication entitled *Breast Implants: An Informational Update.* This publication is revised periodically and includes information on the availability of implants, how to report problems with implants, resource groups for women with implants, and the most frequently asked questions about implants.

COMMONLY ASKED QUESTIONS

1. **How long will breast implants last?** Breast implants are not constructed to last indefinitely. Both gel-filled and saline-filled implants may leak or rupture with time, necessitating their removal. Many patients receive several sets of implants during the course of their life- times. Women who receive implants for reconstruction after cancer surgery can expect a one in three chance of needing a second surgery within 5 years, and women who receive implants for augmentation can expect a one in eight chance of needing surgery within 5 years.[18] The cosmetic result after multiple implant-related surgeries often is suboptimal, and additional breast tissue may be lost with each operation.

   In a series of implants removed for various reasons 1 to 25 years after placement, slightly more than half were frankly ruptured and another 20 percent were leaking.[19] When gel-filled implants rupture, the silicone gel gains entry into the implant-related capsular space. Even intact gel-filled implants may "sweat" silicone fluid into the capsular space. The nature of the lining of the capsule may slow but will not prevent migration of the silicone to deeper tissues.[20] Precipitous deflation of a gel-filled implant seldom occurs. However, rupture of a saline-filled implant may be associated with rapid deflation as the saline is absorbed into the body.

2. **How can I tell if my implant is ruptured?** There may be no signs or symptoms of a ruptured gel-filled implant. Some women note a decrease in breast size, loss of symmetry, pain, burning, sensory changes, or axillary masses. Mammography can diagnose some implant ruptures, but MRI is more sensitive for this use. However, mammography and MRI of the breast detect only gross rupture that would be apparent to the naked eye. Sometimes silicone from the implant may be observed only microscopically.

3. **If my implant is ruptured, should it be removed?** Most surgeons recommend removal of ruptured implants because rupture is considered evidence of device failure. Removal of the ruptured implant may or may not improve the symptoms experienced by the patient, and the cosmetic result of implant removal surgery is not uniformly satisfactory. At the time of removal of ruptured implants, every attempt should be made to remove silicone gel, elastomer shell fragments, and the implant-related capsule. General anesthesia and a major surgical approach usually are required. At the time of removal of a ruptured implant, some patients choose not to replace the implant, while others replace the implant with saline-filled or, in some instances, gel-filled implants. Alternatively, autologous tissue may be moved to the upper chest to create breast mounds with a cosmetically acceptable result. Some insurance companies will not pay for the removal of ruptured implants, especially if implant placement was done for cosmetic reasons. Patients who desire the removal of implants thus are faced with a considerable expense.

   As a result of implant manufacturers' settlement funds, patients may recover some of

Women who receive implants for reconstruction after cancer surgery can expect a one in three chance of needing a second surgery within 5 years, and women who receive implants for augmentation can expect a one in eight chance of needing surgery within 5 years.

At the time of removal of ruptured implants, every attempt should be made to remove silicone gel, elastomer shell fragments, and the implant-related capsule.

the expense of removing ruptured implants. Identification of the manufacturer of the implant can almost always be achieved by noting the distinguishing features of the back patch.[21]

4. **Is it safe to have screening mammography with implants?** Women with implants have the same risk of developing breast cancer that other women have. They must undergo screening mammography in order to receive the benefit of early cancer detection. As was mentioned above, no evidence exists that the compression of mammography will rupture an intact implant. However, a permanently folded implant may have flaws in the elastomer shell that permit the egress of silicone during compression. Special techniques are required to image the breast tissue adequately when implants are present. MRI does not require breast compression but is not the ideal screening technique. Therefore, the physician and the radiologic technologist must be informed that implants are present.

No evidence exists that the compression of mammography will rupture an intact implant.

5. **Will implants increase any risk of arthritis or other connective tissue disorders?** Some women with implants have signs and symptoms of connective tissue disease such as pain and swelling in joints, swollen lymph nodes, fatigue, and muscle weakness. Women with these complaints may or may not have improvement in symptoms after removal of the implants. There are no data at this time to indicate that women with implants are at a higher risk of developing common immune-related disorders such as systemic lupus erythematosus, scleroderma, and rheumatoid arthritis. Investigators note that the time interval between placement of the implants and data gathering may be inadequate to capture all relevant cases of connective tissue disease. Furthermore, research to determine whether these symptoms constitute a unique, previously undescribed disorder associated with breast implants has not been undertaken.

There are no data to indicate that women with implants are at a higher risk of developing common immune-related disorders such as lupus erythematosus, scleroderma, and rheumatoid arthritis.

6. **Will implants increase my risk of developing breast cancer or other cancers?** There is no evidence to date that breast implants increase a woman's risk of breast cancer or other cancers. However, the majority of women undergoing augmentation have not yet reached the peak years of cancer diagnosis. The observation of women after augmentation must be extended for many years to fully exclude the possibility of a link between implants and cancer.

REFERENCES

1. Edwards JCW, Sedgwick AK, Willoughby DA. The formation of a structure with the features of synovial lining by subcutaneous injection of air: An in vivo tissue culture system. *Pathology* 1981; 134:147.
2. Stern DR, Sexton FM. Metaplastic synovial cyst after partial excision of nevus sebaceous. *Am J Dermatopathol* 1988; 10:531.
3. Gonzales JG, Ghiselli RW, Santa Cruz DJ. Synovial metaplasia of the skin. *Am J Surg Pathol* 1987; 11:343.
4. Farkas LG, McCain WG, Sweeney P, et al. An experimental study of the changes following sialastic rod preparation of a new tendon sheath and subsequent tendon grafting. *J Bone Joint Surg* 1983; 55(6):1149–1158.
5. Barland P, Novikkoff AB, Hamerman D. Electron microscopy of the human synovial membrane. *J Cell Biol* 1962; 14:207–220.
6. Hardt NS, Emery JA, Steinbach BG, et al. Cellular transport of silicone from breast prostheses. *Int J Occ Med Toxicol* 1995; 4(1):127–134.
7. Vistnes LM, Ksander GA, Kosek J. Study of encapsulation of silicone rubber implants in animals: A foreign body reaction. *Plast Reconstr Surg* 1978; 62:185.
8. Asplund O. Capsular contracture in silicone gel and saline-filled breast implants after reconstruction. *Plast Reconstr Surg* 1984; 73(2):270–275.
9. McKenney P, Tresley G. Long-term comparison of patients with gel and saline mammary implants. *Plast Reconstr Surg* 1983; 72(1):27–31.

10. Carpaneda CA. Inflammatory reaction and capsular contracture around smooth silicone implants. *Aesthetic Plast Surg* 1997; 21(110):110–114.

11. Hardt NS, Yu LT, La Torre G, Steinbach B. Fourier transform infrared microspectroscopy used to identify foreign material related to breast implants. *Mod Pathol* 1994; 7(6): 669–676.

12. Worton EW, Seifert LN, Sherwood R. Late leakage of inflatable silicone breast prostheses. *Plast Reconstr Surg* 1980; 65(3):302–305.

13. Kossovsky N, Heggers JP, Robson MC. The bioreactivity of silicone. *Crit Rev Biocompat* 1987; 3:53.

14. Hardt NS, Emery JA, LaTorre G, et al. Macrophage-silicone interactions in women with breast prostheses. *Curr Top Microbiol Immunol* 1996; 210:245–252.

15. Hardt NS, Yu L, LaTorre G, Steinbach B. Complications related to retained breast implant capsules. *Plast Reconstr Surg* 1986; 95(2):364–371.

16. Shipley RH, O'Donnell JM, Bader K. Personality characteristics of women seeking breast augmentation. *Plast Reconstr Surg* 1977; 60(3):369–376.

17. Beale S, Lisper H, Palm B. A psychological study of patients seeking augmentation mammaplasty. *Br J Psychiatry* 1980; 136:133–138.

18. Gabriel SE, Woods JE, O'Fallon WM, et al. Complications leading to surgery after breast implantation. *N Engl J Med* 1997; 336:679–682.

19. Robinson OG, Bradley EL, Wilson DS. Analysis of explanted silicone implants: A report of 300 patients. *Ann Plast Surg* 1995; 34:1–7.

20. Emery JA, Spanier S, Kasnic G, Hardt NS. The synovial structure of breast implant associated bursae. *Mod Pathol* 1994; 7(7):728–733.

21. Middleton MS, McNamara MP. Breast implant classification with MR correlation. *Radiographics Online,* accepted 2000.

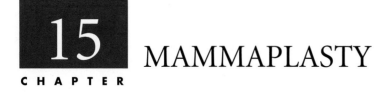

15 MAMMAPLASTY

CHAPTER

INTRODUCTION

Aesthetic revision of the breast, or mammaplasty, includes a variety of surgical techniques aimed at altering the size, shape, and contour of the breast. Elective augmentation mammaplasty is a cosmetic procedure that is performed to enlarge the breasts or improve their silhouette. Women who seek augmentation often are young adults who have normal, though small breasts or older women after childbirth. In the latter case, regression of breast parenchyma postpartum can result in reduced breast volume and more noticeable ptosis. Ptosis refers to descent of the nipple to a position below the inframammary crease. Implants often are desired in this situation to "fill out" loose skin. Occasionally, women request alteration of the size or shape of their nipples and/or areolae to conform to a more "ideal" image. Indicated breast augmentation is performed to correct marked asymmetry in patients with congenital hypoplasia of one breast. Mammaplasty techniques with or without augmentation also are employed to modify misshapen breasts, such as those with a tubular contour.

Numerous techniques have been described for reconstruction of the breast after surgical treatment of breast cancer. Depending on whether the primary therapy consists of simple or modified radical mastectomy, reconstruction may involve the use of implants, myocutaneous flaps, or tissue transfers.

Reduction mammaplasty includes several techniques to decrease the size of the breasts and improve their contour in women with macromastia and/or marked ptosis. These procedures are considered to be indicated (as opposed to purely elective) in most cases because the symptoms of neck, back, and shoulder pain usually are relieved after surgery.

This chapter discusses the most relevant points concerning augmentation and reduction of the female breast and some of the options for breast reconstruction after surgery for breast cancer. For more in-depth discussions of these topics, the clinician is directed to the suggested readings at the end of the chapter.

BREAST AUGMENTATION

Despite the fact that most insurance companies do not cover it, augmentation mammaplasty has become a commonly performed procedure in the United States. Women choose to undergo breast augmentation for a variety of reasons. Some women with small breasts describe extreme difficulty finding bras, bathing suits, and clothes that fit well. Others seek to improve their body image and enhance their sense of femininity. Still others feel that implants will make them more attractive to potential mates. Whatever the reason, the decision to pursue breast augmentation is a very personal one.

When a patient comes to a plastic surgeon, she often has already decided to proceed with surgery. Unfortunately, she may then be less likely to absorb the information offered about the risks or long-term problems that can be associated with breast implants. When consulted before surgery, a primary care clinician has a unique opportunity to help these women reach an educated decision. If the woman is given adequate information about potential complications before the fact, she is likely to be more accepting of problems if they arise.

When consulted before seeking breast augmentation, a primary care clinician has a unique opportunity to help these women reach an educated decision.

After discussing the patient's preferences with her, the plastic surgeon is challenged with the task of meeting her expectations. The surgeon must decide on the optimal location for the skin incision, the type and size of implant to use, and the location for implant placement (subglandular versus submuscular). Patient variables also must be considered, including the patient's overall body habitus, the size and symmetry of her breasts, and the degree of glandular ptosis present. While most common in obese women, ptosis also occurs after weight loss and in association with atrophy in the postpartum and postmenopausal periods.

Placement of breast implants may be performed in the outpatient setting under general anesthesia or using conscious sedation and local anesthesia. With the latter technique, the second through eighth intercostal nerves are blocked individually, followed by local infiltration of the incision site, inframammary crease, and soft tissue of the inferomedial origin of the pectoralis major muscle.[1]

The patient's arms are secured in a position that allows exposure of the incision site. The skin incision may be axillary, inframammary, or periareolar (see Fig. 14-33), depending on the patient's preference, the shape and size of her breasts, and the planned location for the implants. Periareolar incisions are the most versatile, accommodating all types of implants and the subglandular and submuscular implant locations.[1] During mammaplasty, the inframammary crease should be lowered sufficiently to keep the midpoint of the implant centered on the nipple.[1] The periareolar incision facilitates this maneuver. It also is the incision of choice for the correction of tubular breast hypomastia because it allows excision of periareolar skin and underlying parenchyma when necessary.[1]

Breast implants may be placed through periareolar, inframammary, or axillary incisions.

Women with moderate preoperative breast volume and some degree of ptosis fare well with an inframammary incision because the scar remains hidden in the inframammary crease. This incision is suboptimal in women with very small breasts because it is more easily visible. The transaxillary approach is ideally suited for patients with small breasts and minimal ptosis and women who primarily desire an improved contour of the upper breast. It is not appropriate for the placement of subglandular implants, correction of tubular breasts, and secondary procedures that require the excision of an implant capsule.[1] Endoscopy sometimes is used adjunctively when an axillary approach is taken.

After a pocket for the implant in the subpectoral or subglandular location (Fig. 14-34) has been developed, a sizer is introduced. Inflation of the sizer determines the implant volume necessary to achieve optimal breast size and contour. Care is taken not to cause convexity of the upper breast or an unnaturally wide shape. If a submuscular location is planned, the inferomedial edge of the pectoralis major muscle is detached partially from its sternal origin to create the implant pocket.[1,2] The patient is brought to a sitting position during sizing to determine the best implant volume.

The inflation volume of saline implants is adjustable.

The implant location is determined after consideration of the patient's presurgical breast shape and personal preference. Several advantages of subpectoral implants (Fig. 15-1) have been identified. This location allows palpation of more breast parenchyma during clinical examination or self-examination and visualization of more breast tissue on mammography (for a description of mammographic technique in patients with implants, see Chap. 13). Capsular contracture is less likely to occur and may be less obvious when it does develop.[1,3,6] The superior portion of the implant is covered by muscle so that ripples in the implant shell are less likely to be noticeable. Despite these benefits, subpectoral implants are not ideal for all augmentation candidates. For example, when postpartum atrophy causes loose skin, subglandular implants may produce a more desirable cosmetic effect. The pocket for the insertion of subglandular implants is easier and quicker to create, and some patients prefer the appearance or "feel" of subglandular implants.

When the U.S. Food and Drug Administration (FDA) imposed a moratorium on silicone gel-filled implants in 1992, saline implants became the only prostheses used for primary augmentation procedures. Silicone implants still may be used for secondary procedures such as revision after the removal of a ruptured implant, correction of a congenital abnormality, and reconstruction after mastectomy.

Silicone implants still may be used for secondary procedures such as revision after the removal of an implant, correction of a congenital abnormality, and reconstruction after mastectomy.

Comparison of saline and silicone implants demonstrates the advantages and disadvantages of each type (Table 15-1). Both types are available in various sizes. However, saline implant volume is adjustable, making it possible to insert these prostheses through a smaller incision. Silicone implants come in fixed sizes. Both types of prostheses are available in different shapes (e.g., round versus teardrop) and shell surface textures (e.g., rough versus smooth). Teardrop-shaped implants usually are reserved for augmentation in the setting of breast reconstruction. Textured implants were developed in an effort to decrease capsule formation around the implant shell, thus reducing the likelihood of capsular contracture. Although it may be delayed, capsular contracture occurs even with textured implants. Textured saline implants may be more prone to develop ripples than are smooth saline implants,[1,4] making smooth implants a better choice in very thin patients. Overfilling of the implant has been shown to decrease ripple formation.[4] Some patients prefer silicone to saline implants because they feel more "natural" and are less likely to ripple.

Spontaneous rupture occurs with both saline and silicone implants and usually indicates implant replacement.

Spontaneous rupture can occur with either type of implant, but deflation is much more common with saline prostheses. Overfilling of saline implants has been proposed to decrease the likelihood of spontaneous deflation,[1] but this practice has

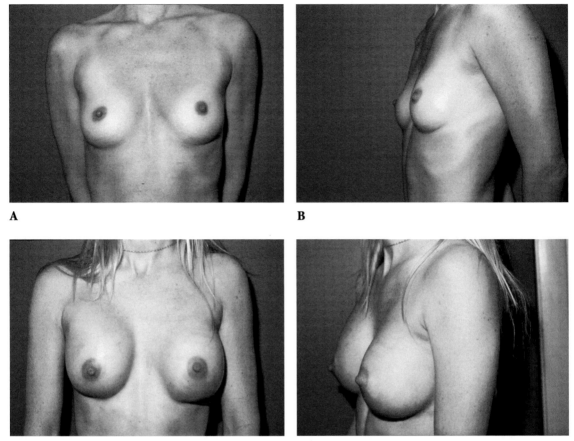

A   **B**

C   **D**

FIGURE 15-1 *A* and *B.* Preoperative appearance of a young woman requesting augmentation. *C* and *D.* Postoperative appearance after subpectoral placement of saline implants (approximately 250 mL) via an inframammary incision. (Courtesy of Hollis Caffee, MD, Professor and Chief, Department of Plastic and Reconstructive Surgery, University of Florida College of Medicine.)

TABLE 15-1   COMPARISON OF SILICONE AND SALINE IMPLANTS

	SILICONE	**SALINE**
Volume	Fixed	Adjustable
Shape	Round or teardrop	Round or teardrop
Texture	Smooth or rough	Smooth or rough
Ripples	Rare	Common
Spontaneous rupture	Less common	More common

not been convincingly effective.[4] The saline released during implant deflation is reabsorbed rapidly. Silicone, by contrast, is not degraded. It has been found in sites distant from the breast even when a silicone-filled implant appears intact. Rupture is described as intra- or extracapsular, depending on whether the extruded silicone is confined by the implant-related capsule (as is discussed below). The FDA considers any rupture to represent device failure and recommends implant removal, with or without replacement, whenever rupture occurs. Some surgeons believe that revision is not absolutely required for asymptomatic patients with an intracapsular rupture. If conservative follow-up is offered, the patient should be advised that few data are available concerning the possible effects of disseminated silicone. Complete removal of extruded silicone liquid or gel at the time of reoperation can be difficult, especially with an extracapsular rupture.

The immediate postoperative complications associated with breast augmentation are uncommon and include hematoma formation and wound infection (Table 15-2). Hematoma formation occurs with approximately 1 percent of implants[1] when meticulous attention is given to hemostasis during surgery. To prevent infectious complications, intravenous antibiotics are administered before breast augmentation. Some surgeons also instill antibiotics within the lumen of saline implants and/or within the implant pocket.

Later complications include asymmetry, spontaneous deflation or rupture, implant migration, loss of skin or nipple sensation, and capsular contracture (Table 15-2). Patients with marked asymmetry before augmentation are more likely to accept asymmetry postoperatively, and adequate counseling helps prevent patient dissatisfaction. Spontaneous deflation of saline implants has been reported to occur in 2 to 76 percent of patients.[1,4,5] Patients may prefer silicone to saline implants because they are less likely to rupture spontaneously. However, as was mentioned above, when rupture of a silicone implant occurs, the extruded silicone can be difficult to remove.

Patients may be reluctant to undergo mammographic screening because of concern that the compression will cause implant rupture. Mammography is unlikely to

TABLE 15-2 COMPLICATIONS OF MAMMAPLASTY PROCEDURES

PROCEDURE	COMPLICATIONS
AUGMENTATION	
Immediate	Hematoma, wound infection
Late	Asymmetry, rupture, migration, diminished sensation, contracture
BREAST RECONSTRUCTION	
With implant	Same as above
With flap	Fat necrosis, hematoma, infection, prolonged healing, donor site problems
With latissimus flap	Large scars, rarely shoulder weakness
With TRAM flap	Abdominal weakness, hernia, large scars
REDUCTION	
Immediate	Hematoma, wound infection
Late	Hypertrophic scarring, asymmetry, nipple necrosis, or diminished sensation

cause rupture of an intact implant. However, mammography may accelerate the deflation of a leaking implant or force silicone out of the intracapsular space once rupture has occurred.

Cephalad migration of implants occasionally occurs with subpectoral implants placed through axillary incisions. To prevent such movement, the patient may be instructed to wear an adjustable strap across the upper pole of the breasts for up to 6 weeks.[1] Loss of skin or nipple sensation can occur with periareolar incisions and with nipple or areola revision.

After the placement of any foreign material within the breast, a specialized scar, or capsule, forms. This scar develops to reduce surface friction between the implant shell and the breast tissue and is similar to synovium (see Chap. 14). A variable amount of myofibroblastic infiltration of the capsule occurs in response to inflammation from hematoma formation, infection, trauma, silicone, or other, undetermined causes.[6] The resultant capsular contracture changes the shape and firmness of the augmented breast. Contracture with subpectoral implants pushes them superiorly and causes a more convex shape in the upper pole.[1] With subglandular implants, contracture does not change the position of the implants, but a shelflike deformity is seen.[1] Some surgeons advocate frequent massage of the implanted breast to help prevent contracture. When it occurs, contracture can be painful. Closed capsulotomy is the first step in the treatment of capsular contracture. With this procedure, manual application of local pressure is used to break the connective tissue bands. This technique fails more commonly with submuscular implants, and open capsulotomy may be necessary. Careful incision of the capsule at many sites is required to relieve constriction of the implant shell.

Explantation with or without secondary reimplantation is an alternative for the correction of recurrent capsular contracture, implant rupture, or substantial asymmetry. Both the implant and its capsule are removed at the time of revision. Either silicone or saline prostheses may be selected for reimplantation, and the location of the implant often is changed. Implant removal without replacement sometimes yields an adverse aesthetic outcome. However, concurrent mastopexy in these patients may improve the final result considerably.[7]

Women who become pregnant after augmentation mammaplasty should be counseled that breast-feeding is still a desirable option. These patients often harbor concerns that nursing will alter the cosmetic appearance of the breasts. Little information about this issue has been collected.

Breast-feeding is still possible after augmentation mammaplasty.

The number of women who experience complications of breast augmentation is difficult to assess because patients who seek revision of their implants often choose a new surgeon.[2] Even though up to 30 percent of patients seek surgical correction of contractures or asymmetry, over 90 percent of patients who undergo augmentation mammaplasty are satisfied with their decision.[1,2,4]

BREAST RECONSTRUCTION AFTER MASTECTOMY

Surgical treatment of breast cancer may include subcutaneous mastectomy, breast conservation therapy (i.e., lumpectomy plus radiation therapy), or modified radical mastectomy. The options appropriate for an individual patient depend on the extent of disease (see Chaps. 7 and 8) as well as the patient's personal preference. Factors that enter into a woman's decision-making process include how much her breasts contribute to her overall body image and self-esteem, the degree to which she wishes to prevent local recurrence, and how she feels about wearing an external prosthesis.

Because this society places a great deal of emphasis on the breast as a symbol of femininity and sensuality, some women with invasive breast cancer feel strongly that they should retain as much breast tissue as is safely feasible. For them, breast conservation therapy is preferred to modified radical mastectomy with reconstruction. By contrast, the possibility of local recurrence may be so loathsome that a woman prefers extirpative surgery. If reconstruction is chosen, it may be performed at the time of mastectomy or after initial healing has occurred. Extensive preoperative counseling, including input from a plastic surgeon, will allow the formulation of the most agreeable plan. External prosthetic devices worn in the brassiere are weighted and sized to match the contralateral breast. They function very well in most cases. However, they may become dislodged during activity and cannot be worn with some types of clothing. Generally, women who wear a prosthesis for some time after mastectomy and then choose to undergo reconstruction are more likely to be satisfied with the cosmetic result.[3] These women compare the aesthetics of the reconstructed breast with that of the mastectomy scar. Women who undergo immediate reconstruction tend to compare the appearance of the new breast to that of the original breast and therefore are less content. A potential reconstruction candidate should be counseled that several operations may be necessary to achieve the best final result.

When a subcutaneous, or "skin-sparing," mastectomy is performed to treat in situ cancer, a saline or silicone implant is used to replace the excised breast tissue.[6] In an effort to maintain symmetry, a smaller contralateral implant may be required. In very thin patients, insufficient skin may be present to accommodate the implant easily. Capsular contracture is more likely to occur when the implant is placed under such tension. Submuscular implantation is indicated in this situation with or without use of a tissue expander.[8] A tissue expander is an adjustable implant that contains a valve through which saline is instilled over a period of months. The patient returns to the physician's office regularly for progressive inflation of the expander. The skin stretches slowly over time, and when the expander reaches a volume approximately 30 percent greater than that desired for the permanent implant, the expander is removed.[3] The selected implant then is placed, and a more aesthetically appealing result is achieved. Currently, expanders are available that have removable instillation valves. When the skin has been stretched sufficiently, a small incision is created under local anesthesia through which the valve is removed. The expander then serves as the permanent prosthesis.

Tissue expanders help prevent capsular contracture in thin patients who have insufficient skin to cover an implant without tension.

When reconstruction follows modified radical mastectomy, the insertion of an implant may not restore symmetry sufficiently. In these cases, transfer of a myocutaneous flap has been successful. The two most commonly performed procedures are the latissimus dorsi flap and the transverse rectus abdominis myocutaneous (TRAM) flap. The latissimus dorsi flap technique involves an oval skin incision just behind the posterior axillary line. The underlying fat and muscle are elevated with the skin and tunneled beneath the axillary skin to reach the anterior chest. The flap is positioned around and overlying a prosthesis to achieve the optimal results.[8] Because an implant is present, capsular contracture necessitating reoperation can occur. A variation of this flap procedure is the latissimus dorsi "J" reconstruction, in which an additional vertical ellipse is taken to include redundant fat in the posterior axillary fold. This technique obviates the need for implant placement because a sufficient breast mound is created from the autogenous tissue. The only major drawbacks to these procedures are the scars that are created.

The TRAM flap involves a large transverse abdominal incision between the anterior superior iliac spines. The rectus muscle on one side is released from its insertion at the pubic bone, and the overlying skin and fat are transferred with the muscle to the chest. Because of the volume of transposed tissue, placement of an implant in addition to the TRAM flap is not necessary. Abdominal wall weakness and hernia formation are possible complications. With either type of flap, wound hematoma or infection, fat necrosis, and a prolonged recovery course may occur. Also, problems with healing of the donor site wound are common. Mastopexy of the contralateral breast may be required to achieve optimal symmetry. Table 15-2 lists the most commonly encountered complications of breast reconstruction surgery.

After complete healing of the reconstructed breast, attention may be turned to fashioning a nipple and an areola. Commonly, pigmented skin from the groin or medial thigh is taken as a full-thickness graft and transplanted to a deepithelialized site on the breast mound to create an areola.[3,8] Alternatively, an areola may be simulated by the placement of a tattoo. Nipple projection may be created by transplanting a portion of the contralateral nipple ("nipple sharing") or creating a subcutaneous tissue flap.[8]

BREAST REDUCTION

Patients with macromastia frequently complain of symptoms related to the size and heaviness of the breasts: neck, shoulder, and upper back pain; inframammary moniliasis; and/or skin maceration (Fig. 15-2). These women have deep indenta-

Indications for reduction mammaplasty include neck, shoulder, and upper back pain; inframammary moniliasis; and skin maceration.

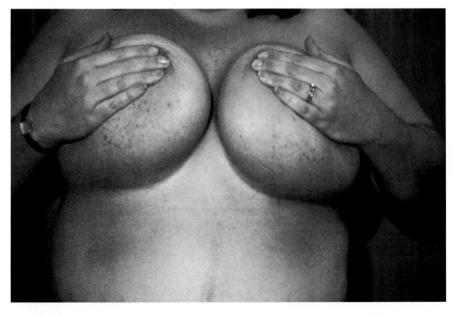

FIGURE 15-2 This patient with large breasts complained of skin changes beneath her breasts, including macerated skin and brown discoloration. (Courtesy of Hollis Caffee, MD, Professor and Chief, Department of Plastic and Reconstructive Surgery, University of Florida College of Medicine.)

tions in their shoulders from their bra straps and an exaggerated kyphosis. Less often they report embarrassment and self-conciousness as problems associated with their large breasts. They may report little or no change in breast size with overall weight loss and seek referral to a plastic surgeon for assistance. After reduction mammaplasty, these patients usually report a marked improvement in symptoms and offer enthusiastic confirmation that their decision to have surgery was correct.[9,10]

Of key importance in assuring patient satisfaction with any breast surgery is appropriate preoperative counseling. The possibility of hematoma formation, wound infection, hypertrophic scarring, nipple necrosis, marked asymmetry, and loss of nipple sensation must be described in detail before surgery is performed (Table 15-2).[9,10] Depiction of the size and location of the expected scars, using photographs

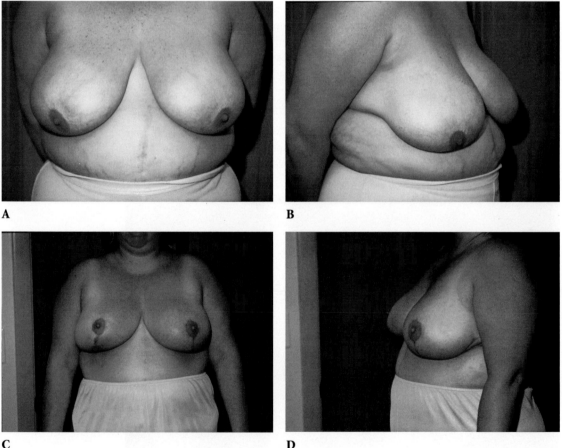

A   **B**

C   **D**

FIGURE 15-3 *A* and *B.* Preoperative appearance of a woman requesting reduction mammaplasty. Note the marked ptosis with the nipples pointing downward and nipple location well below the inframammary crease. *C* and *D.* Postoperative appearance after inverted-T-scar reduction mammaplasty. (Courtesy of Hollis Caffee, MD, Professor and Chief, Department of Plastic and Reconstructive Surgery, University of Florida College of Medicine.)

to demonstrate the typical pre- and postoperative appearance, will help the woman have realistic expectations after surgery.

The goal of surgery is to move the nipple and areola to approximately the level of the inframammary fold while excising wedges of excessive skin and breast tissue to create a new breast mound. To achieve this outcome, one of several incision types may be used. The "inverted-T-scar" technique is the one that is employed most commonly (Figs. 15-3 and 15-4).[9,10] The patient is examined while standing, and a "keyhole" incision is mapped out on her breast skin. Careful marking of the skin is crucial to obtain symmetric results. Often the areola is made smaller during the course of the procedure. The nipple–areola complex is moved cephalad either by transposition on a pedicle containing skin, fat, and breast parenchyma or as a free full-thickness graft. When it is moved using a pedicle, the nipple retains some connection with the underlying ductal system. In young women, this may be important if future childbearing and breast-feeding are desired.[11] When it is moved as a free graft, the nipple is severed from all ductal connections and successful lactation is not possible. This technique is considered best for the reduction of extremely large breasts. Unfortunately, loss of sensation, nipple projection, and some pigmentation of the nipple–areolar skin then occurs. When a pedicle flap is used, the connection may be inferior, central, or superior, depending on the preference and experience of the surgeon. Possible benefits of the superior pedicle approach are improved long-term projection of the breast and operative efficiency.[9,10]

Another method of reduction mammaplasty is the "vertical-scar reduction" technique.[12] This more recently described procedure involves skin excision in only one

The inverted-T-scar technique is the most frequently performed breast reduction procedure.

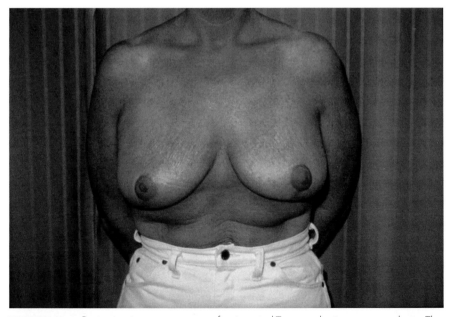

FIGURE 15-4 Postoperative appearance after inverted-T-scar reduction mammaplasty. The scar is barely visible in this photograph but will fade even more with time. (Courtesy of Hollis Caffee, MD, Professor and Chief, Department of Plastic and Reconstructive Surgery, University of Florida College of Medicine.)

direction, resulting in a smaller scar. Although it is quicker to perform and can yield excellent aesthetic results, this technique is less precise and more dependent on the surgeon's intuition and expertise. Also, it is best suited to patients who require only moderate reduction.[12]

Reduction mammaplasty is covered under most insurance plans. However, some plans require detailed documentation of preoperative symptoms accompanied by photographs demonstrating breast size, shoulder furrows, and/or skin maceration.[13] A minimum weight of excised breast tissue also may be required to meet the criteria for "indicated" instead of "cosmetic" surgery.[13]

REFERENCES

1. Hidalgo DA. Breast augmentation: Choosing the optimal incision, implant, and pocket plane. *Plast Reconstr Surg* 2000; 105(6):2202–2216.
2. Cunningham BL, Lokey A, Gutowski KA. Saline-filled breast implant safety and efficacy: A multicenter retrospective review. *Plast Reconstr Surg* 2000; 105(6):2143–2149.
3. McInnis WD. Plastic surgery of the breast. In: Mitchell GW, Bassett LW, eds. *The Female Breast and Its Disorders.* Baltimore: Williams & Wilkins; 1990:196–217.
4. Cocke WM. A critical review of augmentation mammaplasty with saline-filled prostheses. *Ann Plast Surg* 1994; 4(32):266–269.
5. Lavine DM. Saline inflatable prostheses: 14 years' experience. *Aesthetic Plast Surg* 1993; 17:325.
6. Wood RJ, Jurkiewicz MJ. Plastic and reconstructive surgery. In: Schwartz SI, Shires GT, Spencer FC, et al, eds. *Principles of Surgery,* 7th ed. New York: McGraw-Hill; 1999: 2129–2134.
7. Netscher DT, Sharma S, Thornby J, et al. Aesthetic outcome of breast implant removal in 85 consecutive patients. *Plast Reconstr Surg* 1997; 100(1):206–219.
8. Wickman M. Breast reconstruction—past achievements, current status and future goals. *Scand J Plast Reconstr Surg Hand Surg* 1995; 29:81–100.
9. Short KK, Ringler SL, Bengston BP, et al. Reduction mammaplasty: A safe and effective outpatient procedure. *Aesthetic Plast Surg* 1996; 20(6):513–518.
10. Hidalgo DA, Elliot LF, Palumbo S, et al. Current trends in breast reduction. *Plast Reconstr Surg* 1999; 104(3):806–815.
11. Brzozowski D, Niessen M, Evans HB, Hurst LN. Breast-feeding after inferior pedicle reduction mammaplasty. *Plast Reconstr Surg* 2000; 105(2):530–534.
12. Riascos A. Vertical mammaplasty for reduction. *Aesthetic Plast Surg* 1999; 23(3):213–217.
13. Seitchik MW. Reduction mammaplasty: Criteria for insurance coverage. *Plast Reconstr Surg* 1995; 95(6):1029–1032.

SUGGESTED READING

Berger K, Bostwick J. *What Women Want to Know about Breast Implants.* St. Louis: Quality Medical Publishing; 1998.

Bruning N. *Breast Implants—Everything You Need to Know.* Alameda, CA: Hunter House; 1992.

McCraw JB, Cramer AR, Horton CE. Breast reconstruction following mastectomy. In: Bland KI, Copeland EM, eds. *The Breast.* Philadelphia: Saunders; 1991:656–693.

INDEX

NOTE: Page numbers in italics indicate figures; those followed by *t* refer to tables.

A

Abscesses, 31–32, *32, 33*
   mammographic appearance of, 167, *169*
   during pregnancy, 94*t*
AC regimen
   for early breast cancer, 83
   for metastatic breast cancer, 91
   for stage IIIA breast cancer, 90
   for stage IIIB breast cancer, 90
Adenomas. *See also* Fibroadenomas
   lactating
      mammographic appearance of, 158
      during pregnancy, 94
   microadenomas, surveillance of prolactin levels with,
      69
   tubular, mammographic appearance of, 158, *159*
Adenosis, 35, *36*
   sclerosing, 25, *26*
Advanced breast cancer. *See* Late breast cancer
Age
   as cancer risk factor, 20–21
   at first term birth, breast cancer risk related to, 23
   postoperative radiotherapy for early invasive breast
      cancer and, 80–81
Alcohol intake, as cancer risk factor, 24

American Cancer Society (ACS), mammographic
      screening guidelines of, 126
American College of Radiography (ACR),
      mammographic screening guidelines of, 126
Aminoglutethimide, for male breast cancer, 122
Ampullae, *2, 3*
Anatomy, 1, *2, 3, 4*
Androgens, for male breast cancer, 122
Antibiotics
   for mastitis, postpartum, 31
   prophylactic, for breast augmentation, 220
Areola
   anatomy of, 1
   yeast infections of, 114, *115*
Arthritis, breast implants and, 214
Asymmetric density, on mammograms, 41, *41*
Axillary lymph node dissection
   for early breast cancer, 81–82
   for male breast cancer, 122
Axillary tail of Spence, 1

B

Biopsy
   core, 47, *48,* 49, 140–143, *141, 142,* 146–147
      advantage over fine-needle aspiration, 142

ISBN 0-8385-0514-7

Mozart

Mozart

RICHARD BAKER

Macdonald

I would like to express my gratitude to Timothy Joss for his far-reaching research assistance and to Margaret Dowson who deciphered my manuscript and typed it perfectly.

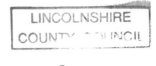
A Macdonald Book

First published in Great Britain by
Thames & Hudson Ltd, 1982
This revised edition published by
Macdonald & Co (Publishers) Ltd, London & Sydney, 1991

Jacket and book designed by Vaughan Allen

ISBN 0 356 19695 X

Typeset in Scantext Baskerville by Leaper & Gard Ltd, Bristol
Printed and bound in Great Britain by
BPCC Hazell Books
Aylesbury, Bucks, England
Member of BPCC Ltd.

Macdonald & Co (Publishers) Ltd
Orbit House
1 New Fetter Lane
London EC4A 1AR
A member of Maxwell Macmillan Pergamon Publishing Corporation

CONTENTS

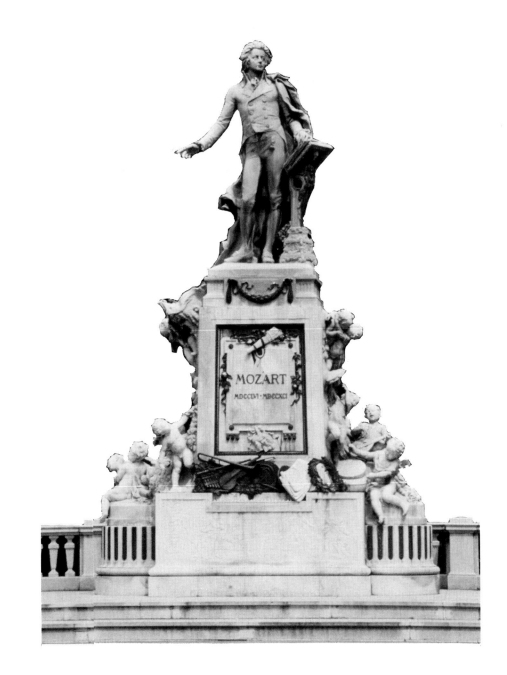

FOREWORD

*I*n every age, to a greater or lesser extent, the paymaster has called the piper's tune and musicians have always had to please someone if they are not to starve. Nowadays state agencies and civic authorities, benevolent trusts and commercial firms have taken over from wealthy individuals as patrons of music. Such organisations, given a glimmer of sense, can often show a remarkably tolerant face to experiment; indeed, the more avant-garde the opus, the more credit the patron will hope to gain for far-sighted disinterest.

It was not always so. Those who kept Handel and Haydn alive were not prepared to wait for posterity's judgment; they wanted to be pleased as instantly by the music as by their food and tended to judge both by much the same criteria. Novelty? Well, just a *soupçon* perhaps, but not too much and not too often.

Of course there were liberal patrons. But even the best of them demanded an attachment which could seem like slavery to an artist of spirit. Mozart was such an artist. He rebelled against the respectable chains his father had learned to wear. Yet for most of his life – such were the conditions prevailing at the time – he was searching for a steady appointment at court which would spare him the anxieties of a freelance existence.

Beethoven was Mozart's junior by only fourteen years, but he belonged to a different age. The irreverence which Mozart generally confined to private letters erupted in Beethoven's open refusal to doff his hat to authority; the revolutionary spirit was abroad, and the Romantic tide was starting to flood, bringing with it the cult of the individual. Though Mozart bridled at the old system, he had to live with it, and that included working within the established musical language of the day. No furious smashing of piano-fortes for him, no bursting the barriers of symphonic form with choral finales. Instead, a disciplined approach which kept the strongest emotions within the context of musical good manners. 'The passions, whether violent or not,' wrote Mozart on the subject of opera, 'should never be so expressed as to reach the point of causing disgust; and music, even in situations of the greatest horror, should never be painful to the ear but should flatter and charm it and thereby always remain music.'

To make conscious use of music as a vehicle for conveying the composer's own feelings in the fashion of Berlioz or Tchaikovsky would have been even more unthinkable in Mozart's time. There was then a European fraternity of creative musicians who drew on a common melodic tradition; no great store was set on originality and indeed one musicologist has estimated that 80 per cent of Mozart's tunes occurred also in the music of his con-temporaries.* Gradually this fraternal spirit was eroded, giving way to a competitiveness which demanded marked individual styles, almost a kind of brand warfare. Composers in Mozart's day experienced none of the anguish of 'finding their own voice' which besets serious composers of the twentieth century. Such atomisation simply did not exist, for the composer was merely required

---

*B. Szabolcsi: 'Folk Music – Art Music – History of Music', *Studia Musicologica* (Budapest), vii (1965), 171–9.

to produce to order a certain quantity of an established commodity.

Yet for many people Mozart is the greatest of composers. No words can do justice to his simplicity or his sublimity; he is, like Shakespeare, ageless. But for all his transcendent genius, it is helpful to see him too as a child of his time. The power of Mozart was after all generated by an eighteenth-century dam.

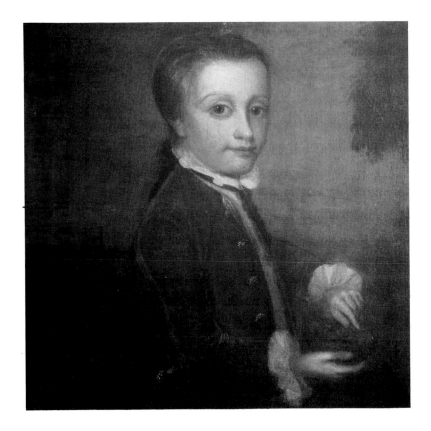

CHAPTER   ONE

THE WORLD MOZART
ENTERED

A modern visitor aware of the grace of Mozart's music
may well be surprised by the solid grandeur of his
native city. The great Cathedral of St Rupert, dedicated with a week of celebration in 1628, has a massive
dignity not always associated with the Baroque; the towers
and spires and courtyards are on a splendid scale, and the
Archbishop's Palace, which occupies a large area in the
centre of the old city, is fit for a monarch. Appropriately,
since the Prince-Archbishops of Salzburg had exercised
temporal as well as spiritual sway over the city and district
since Bishop Rupert was sent there as a missionary in the
year 696.

The city, like Edinburgh, is dominated by a medieval
castle, the Hohensalzburg, and a hilly ridge runs from the
fortress along the southern edge of the city to the Mönchs-
berg. In ancient days this no doubt formed an admirable
defensive feature, but it also had the effect of compressing a
mini-metropolis into a small space bounded on its northern
flank by the River Salzach. Archbishop Wolf Dietrich, who
inaugurated the building of the Cathedral and the Palace,
extended the city across the river by building what is now
the Mirabell Palace on the other side for his mistress; but

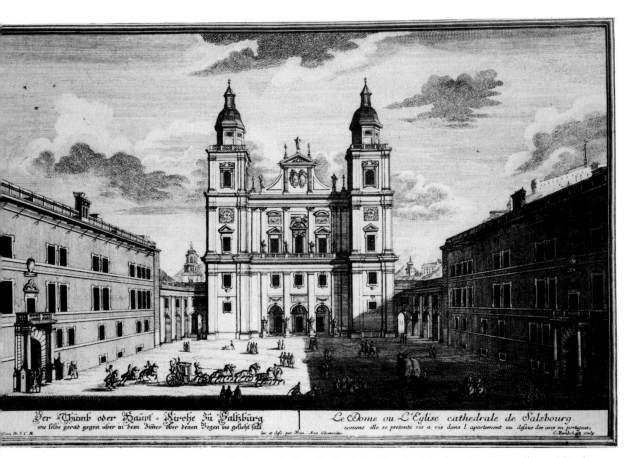

In Mozart's day, the Catholic Church wielded temporal as well as spiritual power in many parts of Europe. The grandeur of Salzburg Cathedral (above), built in the early 17th century, reflects the central importance of religious institutions at that time.

for all its spreading growth, then and later, there is still something claustrophobic about Salzburg.

Or is that feeling merely inspired by the knowledge that Mozart was eager to leave the place?

He was born at a time when conditions were changing for the musician. His father Leopold, an able man who graduated with distinction from a Jesuit school in Augsburg and continued a good all-round education at Salzburg University before abandoning his general studies in favour of music, settled for what was still the most frequent employment for musicians – a permanent post in a noble household. He served five successive Prince-Archbishops of Salzburg for a total of forty years, never quite achieving the coveted title of Kapellmeister, Master of the Music. But his conditions of service did not prevent him publishing, in 1756, the year of his famous son's birth, a 'Violin School' which achieved an international reputation and is still studied today. Leopold was very well aware that a world existed outside Salzburg and was almost too eager that his son should succeed in it.

A number of eighteenth-century composers managed to break away from their aristocratic patrons and make their own terms with the musical public. This was partly because a new middle-class audience was growing up. Subscription concerts had begun in large cities like London, Hamburg and Paris, where the famous Concert Spirituel was established in 1725; numerous music societies were being formed, musical periodicals started to appear in the early years of the century and publishers like Haydn's Artaria were beginning to assert an influence which was to become dominant in later times.

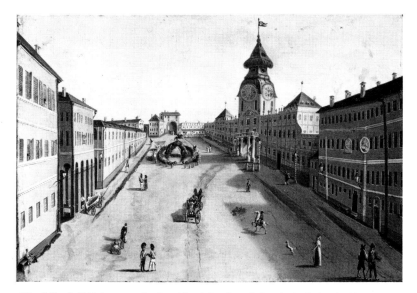

The Mirabell Palace, on the far side of the river Salzach, built by Archbishop Wolf Dietrich for his mistress.

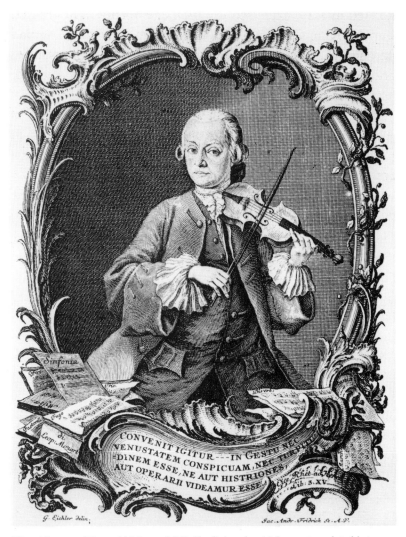

The titlepage of Leopold Mozart's Violin School *which was translated into several different languages and earned him international acclaim.*

Various opportunities, then, were presented to the musician in the mid-eighteenth century. In his early years Handel made a living as an organist in Halle, produced his first operas in Italy with the help of aristocratic patrons, and became briefly Kapellmeister to the Elector of Hanover. Then he decamped to London where he entered into contracts with theatres, continued to produce works for the stage under the auspices of the Royal Academy of Music, formed in 1719, exercised the privilege of copyright granted him by King George I in 1720 and, apart from a few bad patches, made enough money to give charity performances and become a regular subscriber to the Musicians' Benevolent Fund from its inception in 1738.

Bach, after a spell as Kapellmeister to Prince Leopold of Anhalt-Cöthen, became Cantor of St Thomas's School in Leipzig and spent the rest of his life as a city council employee. He was required to inform the Burgomaster if he wished to leave Leipzig and had to promise not to make church music 'too long or too operatic', but he was able to enhance his modest salary with various 'perks' and to extend his scope by working for the University and directing the Telemann Singing Society. This was a 'collegium musicum', another increasingly popular means of taking music outside the precincts of church and castle.

Haydn in his late twenties entered the service of the Esterházy family, becoming Kapellmeister in 1766. Though he intensely disliked the isolation of Prince Nicolaus' country estate at Esterháza, where the musicians had to spend much of their time, it was there that Haydn produced some of his finest and most inventive music. His meeting with the publisher Artaria took place in 1780, after which date his Esterházy contract allowed him to travel and to promote his compositions as he wished. 'The free arts and the beautiful art of composition', wrote Haydn in 1778, 'tolerate no shackling. The spirit and the soul must be free if one would gather one's deserts.' Haydn fortunately lived long enough to reap an appropriate reward. In 1790 he retired from service to the Esterházy family with a pension which was subsequently increased in stages, made his immensely successful journeys to London and settled in Vienna where he lived in old age, having learned how to preserve his economic independence. (But long before leaving his aristocratic patrons, they had rewarded him with marks of high esteem, none apparently more telling than Prince Esterházy's order to the wine superintendent 'to deliver one quart of officers' wine' to Haydn daily).

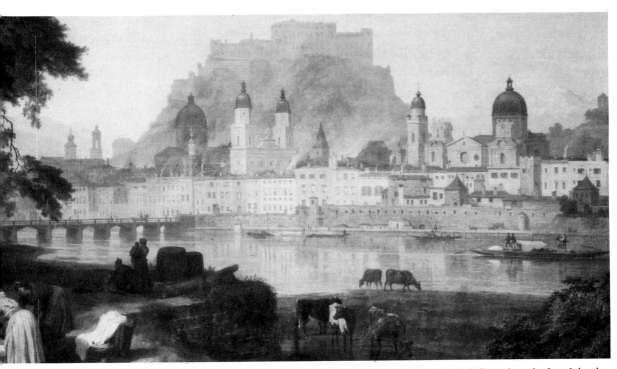

The city of Salzburg is hemmed in on three sides by hills and on the fourth by the river Salzach. The medieval castle, perched high on an outcrop of rock, dominates the city.

Mozart's forerunner in restoring truth and dignity to the musical stage, Christoph Willibald Gluck, married a rich woman, which has always been one way to balance a budget. He too worked for a variety of employers, from princely households to the management of the Paris Opera. His last years brought disappointment and ill-health, but he rode out daily in his own carriage from a fine house in Vienna, where he was highly respected as a leading practitioner of the craft of music.

In the more limited community of Salzburg, Leopold Mozart, a reserved man conscious of his status and not given to indiscriminate friendship with his musical colleagues, considered himself the equal of successful merchants and other professional people. Thus he established friendly relations with, among others, the families of the Court Surgeon Andreas Gilowsky, the Chancellor Franz von Mölk, the Prince's personal physician Dr Silvester Barisani and Georg Josef Robinig, a hardware dealer and Barisani's landlord.

As an educated man whose subjects of study had included Dialectics and Physics, Leopold would have been open to the prevailing mood of 'the age of enlightenment', with its rational critique of all feudal institutions, its belief in social and political rights and in progress towards a more equitable society. The untrammelled human mind was to be the arbiter of truth, including the doctrines of religion, and a scientific, objective approach was called for in the study of music as of other matters. Johann Adolf Scheibe, who is chiefly remembered as the author of an attack on Bach, the last great master of abstract polyphony, defined the appropriate attitude of a mid-century composer thus: 'Musicians must think naturally and possess enlightened reason ... reasonable thinking and knowledge of the science of beauty create good taste in music.'

There was another force acting upon the Mozarts, father and son, which encouraged a rational, egalitarian approach to life and art. Freemasonry was established in Germany in the 1720s and spread rapidly among the bourgeoisie, though its influence was widespread too in aristocratic circles and even among the clergy, in spite of Pope Clement XII's edict of 1738 forbidding Catholics to join. Particularly strong in south Germany and Austria were the Masonic adherents known as 'Illuminati', whose aims were strongly ethical in character. Adam Weishaupt, their founder, went so far as to declare that 'Accumulated property is an insurmountable obstacle to the happiness of any nation', while a general Masonic aim was to 'combat superstition and fanaticism in the persons of the monkish orders, the main supporters of both these evils', who were, it was alleged, possessed of 'a superfluity of goods'. Freemasonry was naturally regarded with a suspicion which often amounted to outright hostility by many church and state authorities, among them the ecclesiastical principality of Salzburg.

There the Illuminati met by night in a lonely grotto at nearby Aigen, now known as the 'Illuminaten-Höhle'. Mozart attended some of these meetings, giving rise to the supposition that he may have been an Illuminatus. Certainly, both he and his father became Freemasons, a move which bore fruit in a number of works, above all *The Magic Flute*, whose story reflects Masonic rituals. In the later years of the eighteenth century, when democratic ideas exploded in the violence of the French Revolution, Freemasonry together with other 'enlightened' notions sharply lost favour in Austrian ruling circles, but at the time when Leopold Mozart entered court service at Salzburg, even the Prince himself, Baron Leopold Firmian, was suspected of Freemasonry (though it is difficult to see how this could be reconciled with his expulsion of 20,000 Protestants).

Firmian's successor, Count Jakob Ernst, was much given to entertainment, as was the man who followed him as Prince-Archbishop, Count Andreas Dietrichstein. Count Sigismund Schrattenbach, who took office in 1753, was a

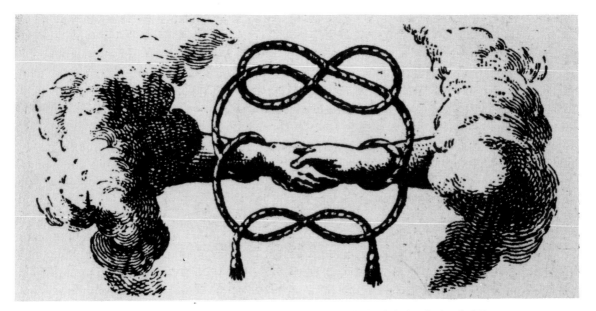

This image of clasped hands, symbolic of the brotherhood of Freemasonry, was printed on copies of a song which formed part of the closing ritual of the Viennese Masonic Lodge Zur gekronten Hoffnung *(Crowned Hope). It was for this lodge that Mozart composed the Masonic cantata (K623).*

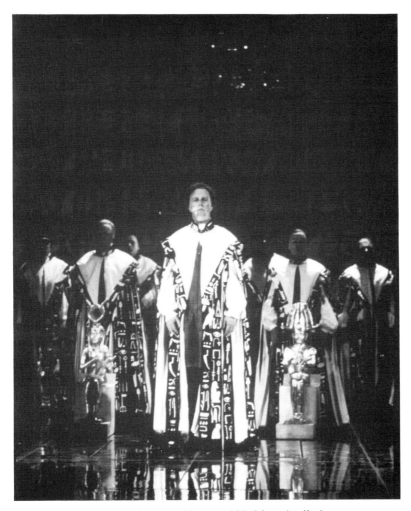

*Mozart wrote a number of works which reveal his Masonic allegiance,
pre-eminently* The Magic Flute *(K620). This scene from the 1988 production
by the English National Opera shows Sarastro and the brotherhood.*

reformer who set about raising the moral tone in Salzburg,
but fortunately for the Mozarts he was fond of music and
treated them with easy-going indulgence.

Mozart's sister Maria Anna ('Nannerl'), who was born in
July 1751 and outlived her brother by nearly forty years,
listed in her memoirs the number of musicians in the
employ of the Salzburg court. Apart from the Kapellmeister
and his deputy there were five violinists, two cellists, one

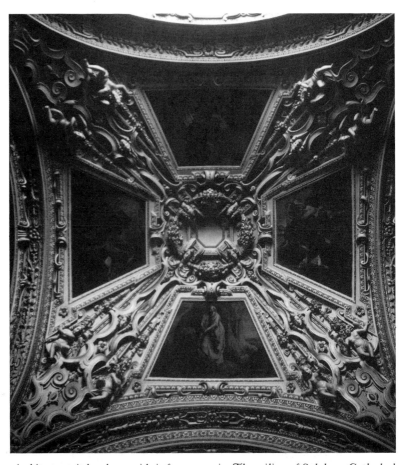

Architecture, it has been said, is frozen music. The ceiling of Salzburg Cathedral echoes the balance between decoration and classical symmetry which is also to be found in the compositions of baroque composers.

viola player, two bassoonists, three horn players, three oboists, three flautists, one trumpeter and two organists – a chamber orchestra of moderate size. Music for the Cathedral was always in demand, and so was background music for the dinner table, as well as music for more formal concerts and theatrical performances. Leopold Mozart, apart from his skill as a violinist, was adept, we are told, at composing works in every genre. Since music was at that time one of the chief means of entertaining and impressing state visitors, and since Leopold was allowed to write and perform for house-

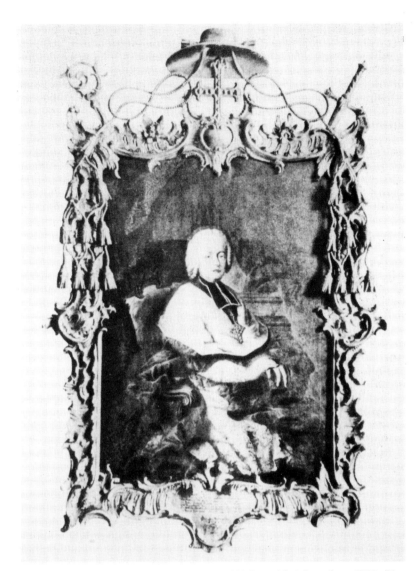

Count Sigismund Schrattenbach, Prince-Archbishop of Salzburg from 1753–71, was fond of music and proved a benevolent employer.

holds other than the Archbishop's, he was a successful and very busy man when, on 27 January 1756, his wife Anna Maria gave birth to the second of their seven children; no others survived. He was christened Joannes Chrysostomus Wolfgangus Theophilus. Theophilus in its Latin form is Amadeus, a name which means 'beloved of God'.

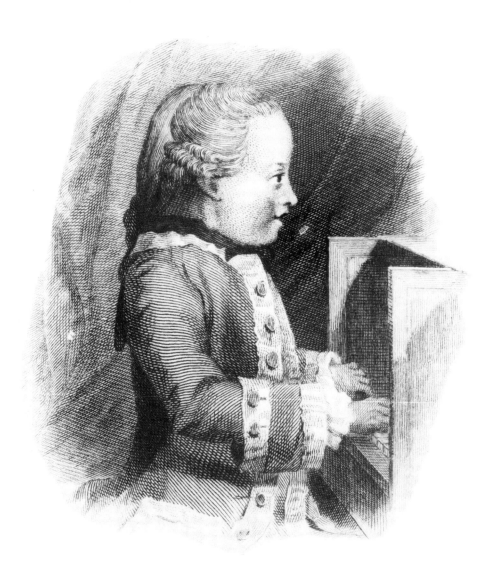

CHAPTER TWO

A PRODIGY OF NATURE
1756–71

The tourists who inspect Mozart's birthplace, No. 9 Getreidegasse, walk in droves through a solidly built town house in a narrow, traffic-free street of prosperous shops. The house, formerly No. 225 and part of an elegant square which no longer exists, was the property of Johann Lorenz Hagenauer, a wholesale grocer, who leased his third floor to the Mozarts. Their quarters were modest but comfortable and it was there, in a low-ceilinged room with a small window giving onto an inner courtyard, that the new baby was born.

Leopold lost no time in teaching his children music and in 1760 he made a note alongside the first eight pieces in Nannerl's music book that 'the preceding eight minuets were learnt by Wolfgangerl in his 4th year'. The young boy's musical talent was not surprising, for his maternal grandfather, like his father, showed much aptitude for the art. From his grandfather, too, Wolfgang inherited a love of merriment which was not conspicuously present in Leopold, and all who knew the great composer as a young boy remembered his sense of fun.

'Before he began music,' recalled Johann Andreas Schachtner, the court trumpeter, shortly after Mozart's

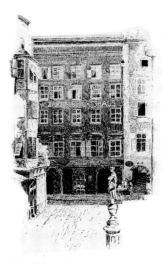

No. 9 Getreidegasse once formed part of an elegant Italianate square, the Lochelplatz, which sadly has now disappeared.

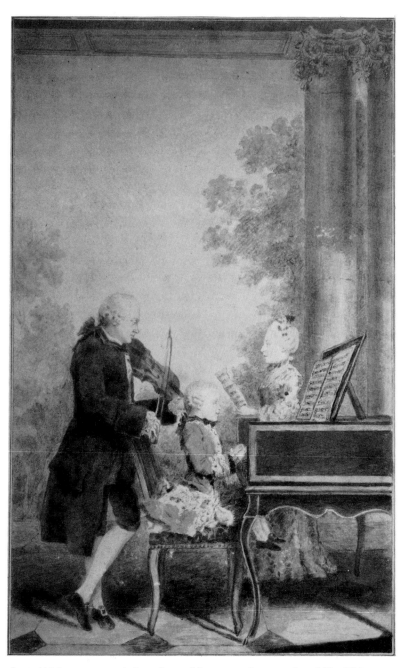

Leopold Mozart was a dedicated, possibly over-zealous, teacher of his children, both of whom showed precocious talent.

death, 'he was so ready for any prank spiced with a little humour that he could quite forget food, drink and all things else.'

The liveliness of his mind greatly impressed his sister Nannerl. 'He was desirous of learning everything he set eyes on,' she wrote in later years. 'In drawing and adding he showed much skill, but, as he was too busy with music, he could not show his talents in any other direction.' Soon, it seems, music invaded his whole life: even children's games, according to Schachtner, 'had to have a musical accompaniment if they were to interest him; if we, he and I, were carrying his playthings from one room to another, the one of us who was empty-handed always had to sing or fiddle a march the while.' Wolfgang even invented a musical bedtime ritual which, according to Nannerl, he kept up until he was ten years old: 'He composed a melody which he would sing out loud each day before going to sleep, to which end his father had to set him on a chair. Father always had to sing the second part and when this ceremony, which might on no occasion be omitted, was over, he would kiss his father most tenderly and go to bed very peacefully and contentedly.'

It is clear that Mozart loved his parents, and particularly his father, very dearly. Affectionate as he was, he required constant assurances of love from others and if anyone teased him on the subject 'bright tears welled up in his eyes, so tender and kind was his heart'. Schachtner perceived that there were dangers in a temperament so mercurial: 'He was of a fiery disposition; no object held his attention by more than a thread. I think that if he had not had the advantageously good education which he enjoyed he might have become the most wicked villain, so suscept-ible was he to every attraction, the goodness or badness of which he was not yet able to examine.' The eagerness with which the eight-year-old Mozart left the harpsichord when a favourite cat came into the room, and the facility he showed for picking up card tricks and fencing tips from visitors, when recovering from illness, though scarcely

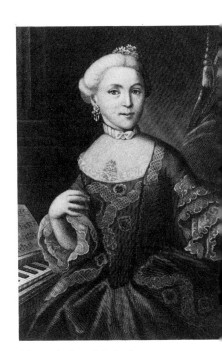

Mozart's sister Maria Anna Walburga, nicknamed Nannerl, was a sympathetic companion with a lively sense of humour.

justifying the epithet 'wicked', bear witness to a nature wide open to distraction.

An understanding of Mozart in childhood is very relevant to his later development, for in the view of his sister: 'He was, apart from his music, almost always a child, and thus he remained. This is a main feature of his character on the dark side. He always needed a father's, a mother's, or some other guardian's care: he could not manage his financial affairs.' It was this irresponsible aspect of Mozart's character, almost to the exclusion of any other, which was emphasised in the film *Amadeus* (1984), but it is impossible to believe that he was, in reality, the giggling ninny portrayed in that film. Nannerl went on to say in her memoirs that her brother married a girl quite unsuited to him, and this led to the great domestic chaos at and after his death. In fact, subsequent research indicates that Constanze was in many respects a good wife, and after Mozart's death she did all she could to promote interest in his works.

It is difficult to see how any wife could have matched the protective pride of the young Mozart's parents, from whom he inherited high intelligence but, it seems, little in the way of good looks. Leopold and Anna Maria had been known as the handsomest couple in Salzburg and Nannerl was considered a beauty. Wolfgang, however, was described by his eldest sister, for all her devotion, as 'small, thin, pale in colour and entirely lacking in any pretentions as to physiognomy and bodily appearance.'

However, there is nothing to suggest that he was unfit for the rigours of Leopold's educational regime, which embraced many subjects apart from music, and the available evidence suggests that he enjoyed his early childhood. Though severe and demanding, Leopold greeted the growing evidence of Wolfgang's altogether exceptional talent with deep emotion, as the following incident shows.

Leopold was rehearsing some trios with two favoured colleagues from the court orchestra, Wentzel and Schachtner, when Wolfgang asked to be allowed to play

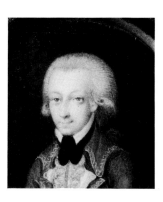

The young Mozart. His eyes have a visionary look, but the face is thin and pale. The relentless programme of exhibition performances organised by his father, and the ceaseless travel involved, adversely affected the young boy's health.

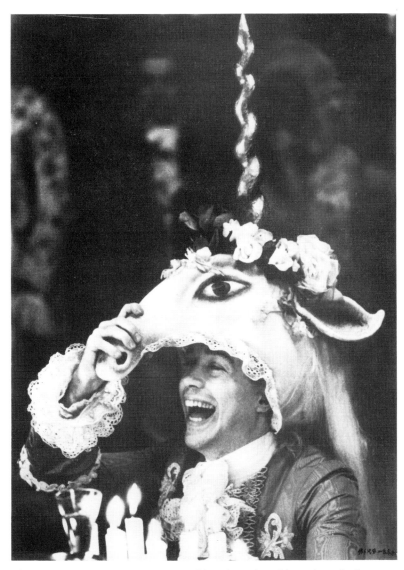

Tom Hulce in the title role of the 1984 film adaptation of Amadeus *by Peter Shaffer. Constanze Mozart commented that her husband 'was always so gay', and the composer's extrovert nature was stressed in the film.*

second violin. Leopold refused, saying that he had not yet had the least instruction in the instrument. (Though Wolfgang must have been very young at the time, this statement may not have been absolutely true because we are told the boy was holding 'a little violin' at the time of the incident and went off with it in a sulk). Schachtner thereupon suggested he should be allowed to play second violin along with him. 'Very well,' said Leopold, 'but play so softly that we can't hear you or you will have to go.' 'And so it was,' Schachtner recalled to Nannerl, 'that Wolfgang played with me. I soon noticed with astonishment that I was quite superfluous. I quietly put down my violin and looked at your papa; tears of wonder and comfort ran down his cheeks.'

In 1761, Leopold was able to write alongside an Andante and Allegro composed between February and April of that year: 'Compositions by Wolfgangerl in the first three months after his fifth birthday.' More wonder and comfort for the proud father, who was already planning to make the great world aware of his clever offspring.

It would not have occurred to Leopold that there was anything wrong about exploiting the talents of Nannerl and Wolfgang. As Henry Raynor says in his book on Mozart:* 'Childhood as something different in nature from adulthood was the discovery of the early romantic movement. Leopold never realised, any more than did anyone in the eighteenth century, that children are not simply small adults.' Accordingly he planned a series of tours which would capitalise on the fashionable interest in prodigies of nature, convincing himself that, quite apart from any economic benefit which might accrue, it was his duty to 'prove the miracle' of his son's genius to the world in an age 'when everything called a miracle is ridiculed'.

To travel at all in those days required courage and endurance almost beyond our imagination, and it seems that conditions in Germany and Austria were the worst in Europe. Both the singer Michael Kelly and the musical scholar Charles Burney complained bitterly of the extortionate levies to which they were subjected – for the hire of vehicles and horses, tolls, turnpikes and the greasing of wheels, not to mention the greasing of palms of ostlers 'who will steal any part of the luggage they can lay hold of'.

---

*Macmillan, 1978

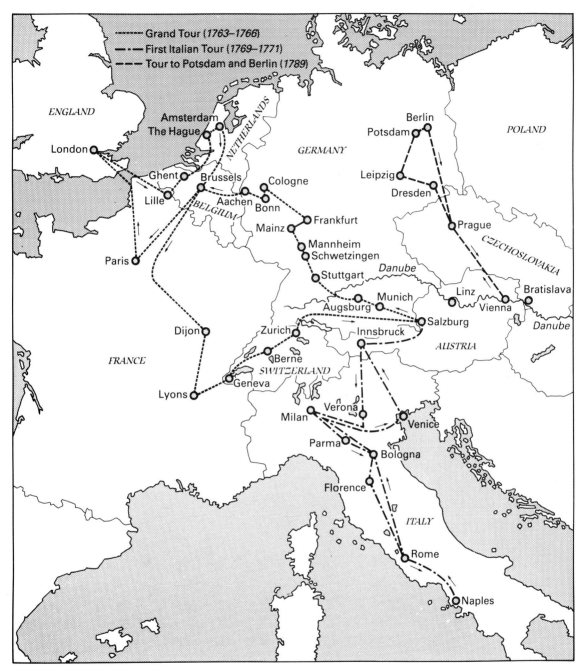

This map indicates the chief towns and cities visited by Mozart during three
important tours. The Grand Tour and first Italian tour began from Salzburg, the
German one from Vienna.

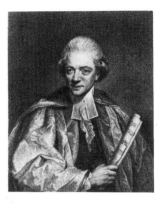

Charles Burney, the musical scholar whose writings provide an excellent insight into eighteenth-century travel.

Burney, like the Mozarts on their first journey, travelled by public conveyance and 'did not meet with a chaise or carriage that had a top or covering to protect passengers from heat, cold, wind or rain; and so violent are the jolts and so hard are the seats of German post-wagons, that a man is kicked rather than carried from one place to another'. Michael Kelly, too, recalled a horrific journey by post-wagon: 'A complete bone-setter it was! While undergoing its operations nothing could have so ably aided its torments as the unconquerable phlegm of the postillion. Whatever one suffers, whatever one says, there he sits, lord of your time.'

Germany and Austria at that time consisted of a large number of small quasi-independent states like Salzburg, so the Mozarts had a wide choice of potential markets. Leopold chose Munich, in Bavaria, as his first objective, partly because the Elector Maximilian Joseph III, who lived there, was a musician himself, and partly because the distance was not too great for what amounted to a trial run. Soon after Wolfgang's sixth birthday, the whole family set out for the Munich carnival season of 1762; few details of the visit have come down to us, but we know the Mozarts were well received and that Leopold made money.

He was sufficiently encouraged to plan a much more ambitious journey in the autumn to Vienna, then of great importance as the seat of the Imperial court and the capital of the Holy Roman Empire. There the powerful Empress Maria Theresa ruled with her consort, the Emperor Francis I; the Seven Years' War which was to establish Frederick the Great's Prussia as a strong north German counterpoise to Austria was nearing its end, and so the court was no doubt glad of entertainment and distraction – not that war in those days seems to have seriously interfered with the social round among the upper classes.

The family went first to Passau, where the important Count Thun-Hohenstein was impressed but ungenerous, and from there to Linz. Here Wolfgang gave his first public concert, in October 1762. Fortunately, as Leopold wrote to his landlord Lorenz Hagenauer, 'young Count Pálffy [nephew of the Hungarian Chancellor] happened to be passing through Linz as our concert was about to begin … he listened with astonishment and spoke later with great excitement of the performance to the Archduke Joseph, who

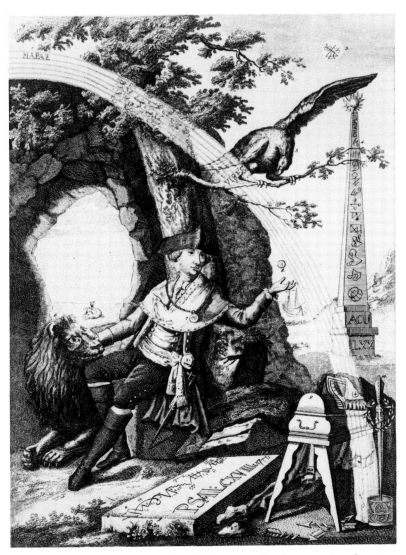

En route to Vienna, Leopold and his children stopped at Passau, where Count Thun Hohenstein expressed his admiration for their talents but kept his purse buttoned. The Count, a fellow Mason, is depicted here surrounded by Masonic symbols.

passed it on to the Empress.' So the ground was prepared for the Mozarts' reception at court.

From Linz they continued their journey by mail boat down the Danube, experiencing violent storms. Let us hope they were better protected than Charles Burney who, in the course of his European journey a few years later, travelled down the Elbe in a boat which was 'long, narrow and quite open at the top. There was straw to lie on, but nothing to cover me or my baggage ... about midnight it began to

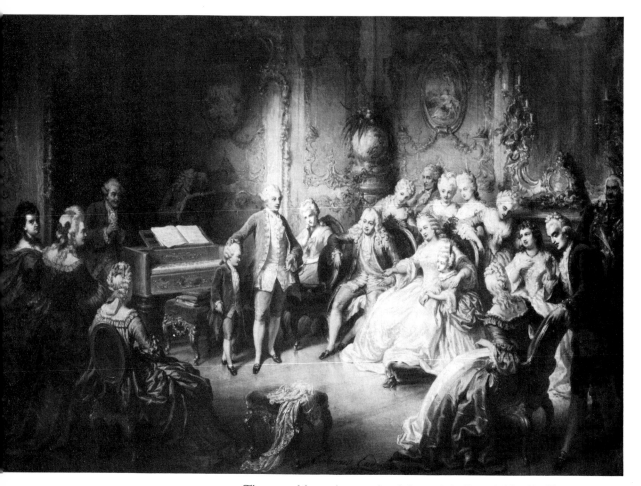

The young Mozart impressed and charmed the Imperial family. Totally uninhibited even in such grand surroundings, he gave the Empress a kiss and asked the young Marie Antoinette, later Queen of France, to marry him.

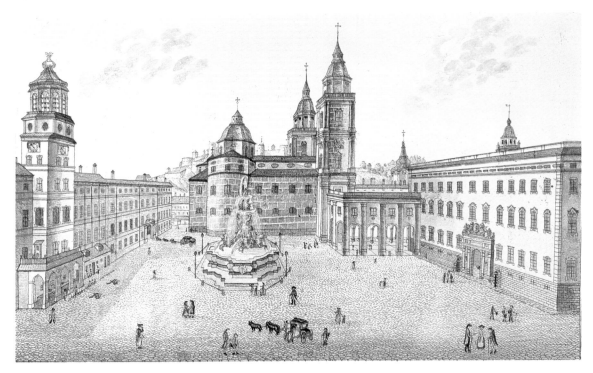

A contemporary view of the Residenzplatz, Salzburg's central square, showing (centre) the Cathedral and (right) the Archbishop's Palace, both built by Archbishop Wolf Dietrich.

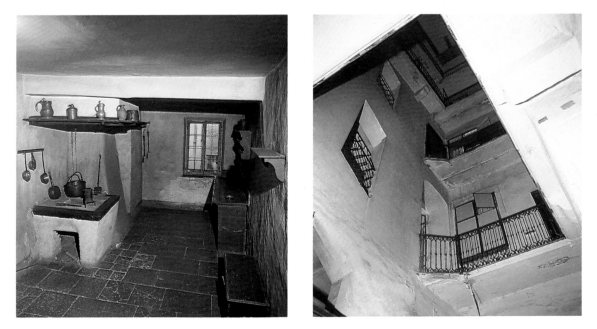

Views of the kitchen and central courtyard of the house where Mozart was born, in Salzburg's Getreidegasse: a respectable home where the family enjoyed a comfortable middle-class way of life.

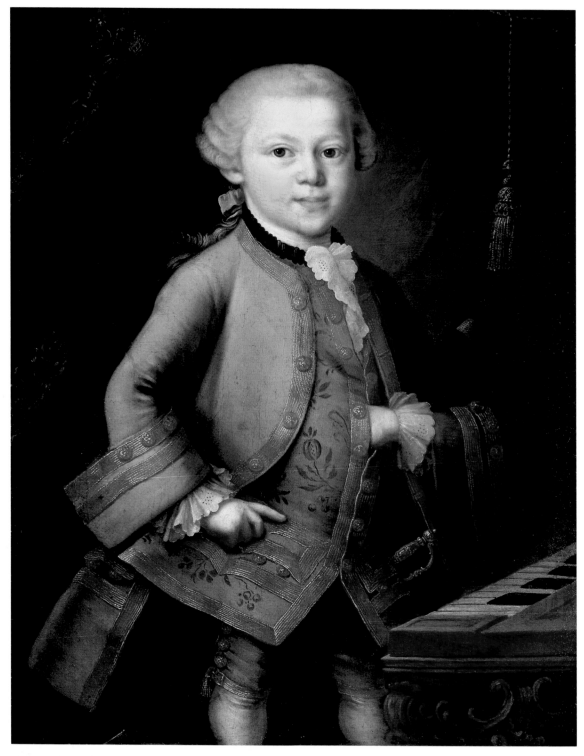

Above and opposite:
These portraits were mementos of the children's appearance together in the Viennese court in 1762. They show the gala
dress which the Empress Maria Theresa gave to Wolfgang and Nannerl to attend a public banquet.

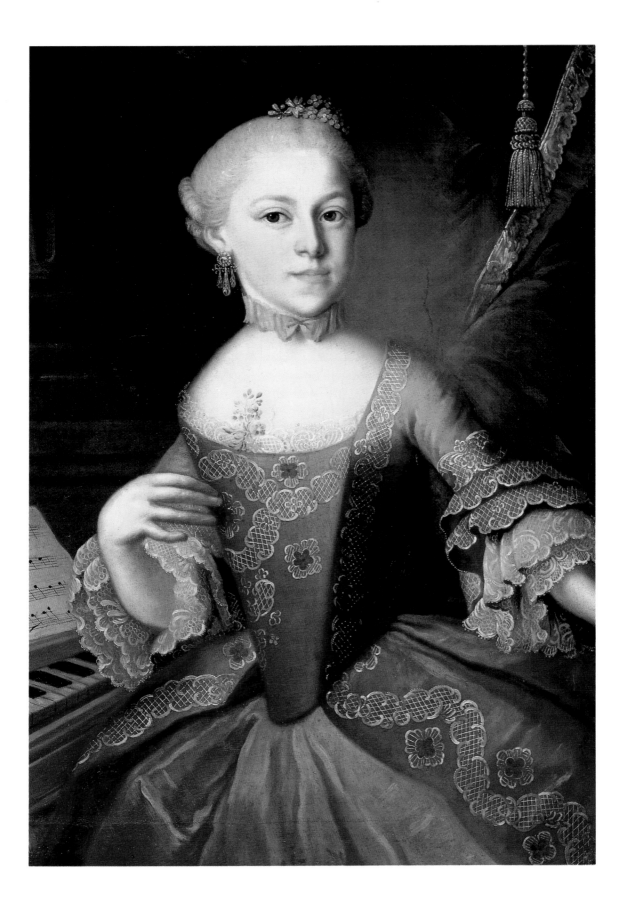

The Palace of Versailles, visited twice by the young Mozart. During his first visit in December 1763, the seven-year-old prodigy and his sister 'took almost everyone by storm'.

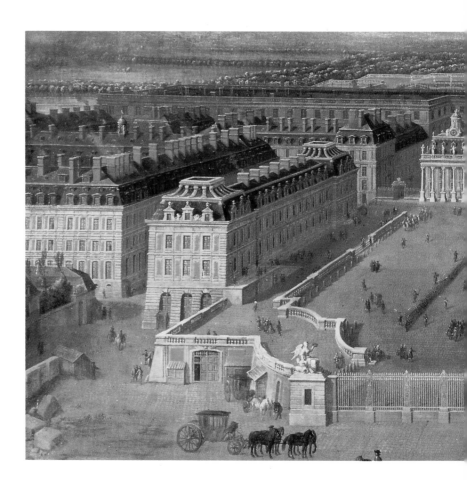

In the summer of 1766 the Mozarts returned to Versailles for three days. Here the ten-year-old Wolfgang seated at the harpsichord makes ready to accompany the singer Pierre Jélyotte in the salon of the Prince de Conti.

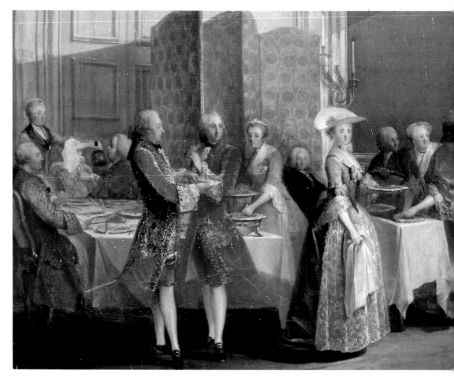

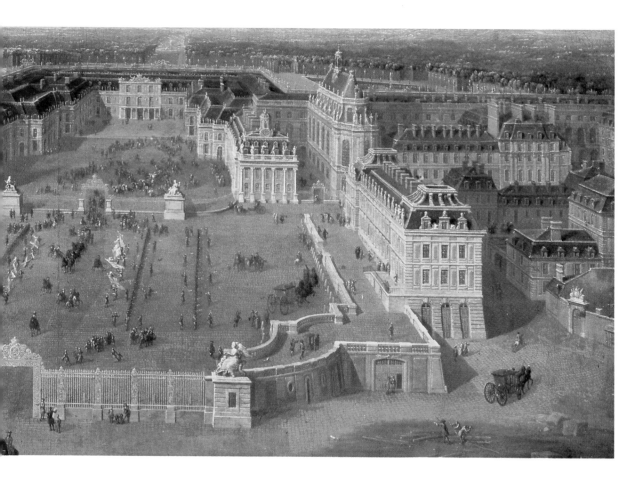

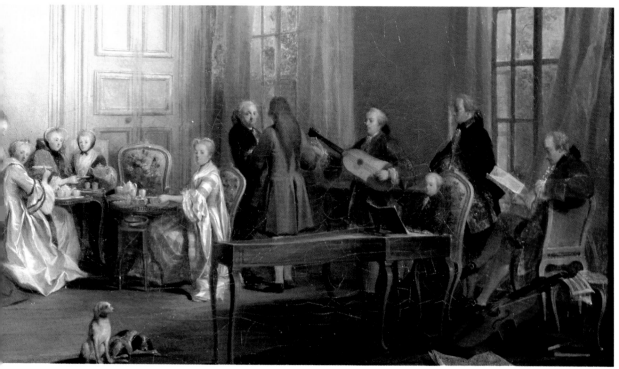

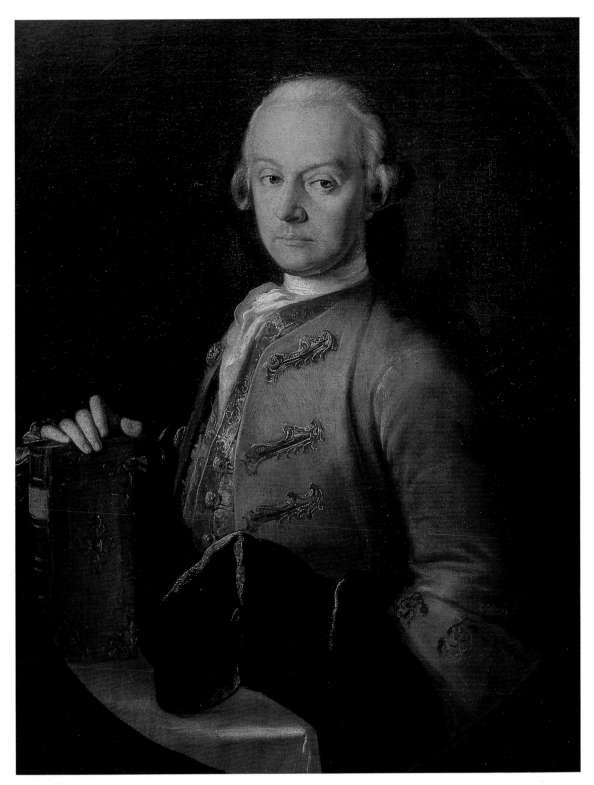

(Above) Johann Georg Leopold Mozart (1719–87) and (opposite) his wife Anna Maria Mozart (1720–78), 'the handsomest couple in Salzburg'.

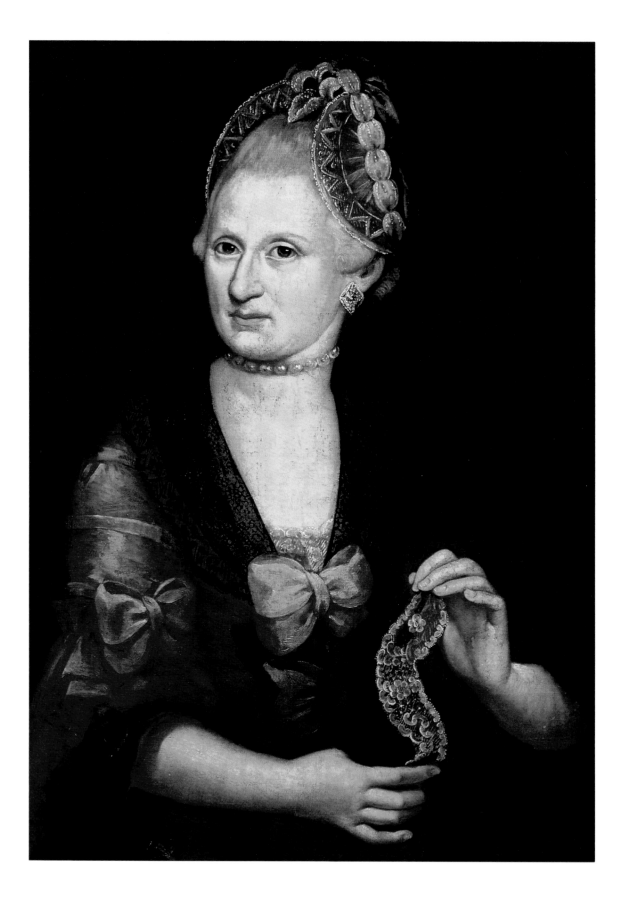

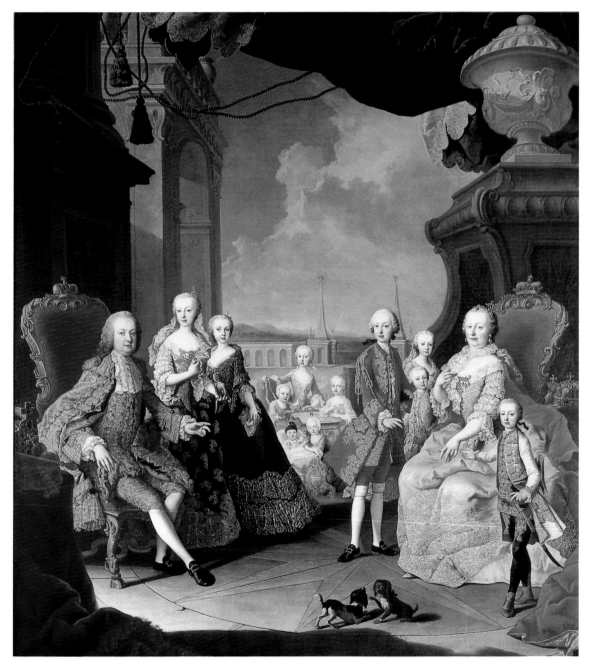

The Imperial Austrian royal family poses in formal style on the terrace of Schönbrunn Palace, Vienna.

rain, after which the wind got up and became quite furious; in this kind of hurricane the boat could make no way. I was now wet, cold, hungry and totally helpless, for the boatman himself was in despair.'

The Mozarts arrived in Vienna safely on 6 October and were very soon engaged in an exhausting round of exhibition appearances at the houses of the nobility. This rose to fever pitch after their reception at the Imperial summer residence, Schönbrunn Palace, on 13 October: 'The nobles,' Leopold told Hagenauer, 'send us their invitations four, five, six, to eight days in advance in order not to miss us.'

Though the Emperor was pleased with the young boy's performance on the harpischord, he was not satisfied until he had produced such party tricks as playing with the keyboard covered over, and with one finger of each hand. Then followed a famous episode related thus by Arthur Hutchings:*

'The Imperial family were evidently charmed by the children, for the Empress Maria Theresa is said to have gone with some of her own children to show the little visitors the adjoining apartments. Wolfgang slipped on a polished floor, and the Archduchess Marie Antoinette, later Queen of France, helped him up and received an immediate offer of marriage in return for her kindness. She was two months older than Wolfgang. Then, according to Leopold, "Wolferl jumped on the empress's lap, threw his arms round her neck and kissed her heartily".'

The visit to Schönbrunn lasted from 3 to 6 pm and one would have thought it enough for that day, especially for young children. However the prospect of six ducats from the Prince von Hildburghausen overruled fatigue and they drove straight to his house for the evening.

Handsome court dresses (which they subsequently wore for a portrait) soon arrived for Wolfgang and Nannerl from the Empress together with a hundred ducats and a pressing

---

* *Mozart: The Man, The Musician* (Thames and Hudson, 1976)

invitation to stay longer. Leopold was only too happy to comply with the Imperial suggestion, for it made his children the fashionable rage of Vienna.

At a concert in November, Leopold was handed the first poetic tribute to his son: 'On the little six-year-old clavier player from Salzburg.' With a reference to another child prodigy who had died young, it reads:

> Child, worthy of our regard, whose ready skill we
> praise,
> Who, small in stature, like the greatest plays;
> For thee the art of sound will hold no pain,
> Full soon wilt thou to mastery attain.
> But may thy frame the soul's exactions bear,
> And not, like Lübeck's child, too soon outwear.

Such fears were well justified, for Wolfgang had already gone down, after his second visit to the Empress on 21 October, with a feverish illness which kept him in bed for some time. Leopold's sympathy was tempered with concern for his pocket: 'In Vienna,' Hagenauer was informed, 'the nobility are afraid of pockmarks and all kinds of rash. So my boy's illness has meant a setback of about four weeks. Although since his recovery we have taken in twenty-four ducats, this is a mere trifle.'

A consoling profit resulted from a visit to Pressburg (now Bratislava) in December and Leopold was able to buy his own carriage, though this did little to soften the bumpy, frozen road 'full of deep ruts and ridges'. When they got back to Salzburg on 5 January 1763 after a brief return to Vienna, Wolfgang was again in bed for a week with rheumatism. However, he used his convalescence to perfect his violin playing, and his father – in spite of several months' absence – was gratified by promotion in February to the rank of vice-Kapellmeister.

We get an impression of Wolfgang's performances at this early age from a newspaper correspondent in Vienna. 'We fall into utter amazement,' he wrote, 'on seeing a boy aged six at the clavier and hear him not by any means toy with sonatas, trios and concertos, but play in a manly way and improvise moreover for hours on end ... I saw them cover the keyboard with a handkerchief and he plays just as well ... Furthermore ... when he was made to listen in another room, they would give him notes ... and he came out with the letter or the name of the note in an instant.'

Such was the degree of public interest that Leopold was very soon planning further travels – this time a Grand Tour which was to take the family away from Salzburg for almost three and a half years. They left on 9 June 1763 in their own carriage which lost a wheel only two days later. The replacement did not fit properly and Leopold and the Mozarts' newly-acquired servant, Sebastian Winter, had to walk at times to ease the weight.

To list their innumerable stopping-places and all the tributes they received is beyond the scope of this book. The family travelled via Munich to Augsburg, where they 'stayed a long time and gained little or nothing'. The children performed at the palace of Schwetzingen, country seat of Karl Theodor, the Elector Palatine and founder of the Mannheim orchestra, then considered the best in Germany. The teenage Goethe heard Wolfgang at one of the Mozarts' four or five concerts in Frankfurt: 'I saw him,' he later recalled, 'when he was a seven-year-old boy. I myself was about fourteen years old and I can still quite clearly remember the little fellow with his wig and his sword.'

There were great hopes of Brussels, where the children did eventually appear before Prince Charles of Lorraine, brother of Emperor Francis I and governor of the Austrian Netherlands, but only after a wait of five weeks while the Prince pursued his customary diversions of hunting, eating and drinking; and the handsome presents bestowed on the family were no substitute for cash in hand.

In mid-November the family arrived in Paris, where they stayed with the Bavarian ambassador. Here again, everything depended on a successful royal reception. Owing to a

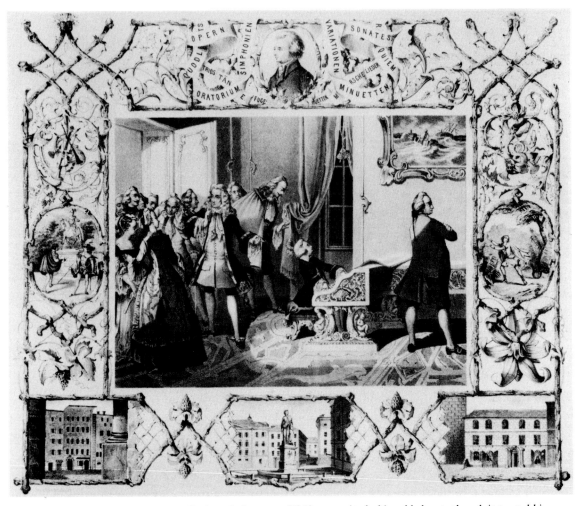

Paris took the young Wolfgang to its fashionable heart, though it treated him coldly when he returned in later years. In this highly romanticised image, which dates from 1860, the young prodigy is made to look more like a juvenile Liszt than Mozart, aged eight.

period of court mourning, they did not go to Versailles until 24 December, where Madame de Pompadour impressed Leopold as 'an extremely haughty woman who still ruled over everything'. The children triumphed. Indeed, as Leopold put it, 'they took almost everyone by storm'.

There was an enforced pause, much regretted by his father, when Wolfgang developed a high fever in February 1764, but Leopold felt he could look forward to 'a good harvest' after 'tilling the soil well'. In March the eight-year-old published his Opus I – two sonatas for the harpischord (K6 and 7),* 'which can be played with violin accompaniment'. These were written no doubt with assistance from his father. Two more sonatas quickly followed and there were two profitable public concerts before the family left Paris in mid-April en route for England. 'I saw how the sea runs away and comes back again,' observed Nannerl in her diary as they waited at Calais for the cross-channel packet.

The Mozarts were in London for fifteen months, from 23 April 1764 to 24 July 1765, lodging with a hairdresser off St Martin's Lane, and subsequently in Chelsea and Thrift (now Frith) Street, Soho. The first of three court appearances took place only five days after their arrival in the English capital and although 'the present was only twenty-four guineas', King George II and Queen Charlotte impressed Leopold by their 'easy manner and friendly ways' and the visit to Buckingham House had the desired effect of making the children fashionable everywhere. 'I have had the shock of taking one hundred guineas in three hours,' Leopold exuberantly informed Hagenauer, his Salzburg landlord, after a benefit concert in June; but he also astutely realised that 'nothing wins the affection of this quite exceptional nation' more surely than charity work, so he let Wolfgang play the organ at a concert in aid of the newly-founded Lying-In-Hospital 'in order to perform thereby the act of an English Patriot'.

Mozart dedicated his Opus 3 (K10–15) – a set of six sonatas 'for the harpsichord which can be played with the accompaniment of violin or transverse flute' – to the Queen and received a present of fifty guineas in reply. Further income was derived from putting Wolfgang on show at the family's Soho lodgings, where, as Leopold said in his advertisement, 'those ladies and gentlemen who did honour him with their company from twelve to three in the afternoon

---

*The K numbers in this book refer to the original edition of Köchel's index, rather than to the less familiar 6th edition published in 1964.

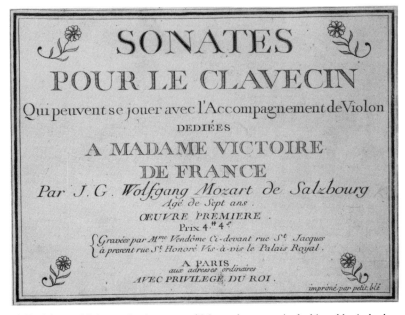

A Parisian publisher took advantage of Mozart's success in fashionable circles by bringing out a set of sonatas which Mozart had composed aged seven, described as his Opus I. In these sonatas, typical of the period, the keyboard player takes precedence over the violinist, whose part is optional.

any day of the week except Tuesday and Friday may, by each taking a ticket, gratify their curiosity, and not only hear this young Music Master and his sister perform in private: but likewise try his surprising musical capacity.'

Among their visitors in June 1765 was a Fellow of the Royal Society, Daines Barrington, who, in a subsequent report, admitted being sceptical at first about the child's extreme youth. Although he had seen Wolfgang run about the room 'with a stick between his legs by way of a horse' and leave the harpsichord to play with his cat, Barrington carefully verified his age before expressing amazement at 'this prodigy of nature'. He submitted the boy to many searching tests, among them the instant composition of operatic arias to express Love and Anger. Mozart responded without difficulty, demonstrating 'a thorough knowledge of the fundamental principles of composition' and great facility in modulation: 'his transitions from one key to another were excessively natural and judicious'. As for Wolfgang's ability as a performer, Barrington declared that 'his execution was amazing, considering that his little fingers could scarcely reach a fifth on the harpsichord.'

Perhaps the most important musical encounter of the London visit was the young Mozart's meeting with Johann Christian Bach, the 'English Bach', son of the great Johann Sebastian and himself a fine composer in the urbane

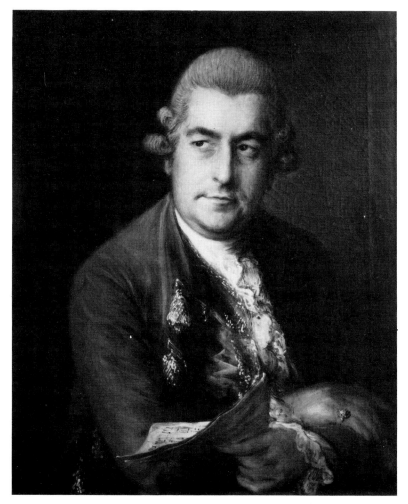

Johann Christian Bach (1735–82), the Queen's music-master and the most fashionable composer in London, whose style of composition and performance the young Mozart sought to emulate.

'galant' style of the day. In her reminiscences, Nannerl describes how this important man shared a keyboard with Wolfgang one day: 'Herr Johann Christian Bach, the Queen's teacher, took Wolfgang between his legs. The former played a few bars, and then the other continued, and in this way they played a whole sonata and someone not seeing it would have thought that only one man was playing.' J.C. Bach was a leading exponent of the newly-introduced fortepiano and may perhaps have sown a seed which was later to grow into Mozart's great series of piano concertos. Certainly he was a strong influence on the boy's childhood compositions, some of which are indistinguishable from those of J.C. Bach.

Before the family left London, Leopold took care to present copies of his son's early works to the British Museum, in order to ensure that posterity would not forget the wonder he had produced.

Most of the remaining months of 1765 and the early part of 1766 were spent in the Netherlands, where the family travelled extensively and responded to an invitation to visit Princess Caroline of Nassau-Weilburg at The Hague. The Princess asked Mozart to write a set of sonatas to mark the coming of age and installation as Stadtholder of her brother, William V of Orange. There were also successful concerts in Amsterdam and many other places. But once again, towards the end of 1765, Leopold's plans had to be shelved because the children were ill, this time with intestinal typhoid. Nannerl at one point was given extreme unction and Wolfgang's life was in danger for some weeks.

In June 1766, the Mozarts were back in Paris, where they stayed for three days at Versailles. From there a slow homeward journey punctuated by frequent concerts and exhibition appearances took them back to Salzburg. Leopold and his family reached home on 29 November 1766.

The long and ambitious venture had been a financial success. The librarian of St Peter's Abbey in Salzburg expressed the belief that 'Herr Mozart's gewgaws, brought home by him, are worth 12,000 florins if they are worth 10

In the course of their visit to London Leopold Mozart presented the British Museum with copies of some of Wolfgang's early compositions, receiving the above acknowledgement from the secretary to the trustees by way of receipt.

kreuzer. In addition, he has bought very many things cheaply in these foreign countries, which he will sell here at a high price, and in this way make even more money on the spot!'

The cost of the enterprise, however, was no less real. It seems not to have occurred to Leopold on this Grand Tour, that 'the boy's triumphs had been achieved at the expense of severe damage to his health. He overlooked the fact that Wolfgang's musical development had not kept pace, could not keep pace, with his intellectual progress. He ignored the boy's nervous fits of weeping caused by homesickness or by news that his childhood friend, Domenicus Hagenauer, had entered a monastery.'

Domenicus Hagenauer, whose father, Johann Lorenz, was the Mozarts' landlord in the Getreidegasse.

After nine months at home, Leopold again got leave of absence from the Archbishop and on 22 September 1767 the family set off to Vienna hoping to take part in the celebrations for the forthcoming marriage of Archduchess Maria Josepha to King Ferdinand of Naples.

As it turned out, the most fruitful result of this journey had nothing to do with the court. The Mozarts were befriended by Dr Franz Anton Mesmer, who was highly fashionable at the time for his 'cures by Magnetism'. He had a large house and a private theatre and for this he commissioned Wolfgang to write a lighthearted rustic entertainment in German, *Bastien und Bastienne*, which fitted his youthful talent and exuberance admirably. (In a later opera, *Così fan tutte*, there is a more famous reminder of Dr Mesmer when Despina, disguised as a doctor, brings Ferrando and Guglielmo back to life by using a magnet).

For the most part, this Viennese visit was not a very happy one. The Princess Josepha died suddenly in October. As Leopold ruefully put it to Hagenauer, 'The prince's bride has become a bride of the Heavenly Bridegroom,' and both the children became ill, though mildly, in the smallpox epidemic which had proved fatal to the Princess. To add to the prevailing melancholy, the Empress Maria Theresa held monthly devotions in memory of her lately deceased husband, and not until the New Year were the Mozarts received at court.

Even then the new Emperor, Maria Theresa's son Joseph II, rewarded them with nothing better than a medal, believing no doubt, as Leopold saw it, 'that he had paid us by his most gracious conversation'. The Imperial passion for economy unfortunately spread to other households; moreover, the gifted boy began to encounter hostility from other musicians who probably disliked precocious gimmickry and perhaps had begun to fear the rivalry of a highly capable twelve-year-old who was no longer merely an amusing novelty.

In March came news from the Archbishop's exchequer in Salzburg that unless Leopold returned within a month he

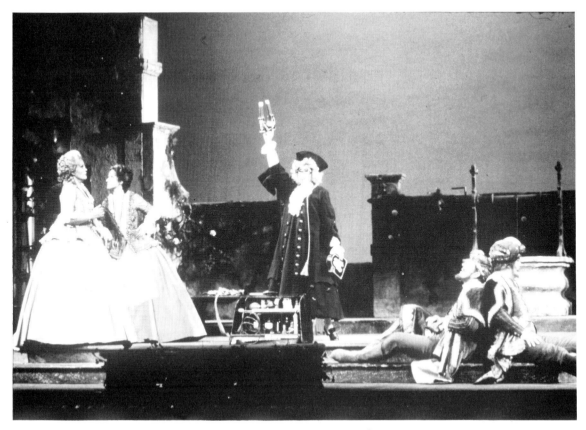

A scene from the 1981 production of Cosi fan tutte *(K588) at the Royal Opera House, in which Despina (centre), in disguise, effects a magnetic cure. Contemporary audiences would have understood the satirical reference to Dr Anton Mesmer, whom Mozart met during a visit to Vienna.*

would receive no further salary, though he could later resume his employment if he chose. Leopold thought it best to remain in Vienna for the time being, since Wolfgang was busily composing a comic opera, *La finta semplice* (The Pretended Simpleton), with the Emperor's approval. Hopes of getting it produced, however, were thwarted by intrigues which drove Leopold to desperation. 'The whole hell of musicians has arisen to prevent the display of a child's ability,' he wrote. 'I cannot even press for a performance since a conspiracy has been formed to produce it, if it must be produced, extremely badly and thus ruin it.'

In his anxiety Leopold went so far as to complain about the theatre authorities in a petition to the Emperor, and in so doing may have overstepped the mark, for the royal family seemed to lose interest. It was therefore with a sense of frustration that the Mozarts returned to Salzburg on 5 January 1769 after an absence of some fifteen months.

The Prince-Archbishop, whose brother had provided interludes of consoling hospitality during the Viennese sojourn, made up for the apparent indifference of the Imperial capital by ordering that *La finta semplice* should be performed on his name day. The Salzburg ruler had earlier put Wolfgang's powers as a composer to the test by shutting him up alone and making him set part of a church service, and towards the end of 1769 Wolfgang was given the title of third Konzertmeister of the Court Chapel. This would have involved composing as well as leading the court orchestra and was no doubt bestowed on the young musician to commit him firmly to Salzburg amid the temptations of the Italian journey his father was now planning. Italian credentials were highly desirable for an eighteenth-century musician, and for a budding opera composer it was necessary above all to succeed in Milan, as J.C. Bach had told Leopold in London.

Once again obtaining leave of absence from the Archbishop, who must have been convinced that the Mozarts' successes abroad reflected credit on him, Leopold and Wolfgang set off accompanied by a servant on 13 December. Though he was now fourteen years of age, Wolfgang's slight build made him look younger – an impression fully exploited by Leopold – and his concerts in northern Italy in early January created immense interest. On the 23rd they arrived in Milan, where they were guests of Count Karl Joseph Firmian, nephew of the former Archbishop of Salzburg who first employed Leopold. Firmian was Governor-General of Lombardy, then under Austrian rule, and it was mainly through his powerful influence that all the right doors opened for the Mozarts, father and son, wherever they travelled on this Italian tour.

Letters home to Wolfgang's mother and sister tell us how things went. Many public and private concerts were arranged in Milan in the first three months of 1770, and for such grand occasions special clothes were required. 'The tailor has just called with cloaks and cowls which we have had to order,' Leopold informed his wife in February; 'I looked at myself in the mirror as we were trying them on and thought of how, in my old age, I too have to take part in this tomfoolery.' If Leopold showed little respect in private for the grand people who patronised him, Wolfgang found relief from social solemnities by writing to his sister in a vein of lavatorial humour which continued to amuse him in later life. He told Nannerl of a dwarf he had seen in an opera at

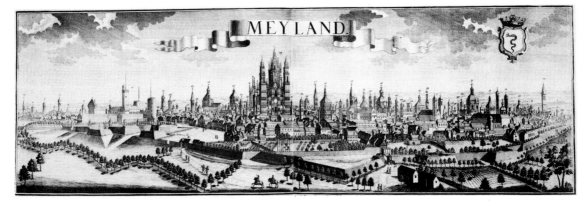

On their first visit to Milan Count Karl Joseph Firmian, the Governor General of Lombardy, arranged for Leopold and Wolfgang to stay in the San Marco Monastery. On subsequent visits father and son stayed in excessively noisy lodgings near to the theatre, which Wolfgang complained about in letters to his sister.

Mantua 'who jumps well but cannot write as I do, I mean as sows piddle'; and there was another in Cremona 'who, whenever he jumped, let off a fart'.

Apart from making Wolfgang's performing talent known to everyone who was anyone in Milan, Firmian made sure the boy was commissioned to write an opera for the next Christmas season. Thus it was with high hopes for the future as well as numerous letters of introduction that Leopold and Wolfgang set off for the south in March.

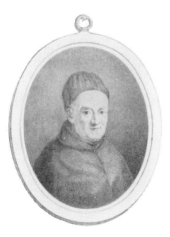

Padre J.B. Martini, who was Maestro di Capella at the Church of St Francis in Bologna at the time of Mozart's teenage visit to Italy, and a musical scholar of high repute.

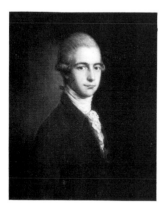

In Italy Mozart met Thomas Linley, pictured here. Kindred spirits, they played sonatas together and corresponded for some time. Mozart is supposed to have wept upon leaving Linley.

In Bologna, Wolfgang's abilities were tested by the influential musical scholar Padre Martini, whose expressions of admiration greatly enhanced the boy's reputation among Italians. In Florence there was a brief encounter with another prodigy, the English violinist Thomas Linley, who was Wolfgang's own age. The pair of them played duets and Wolfgang received a sonnet addressed to him on Linley's behalf. The boys clearly got on well, for Wolfgang later wrote to Linley in affectionate terms.

Soon after arriving in Rome, Leopold began to deliver 'twenty letters of introduction' which produced invitations to numerous palaces. Father and son went to hear the famous choir of the Sistine Chapel perform Allegri's *Miserere*, which was supposed to be their closely guarded exclusive possession; and we are told that Wolfgang, deeply impressed, went home and wrote the whole piece out from memory – though it is just possible he had some prior knowledge of it. In other matters he was less well organised. 'Please try to find the arithmetical tables,' he asked his sister in a letter; 'I have lost my copy and so have quite forgotten them.'

The road to Naples was at that time liable to attacks from brigands, and the city itself was far from salubrious: 'The lazzaroni have their own general,' Nannerl was told, 'who receives 25 ducats from the King every month solely for keeping them in order.' Nevertheless the Mozarts were not deterred from visiting the southern capital where once again they enjoyed a huge success and found time for some sightseeing. Leopold was impressed with the daily 'passeggio' of nobles taking their afternoon carriage drive; Wolfgang enjoyed watching Vesuvius 'smoking furiously' with 'thunder and lightning and all the rest'.

They were back in Rome at the end of June. Wolfgang had an audience with Pope Clement XIV, after he had conferred on him a Knighthood of the Golden Spur, an exceptionally high honour for a musician. 'You can imagine how I laugh when I hear people calling him "Signor Cavaliere",' wrote Leopold to his wife; but for all his

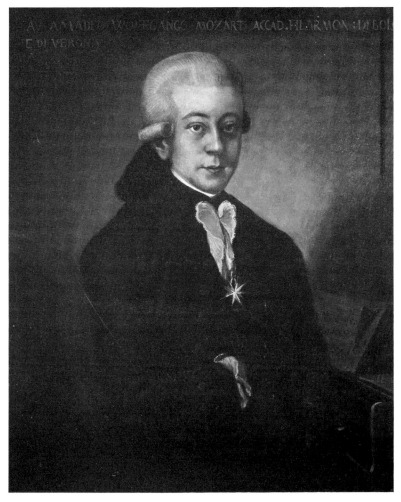

Mozart as a Papal Knight of the Golden Spur. The fourteen-year-old Mozart was the first musician since Lassus in the sixteenth century to receive a first class honour. Three days later he was received in audience by Pope Clement XIV.

amusement he can hardly have been less than gratified.

During a stay of three months in Bologna in the autumn, Wolfgang received the libretto and the list of singers for his Christmas opera *Mitridate, Rè di Ponto* (Mithridates, King of Pontus). In those days to please the 'prima donna' and 'primo uomo' was of the utmost importance and the young Mozart was brilliantly successful in this. By November he was hard at work in Milan and Leopold was able to report that 'the prima donna is infinitely pleased with her arias'.

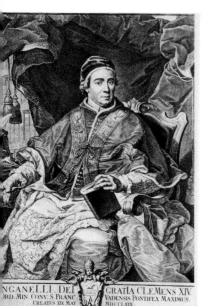

Pope Clement XIV

As for the primo uomo (a male soprano in the fashion of the time), he too was delighted and declared that if a certain duet did not succeed 'he would let himself be castrated again'.

The first performance of *Mitridate*, with Mozart directing a large orchestra from the keyboard, took place on 26 December 1770 to 'extraordinary applause and cries of "Evviva il Maestro! Evviva il Maestrino!"' After this triumph there was a highly successful visit to Venice for the Carnival of 1771 – Wolfgang was asked to write an opera for a future season and was received everywhere. Indeed, they did so much travelling by gondola that, said Leopold, 'during the first days the whole bed rocked in our sleep'. Then it was back via Innsbruck to Salzburg in March.

It was not long before Leopold and Wolfgang again set off for Milan, for the express purpose of carrying out a commission from the Empress Maria Theresa. Archbishop Schrattenbach once again gave permission but withheld

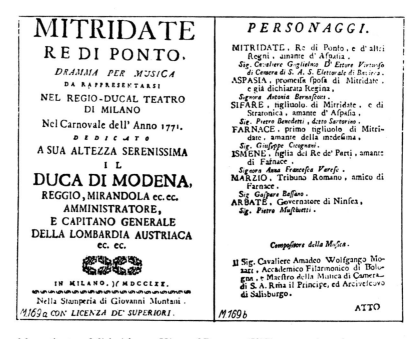

Mozart's opera Mithridates, King of Pontus *(K87) was a triumphant success in Milan. On this playbill, Mozart is described as* cavaliere *and reference is also made to his appointment on the staff of the Archbishop of Salzburg.*

Leopold's salary (it was ultimately paid to him, after Leopold petitioned the Cathedral Chapter 'but without precedent for the future, nor for other court musicians absenting themselves').

After a relatively rapid journey, father and son reached Milan in mid-August and soon Mozart was at work setting the libretto he had been given. *Ascanio in Alba* was completed in a month and given with the utmost success in October during the celebrations for the wedding of the Empress's son, the Archduke Ferdinand, to Princess Maria Ricciarda Beatrice of Modena.

The Mozarts were back in Salzburg again on 15 December 1771. The day after their return, the Prince-Archbishop, Sigismund Schrattenbach, died. Though latterly he had grown impatient with the prolonged absences of Leopold and his brilliant son, he had behaved towards them both with remarkable tolerance; over a period of nine years they had, after all, been away from Salzburg for almost seven. With the accession of Schrattenbach's successor there came a change of attitude which made life more awkward for the adolescent genius.

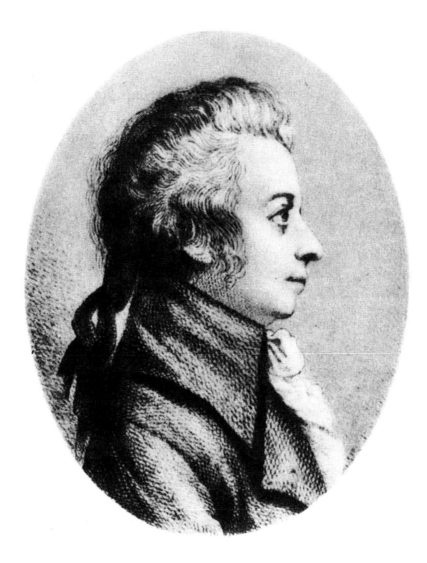

CHAPTER THREE

SERVITUDE AND A BID
FOR FREEDOM
1772–78

Mozart was now sixteen, well past the infant prodigy stage and already an accomplished composer with a large number of works of many different kinds to his credit. Leopold had taken care to give his son a thorough grounding in the theory and practice of composition and no opportunity had been missed during the family's extensive travels to meet and learn from the leading creative musicians of the day. Among them were Fux, Martini, Sammartini, Michael Haydn and, most important of all, Joseph Haydn, whose works were admired and most likely studied by Mozart before they met in 1781.

Wolfgang produced his first symphonies at the age of eight or nine under the influence of established composers in Paris and London in the course of the Grand Tour. Shortly after, he produced his first church music, a motet – 'God is our Refuge' – and a Kyrie (K33) for four voices and strings, while still continuing to compose a great deal of instrumental and vocal music apart from the stage works and other entertainments in operatic style which were his most spectacular success to date.

Archbishop Hieronymus Colloredo, though he has come to be thought of as the villain of the piece in the Mozart

The manuscript of Mozart's earliest piece of Church Music (K20), set to the words from Psalm 46 and composed when he was nine, clearly reveals the helping hand of his father, who took over the task of writing after the bar-lines started to wander. But the musical inspiration belonged to Wolfgang.

story, was, by his own somewhat outdated standards, a fair-minded man. Rather stiff and formal, lacking in personal charm and very careful to preserve the hierarchical structure of a society in which musicians were merely servants, he nevertheless recognised Wolfgang's talent. Shortly after his appointment he commissioned the young man to write a dramatic serenata *Il sogno di Scipione* (Scipio's Dream) for his ceremonial installation in the spring of 1772.

Charles Burney visited Salzburg that summer in the

course of his 'Tour undertaken to collect Materials for a General History of Music' and reported that 'the arch-bishop and sovereign is very magnificent in his support of music, having usually near a hundred performers, vocal and instrumental, in his service. The prince is himself a dilettante and good performer on the violin; he has lately been at great pains to reform his band which has been accused of being more remarkable for coarseness and noise than delicacy and high-finishing.' Perhaps it was as part of the reforming process that Wolfgang was granted a yearly income of 150 florins in August as Konzertmeister or leader of the court orchestra. This was neither very generous nor unduly mean by the standards of the time and many musi-cians would have been content with such an appointment, carrying as it did the right to make extra money through teaching and other engagements, provided the Arch-bishop's requirements were met.

Wolfgang, however, had seen too much of the outside

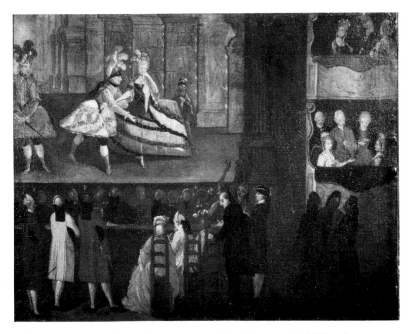

This picture of an eighteenth-century operatic performance in Milan gives some idea of how Mozart's Mithridates *and* Lucio Silla *were first staged.*

LUCIO SILLA
DRAMMA PER MUSICA
DA RAPPRESENTARSI
NEL REGIO-DUCAL TEATRO
DI MILANO
Nel Carnevole dell' anno 1773
DEDICATO
ALLE LL. AA. RR.
IL SERENISSIMO ARCIDUCA
FERDINANDO
Principe Reale d' Ungheria , e Boemia , Arciduca d'Austria
Duca di Borgogna , e di Lorena ec . , Cesareo Reale
Luogo-Tenente , Governatore , e Capitano
Generale nella Lombardia Austriaca ,
E LA
SERENISSIMA ARCIDUCHESSA
**MARIA RICCIARDA
BEATRICE D' ESTE**
PRINCIPESSA DI MODENA.

IN MILANO,
Preffo Gio. Batifta Bianchi Regio Stampatore
Con licenza de' Superiori.

The titlepage of the libretto for Lucio Silla (K135), first performed during carnival season in Milan in 1773. A great success, it was given twenty-six times during the season, but has not survived in the present-day operatic repertoire.

world to want to settle down indefinitely in Salzburg, and his father was eager for him to secure a more spectacular appointment than Colloredo could offer. Italy was particularly attractive, for there the young 'Cavaliere' was treated with respect, instead of having to defer obsequiously to others. Fortunately Wolfgang had been commissioned to write the first opera for the 1772–3 carnival in Milan and in October Leopold and he set off southwards once again.

Lucio Silla was performed for the first time at the Teatro Regio Ducal on 26 December after the Archduke Ferdinand, delayed by official business, had kept everyone waiting for two or three hours. Such was the success of the opera that it was given no less than twenty-six times during the carnival season. *Lucio Silla* has not retained its early popularity, but another work composed during this visit to Milan was the motet 'Exultate, Jubilate', created for the principal male singer at the opera, the castrato Venanzio Rauzzini. This motet includes the lovely 'Alleluia' which has remained one of Mozart's most beloved inspirations.

While father and son were in Italy, Leopold persuaded Count Firmian to back an application to Archduke Leopold of Tuscany for a court appointment there for Wolfgang, and the two Mozarts lingered in Milan hoping for a favourable reply.

Wolfgang's mother and sister received reports of their doings in frequent letters which were partly written in cypher. Since the accession of Colloredo, the Mozarts had reason to suspect that letters might be intercepted and they naturally wished to keep discussion of possible new appointments from the Archbishop. Thus, to cover their delay in returning after the production of *Lucio Silla*, Leopold wrote in plain language to his wife in mid-January complaining that acute rheumatism had forced him to take to his bed. A week later followed another letter with a postscript in cypher which Anna Maria was instructed to cut off from the main text, saying that the story of his illness was a fabrication to put the Salzburg authorities off the scent; in fact they were still awaiting news from Florence. All

Leopold's scheming was in vain, however, for no appointment was forthcoming and in March 1773 the travellers were back home in Salzburg. Shortly after their return they moved from the Getreidegasse to more spacious lodgings in the Hannibal-platz, now the Makart-platz, on the north side of the River Salzach.

Leopold and Wolfgang had little difficulty in obtaining further leave of absence from Colloredo in July since he himself was planning to be away. This time, in the secret

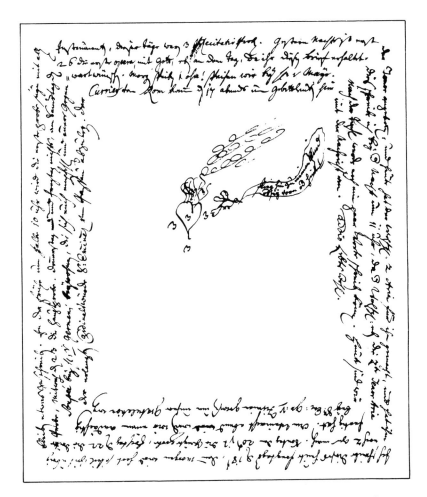

A decorative letter written from Milan by Leopold to his wife. Wolfgang often added obscene footnotes to Leopold's letters home. On this occasion he confined himself to the drawing, which includes an erotic message.

hope of an appointment at the Imperial court, they returned to Vienna, but although they were received by the Empress, there was no vacancy. Wolfgang occupied himself with the composition of a serenade (K185) and a set of six quartets (K168–173), and the Mozarts renewed their friendship with Dr Mesmer. Passing through Vienna on his way back to Salzburg, the Archbishop extended their leave of absence, but he was nonetheless lampooned in Wolfgang's letters to his sister 'from our Residence, Vienna'. Reluctantly he and his father arrived back in Salzburg on 26 September.

Whatever underlying hopes the young Mozart had of employment elsewhere, he now settled down to a period of over a year in Salzburg in the course of which he produced many beautiful works including a string quintet (K174 in B flat), his first truly original piano concerto (K175 in D) and the Symphony in G minor K183, which resembles the great Symphony no. 40 in little more than its key signature but all the same may have surprised Salzburg by its intensity. In those days symphonies were often composed originally as extended opera overtures and subsequently transferred from the theatre to the salon. In that setting they were, like other 'chamber music', thought of as charming entertainment, not to be taken too seriously. Other fine symphonies of this period were the ones in C major K200 and A major K201 – a particularly happy work which has remained popular.

In 1774 the Elector of Bavaria commissioned Mozart to write an opera for the forthcoming carnival season and early in December Wolfgang arrived in Munich with his father to supervise rehearsals. Colloredo was himself going to Munich and so could hardly refuse permission; in the event *La finta giardiniera*, which tells a romantic story about a young countess disguised as a garden-girl, was a huge success which can only have reflected credit on the Prince-Archbishop. There were numerous encores on the first night, 13 January 1775, and the opera was repeated several times in the course of the season. Some of the concerted

Mozart was just eighteen when La Finta Giardiniera (K196) *was first performed in Munich and it continued the composer's run of early operatic triumphs.*

numbers in particular foreshadow the incomparable operas Mozart was to create in the future.

Wolfgang reported his success in letters to his mother, adding: 'We cannot return to Salzburg very soon and Mama must not wish it, for she knows how much good it is doing me to be able to breathe freely.' Colloredo was once again the butt of uncharitable comments from Leopold, who asked Anna Maria to imagine 'the embarrassment of his Grace the Archbishop at hearing the opera praised by the whole family of the Elector and by all the nobles'; he also requested details of any Salzburg gossip about an appointment for Wolfgang in Munich: 'then we shall have something to laugh about, for we know these fools.'

Such rumours proved ill-founded, but, in the course of this Munich season, contemporary observers began to do justice to Mozart's rapidly growing stature as a composer. Of *La finta giardiniera*, the correspondent of an Augsburg journal wrote: 'Flashes of genius appear here and there . . . if Mozart is not a plant forced in the hot-house, he is bound to grow into one of the greatest composers who ever lived.'

Whether Colloredo was quite so far-sighted in assessing his young employee's abilities is doubtful, but he very soon ordered Wolfgang to produce an operatic entertainment for the visit to Salzburg in April 1775 of the Archduke Maximilian. This was a setting of Metastasio's *Il rè pastore*, a story from classical antiquity about a defeated king who lives the life of a shepherd; it contains Mozart's first one-movement overture (in place of the three-movement 'sinfonia' which usually preceded operas in those days) and several beautiful arias and duets.

In the course of Maximilian's visit, Mozart was also called upon as a solo performer in his own instrumental compositions, and there is no evidence to suggest that during the two years he now spent at Salzburg he was not well appreciated. Among the many works he produced at this time were the *Serenata notturna* (K239), five violin concertos of which the last three are well-loved masterpieces, a triple piano concerto (K242) and his first great solo piano concerto, K271 in E flat. And for the wedding in 1776 of Elisabeth Haffner, daughter of the burgomaster of Salzburg, Mozart produced the nine-movement Haffner Serenade.

Wolfgang was still only twenty years of age and relished

any opportunity for enjoyment which came his way. We get one glimpse of him relaxing in a description of a carnival party in February 1776 taken from the diary of Mozart's friend Joachim Ferdinand von Schiedenhofen, who became Court Councillor in Salzburg. 'At seven in the evening to the Master of the Household for supper,' he wrote. 'Then in company to the rout, driving there with the Chief Equerry as a lady, the Marshal as a cavalier, Baron Lilien as a gallant, Count Micha as a courier, Herr Schmid as a hair-dresser, the elder Mozart as a porter and the younger as a hairdresser's boy, Count Überacker as a moor and myself as a lackey...'

The first sign of serious discontent with Salzburg which has come down to us is a letter Mozart wrote in September 1776 to Padre Martini, enclosing some church compositions for his perusal. Mozart complained of the restrictions of duration and personnel placed on his religious works, of the lack of good opera singers, of general parsimony; and he enlisted Martini's sympathy for his father who 'has already served this court for thirty-six years and, as he knows that the present archbishop cannot and will not have anything to do with people who are getting on in years, he no longer puts his whole heart into his work, but has taken up litera-ture which was always a favourite study of his.' It seems that the Mozarts, in common with other resident Salzburg musicians, felt snubbed when the ruler closed his old theatre and ordered the construction of a new one – just opposite the Mozarts' new home as it happened – which would accommodate touring companies to the exclusion of the city's own performers.

In March 1777, the Archbishop rejected a request from Leopold and Wolfgang to go on a concert tour because the Emperor Joseph II was to visit Salzburg in July. On 1 August, the day after the Emperor departed, Wolfgang petitioned Colloredo for release from service on the grounds that, 'The more of talent that children have received from God, the greater is the obligation to make use thereof, in order to ameliorate their own and their parents' circum-

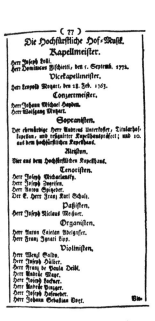

The List of Membership for the Salzburg Court Orchestra, dated 1775.

stances, to assist their parents, and to take care of their own advancement and future ... To profit from our talents is taught us by the Gospel,' the petitioner continued: an invocation of Divine approval echoed by the Archbishop, perhaps sarcastically, in a pencilled footnote to the Council decree agreeing to Mozart's request: 'Father and son herewith granted permission to seek their fortune according to the Gospel.'

Leopold, who had decided to remain behind, was allowed to continue in the Archbishop's service. But on 23 September Wolfgang set off with his mother in search of commissions and with the hope of a more substantial permanent appointment. From the family correspondence we get a vivid picture of what the journey meant both to the travellers and those they left behind at home.

Leopold found it hard to endure the day after the departure of his loved ones – 'that sad day which I never thought we should have to face.' Nannerl 'wept bitterly, complained of a headache and a sick stomach and went off to bed and had the shutters closed. Poor Bimbes [the dog] lay down beside her.' Eventually they found some distraction in the favourite family pastime of 'Bölzelschiessen' [shooting at a pictorial target with an airgun] but the absentees were by no means forgotten. The competitors shot on their behalf, with the result that 'Mama has won eleven kreuzer but Wolfgang has lost four.' Leopold was full of careful advice about good economical lodgings in his native city of Augsburg, but on the way there mother and son paused for three weeks in Munich. Here the Elector did not refuse Wolfgang an appointment outright, saying only that it was too early, that he ought to make more of a name for himself. Wolfgang toyed with the idea of getting ten friends to club together to maintain him for a while on a tight budget in Munich, but Leopold would have none of it: 'You must not make yourself so cheap and throw yourself away in this manner, for we have not come to that yet.'

On 11 October mother and son arrived in Augsburg, where the twenty-two-year-old composer was distracted

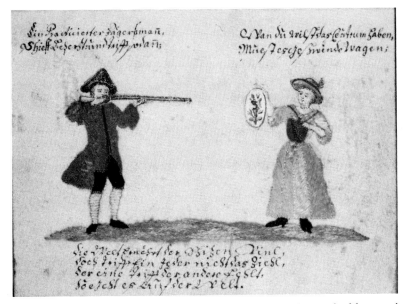

In September 1777, when Wolfgang left Salzburg yet again in search of fame and fortune, this time in the company of his mother, Leopold and Nannerl consoled themselves with air-gun shooting, one of the family's favourite amusements.

from the serious business of making money (constantly urged on him in letters from home) by a lively cousin, Maria Anna Thekla, nicknamed 'the Bäsle' (little cousin). In an exuberant letter, Wolfgang described her to Leopold as 'beautiful, intelligent, charming, clever and gay. Indeed, we two get on extremely well for she, like myself, is a bit of a scamp. We both laugh at everyone and have great fun.' The letter goes on to describe a concert where many of the nobility were present: 'The Duchess Smackbottom, the Countess Makewater, to say nothing of Princess Dunghill with her two daughters who, however, are already married to the two Princes Potbelly von Pigtail. I kiss Papa's hand 100,000 times and embrace my brute of a sister with bearish tenderness.'

Leopold's letters betray an increasing irritation with his son's tendency to be distracted from the matter in hand; exasperation at the younger Mozart's lack of practical sense and his careless approach to correspondence is almost

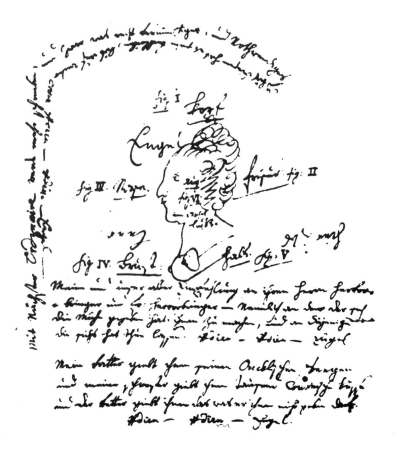

Letter about his cousin, 'the Bäsle', dated 10 May 1779. The writing around the side and at the top reads: 'I shall write more by the next 'Ordinaire' post – and I promise that it shall be something very sensible and important, and we must just be content with that until further notice'. On the drawing itself, Mozart has written 'fig. I: head, fig. II: hair, fig. III: nose, fig. IV: breast, fig. V: neck'. By the forehead is written 'angel'.

always evident: 'Many of my questions receive no answer; on the other hand you will notice that I reply to all yours.'

Apart from 'the Bäsle', Wolfgang's main source of interest in Augsburg was the piano maker Andreas Stein, whose instruments he greatly admired. He played them in public too. As one Augsburg newspaper put it: 'The evening of Wednesday last was one of the most agreeable for the local music lover. Herr Chevalier Mozart, son of the famous Salzburg musician who is a native of Augsburg, gave a concert on the fortepiano in the hall of Count Fugger. As Herr Stein happened to have three instruments of the kind ready, there was an opportunity to include a fine concerto for three claviers.' The programme also included a number of other works by Mozart. 'One thing gave relief to another, so that the numerous assembly was displeased with nothing but the fact that the pleasure was not prolonged still further.' Although his reputation was enhanced, Wolfgang was dissatisfied with the cash profit of his stay in Augsburg, and by the end of October he and his mother were in Mannheim, seat of the Elector Palatine, Karl Theodor, whose large orchestra had an expressive range unrivalled in Europe.

Soon Mozart was attending rehearsals with the orchestra's leader, Christian Cannabich, who – Wolfgang informed his father – 'has taken a great fancy to me. He has a daughter who plays the clavier quite nicely and in order to make a real friend of him, I am now working at a sonata for her.' By no means forgetful of his own abilities and earlier triumphs, Wolfgang was amused by the way the Mannheim musicians reacted to him. 'I thought I should not be able to keep myself from laughing when I was introduced to the people there. Some who knew me by repute were very polite and fearfully respectful; others, however, who had never heard of me, stared at me wide-eyed, and in a rather sneering manner. They probably think I am little and young, nothing great or mature can come out of me; but they will soon see . . .'

Early in November, Mozart made a great impression at a concert in the presence of the Elector and Electress, but the only tangible reward was 'a fine gold watch. At the moment', he told his father, 'ten carolins would have suited me better than the watch which, including the chains and the mottoes, has been valued at twenty. What one needs on a journey is *money*; and let me tell you, I now have *five* watches! I am therefore seriously thinking of having an additional watch pocket on each leg of my trousers, so that when I visit some great lord I shall wear watches on both sides, which moreover is now the "mode", so that it will not occur to him to present me with another one.'

Leopold, now aged fifty-eight, and by his own account in debt despite rigorous domestic economies, categorically agreed. 'It would have been very much better,' he commented, 'if you had received fifteen louis d'or instead of

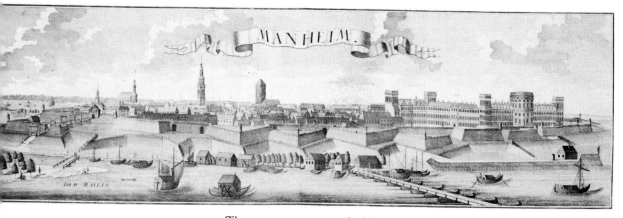

There were many reasons for Mozart to linger in Mannheim, which boasted an art gallery, museums and academies of great renown – but most importantly the court orchestra was reputed to be the best in the world.

a watch ... For the love of God, you really must try to get some money ... you must see to it that the Elector of Mainz hears you play and that you receive a present of money.'

But Wolfgang had decided to remain in Mannheim for the winter. His vague hopes of a court appointment were backed by Leopold in a letter to Padre Martini requesting a testimonial; but nothing happened. It is, after all, possible that the Elector Karl Theodor – who early in January 1778 also became Elector of Bavaria – was reluctant to employ one whose behaviour towards a fellow ruler could be interpreted as desertion. Whatever the reason, Mozart found

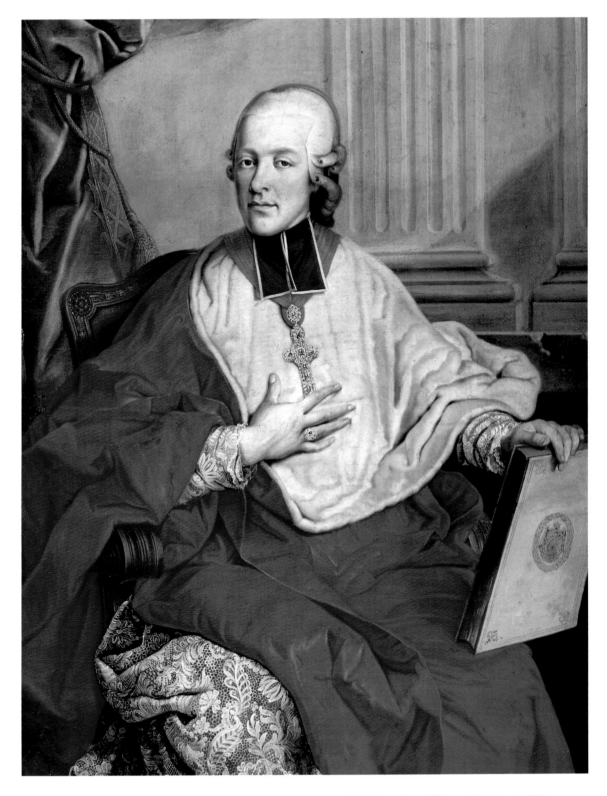

Count Hieronymus Colloredo (1732–1812) was Prince-Archbishop of Salzburg from 1771 until his death. This portrait dates from 1775, when Mozart was Colloredo's restless and increasingly impatient servant.

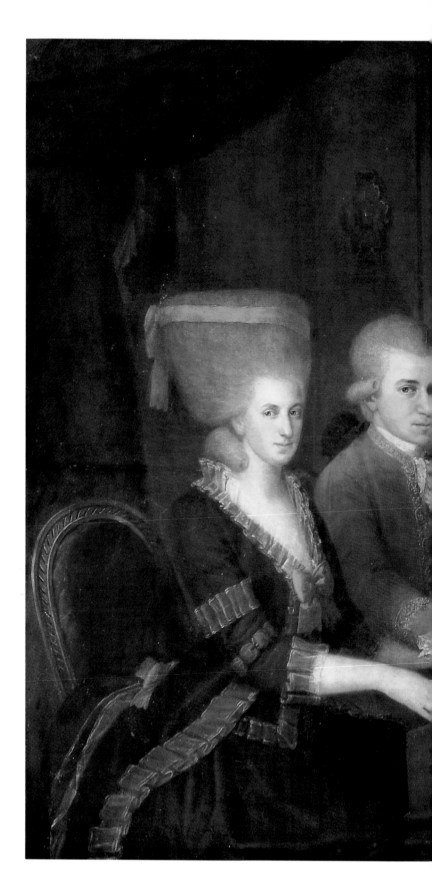

The Mozart family, painted in 1780. The three musicians are seated around the harpsichord, while Anna Maria Mozart, who had died in Paris in July 1778, watches over the group from an oval portrait.

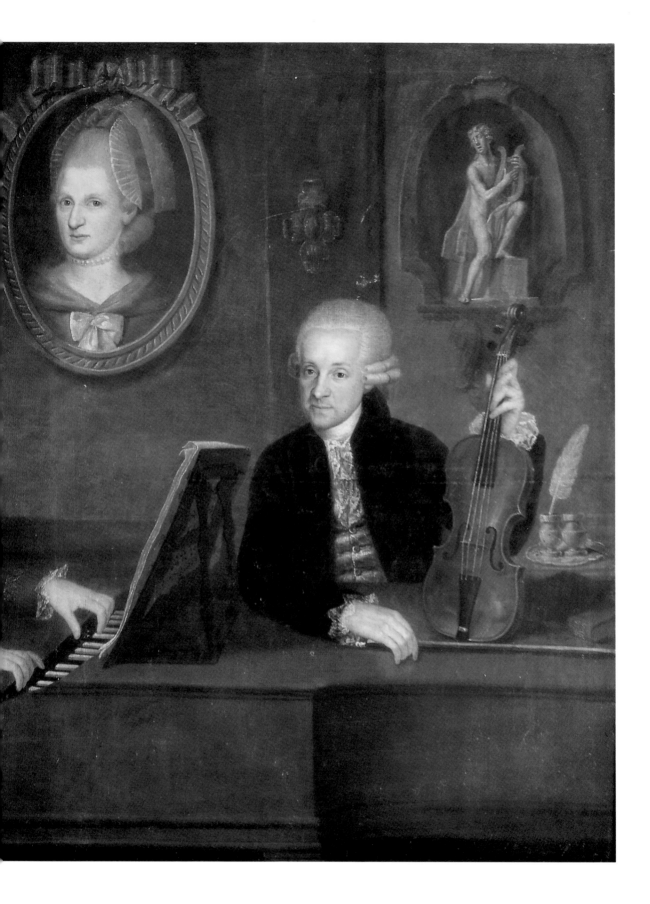

The orangery at Schönbrunn.
This colour engraving entitled
Spring Festival on a
Winter's Day *records a*
concert in February 1786,
when the overture and four
pieces of music from Mozart's
The Impresario *(K486)*
were first performed.

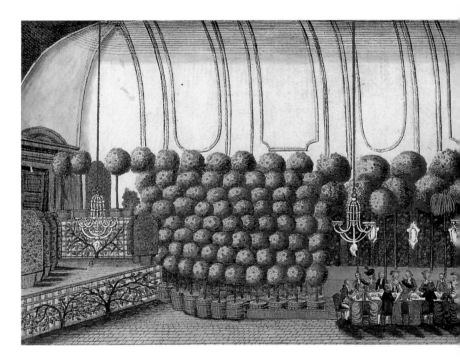

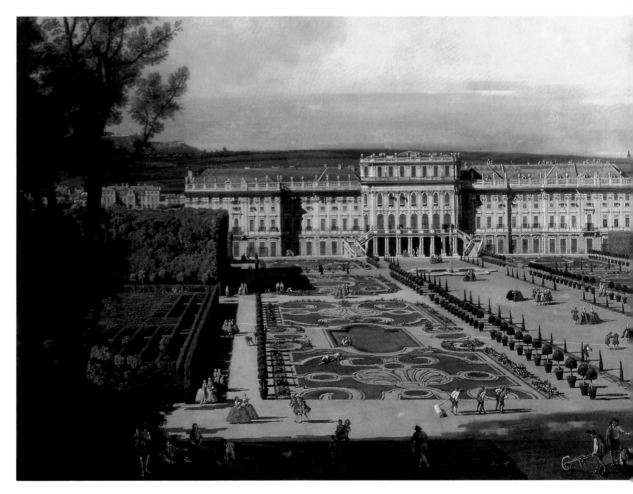

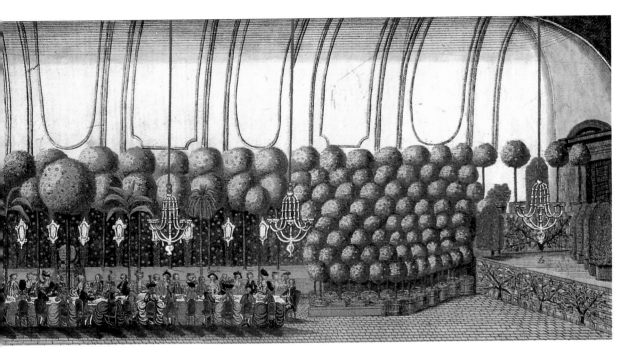

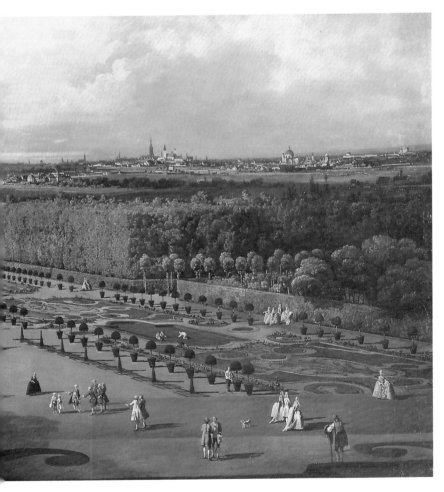

The Palace of Schönbrunn, painted c. 1760, just before young Wolfgang performed for the royal family there, aged six.

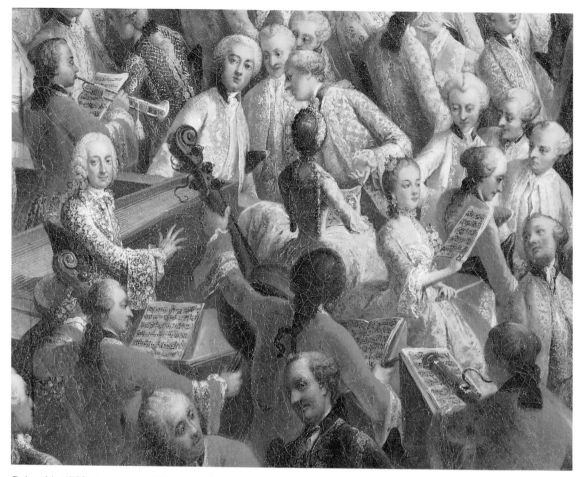

Painted in 1762, during one of Mozart's visits to Schönbrunn, this detail from an oil painting by Eduard Ender illustrates the opulence and sophistication of court life to which Mozart was accustomed from an early age.

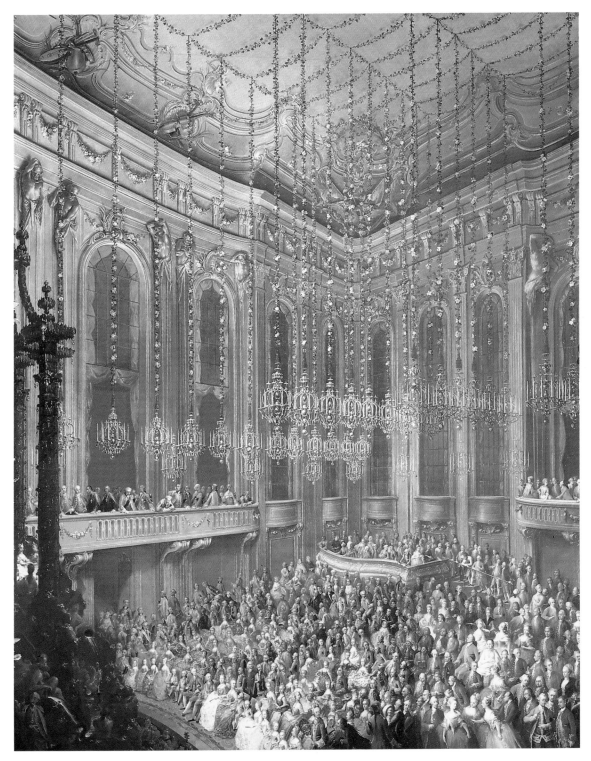

A grand performance in the Redoutensaal to celebrate the wedding of Archduke Joseph to Isabella of Parma, which took place on 10 October 1760. The Redoutensaal in Vienna's Hofburg was the scene of happier moments for Mozart: he attended a masked ball here in 1786, dressed as an Indian guru, and as Court composer often wrote dance music for Redoutensaal festivities.

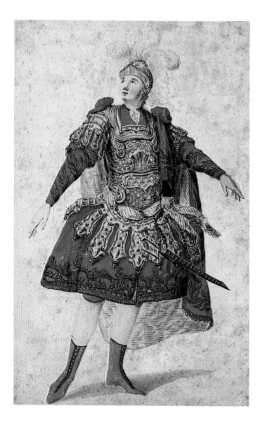

The star performer of Idomeneo *(K366), the tenor Anton Raaff (c. 1711–97), in a heroic role. Though sixty-six years of age when he sang* Idomeneo, *he still commanded the great vocal brilliance necessary to cope with the bravura arias Mozart wrote for him.*

The aquatint of St Michael's Square, Vienna, shows the Burgtheater (centre), built between 1741 and 1756, where Mozart gave numerous concerts, and in which three of his operas were first performed.

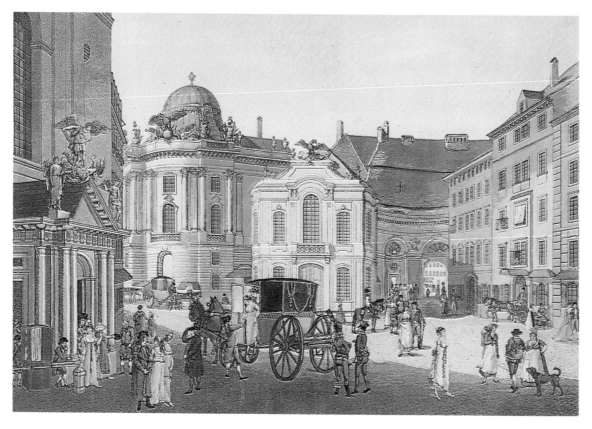

little response from the Mannheim court, though he and
his mother were kindly treated by others.

A Privy Councillor eventually took them into his own
home after Frau Mozart had suffered much discomfort in
dreary lodgings. There, she told her husband, she was often
alone, and had to put up with 'the most horrible cold. For
even if they light a small fire, they never put any more coal
on it, so that when it burns out the room gets cold again. A
little fire of this sort costs twelve kreuzer. So I make them
light one in the morning when we get up and another in the
evening ... as I write I can hardly hold my pen, I am
freezing so ...' Wolfgang was often out with friends,
occasionally with practical results. 'He lunched today with
a wealthy Dutchman,' Anna Maria wrote, 'who is giving
him two hundred gulden for some compositions.'

These were 'three short concertos and a couple of
quartets for the flute', but to his father's unbridled fury
Wolfgang only received 96 gulden, since he failed to
complete the commission. He was never very interested in
the flute; but there was another reason for his inattention to
work.

In January 1778 he became acquainted with a small-part
singer at the court theatre, Herr Fridolin Weber, and was
soon in love with his seventeen-year-old daughter, Aloysia,
who, Leopold learned, 'sings admirably and has a lovely
pure voice. The only thing she lacks is dramatic action;
were it not for that she could be a prima donna on any
stage.' And Mozart promptly formulated plans to further
her career by travelling with the family to Italy. They would
go via Salzburg, an idea which probably raised Frau
Mozart's hopes of an early return home. If so, she reckoned
without the thunderous response of her husband: 'I am
quite willing to believe,' he wrote, 'that Mlle Weber sings
like a Gabrielli; that she has a powerful voice for the Italian
stage; that she has the build of a prima donna but ... what
impresario would not laugh were one to recommend to him
a girl of sixteen or seventeen who has never appeared on a
stage ... as for your proposal (I can hardly write when I

think of it) – your proposal to travel about with Herr Weber *and*, be it noted, his *two daughters* – it has nearly made me lose my reason ... could you *really* make up your mind to go trailing about the world with *strangers*? Quite apart from *your* reputation, what of your *old parents* and your *dear sister*?'

Such wild notions aside, Mozart had been seriously contemplating a visit to the French capital, where he had enjoyed such prodigious success as a child, so he was inclined to respond to his father's brisk injunction: 'Off with you to Paris! Find your place among great people. From Paris the name and fame of a man of great talent resounds throughout the whole world. There the nobility treat men of genius with the greatest deference, esteem and courtesy.' And Leopold was skilful enough to produce an argument which may have clinched the matter. 'Win fame and *make money* in Paris. Then, when you have money to spend, go off to Italy and get commissions for operas. This cannot be done by writing to impresarios. Then you could put forward Mlle Weber's name, which can more easily be done if you do so personally.'

In March, Mozart and his mother set off on the nine-day journey to Paris. They went in their own carriage but only because they had promised to sell it to their coachman on arrival. It was an inauspicious start to the saddest episode so far in Mozart's life.

Very soon Wolfgang began to look up the long list of contacts his father had given him, but in a city the size of Paris it was not that easy, now that they had no private means of transport. 'You say that I ought to pay a good many calls in order to make new acquaintances and revive the old ones. That, however, is out of the question. The distances are too great for walking – or the roads too

Opposite: Aloysia Weber, pictured here as Zemir in Gretry's opera Zemir et Azor. *Mozart was fond of the theatrical Weber family and 'wished nothing more than to make them happy', but it was the talented Aloysia who first won Mozart's heart in the 'golden liberty' of his days in Mannheim.*

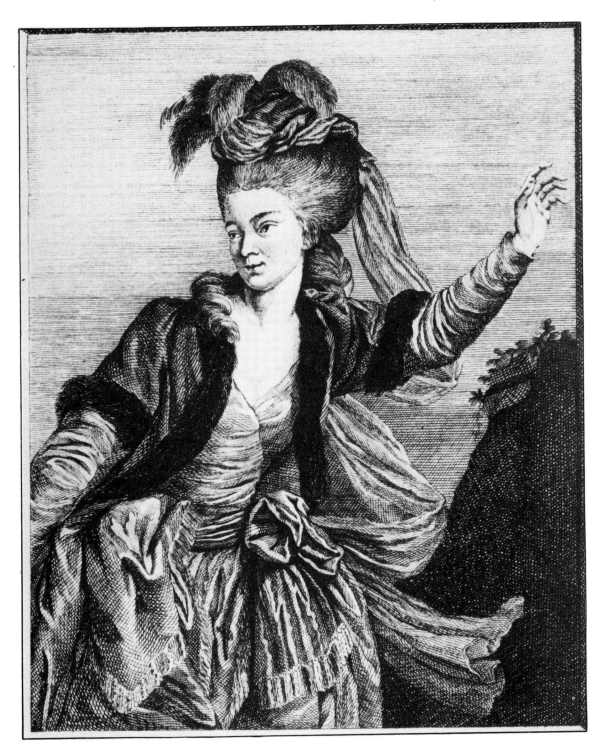

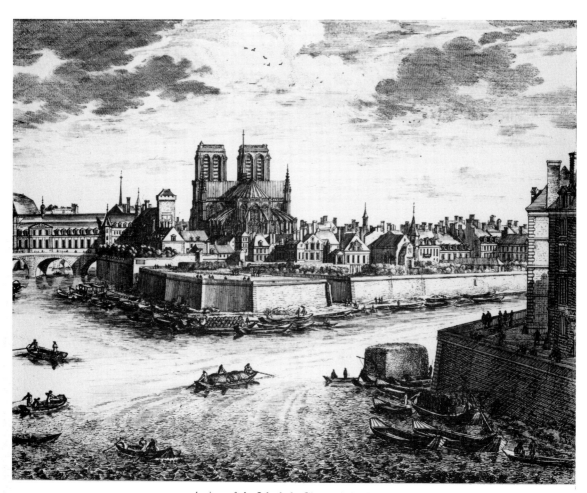

A view of the Isle de la Cité and the Church of Notre Dame in Paris. As an infant prodigy Mozart had been welcomed into Parisian homes but on this visit became despondent and foot-sore tramping the muddy streets for work.

muddy, for really the mud in Paris is beyond description. To take a carriage means that you have the honour of spending four to five livres a day, and all for nothing. People pay plenty of compliments it is true, but there it ends. Paris is greatly changed; the French are not nearly as polite as they were fifteen years ago.'

No doubt the Parisians had found a brilliant little boy of seven far more amusing than an ambitious young man of twenty-two. Fortunately Mozart had at least one influential supporter, Baron Melchior von Grimm, who had done a great deal to promote the interests of the family during their first visit to the French capital. He now sent Wolfgang on the rounds of his aristocratic friends. Let us hope he was sometimes received with more courtesy than the Duchesse de Chabot offered. In her house, Mozart wrote, 'I had to wait for half an hour in a large ice-cold unheated room that hadn't even a fireplace. At last the Duchess appeared. She asked me to make the best of the clavier in that room as none of her own were in good condition. I said that I should be delighted to try it, but that it was impossible at the moment as my fingers were numb with cold. "Oui, Oui, monsieur, you are quite right," was all the reply I got. She then sat down and commenced to draw, having as company some gentlemen who all sat in a circle round a big table while I had the honour to wait. There was total silence and I did not know what to do for cold, headache and boredom. At last I played on that miserable wretched pianoforte. But what vexed me most of all was that madame and her gentlemen never interrupted their drawing for a moment, so that I had to play to the chairs, tables and walls.'

Meanwhile Mozart's mother sat at home in the poor lodgings they had taken for the sake of economy. 'The room is dark,' she told Leopold, 'and looks out on a small closed yard. I can neither see the sun nor tell what the weather is. And for this we have to pay thirty livres a month!' Anna Maria complained to her husband about the food and the high prices in Paris and he sympathised, suggesting she should try to find someone who cooked 'in our German way', but he was unable to help with money. If life was hard in Paris, it was chaotic in Austria, where 'There is no talk of anything but the delivery of horses, and the transport of food ... people are being whipped off the streets and pulled out of their beds to be turned into soldiers. For heaven's sake use patience,' Leopold once again implored his son, 'and exert yourself!'

Since his lodgings had no piano, Wolfgang was already spending his days at the house of Jean le Gros, director of the Concert Spirituel. He planned a sinfonia concertante for four Mannheim players who were in Paris (their instruments were flute, oboe, horn and bassoon) but if Mozart ever wrote it, Le Gros failed to have it copied and it was not included in the concert where it was supposed to be performed. 'Something is going on behind the scenes,' was Mozart's suspicion: 'If this were a place where people had ears to hear, hearts to feel and some measure of taste for music, these things would only make me laugh heartily; but as it is, so far as music is concerned I am surrounded by brute beasts.' One of his trials was giving lessons in composition to the daughter of the Duc de Guines, 'a stupid and lazy girl' who 'had not an idea in her head'; what is more, he was kept waiting for his fees. Music lovers, however, gained from this unhappy experience since Mozart composed for father and daughter the Flute and Harp Concerto (K299), which is among his most beloved works.

In April 1778, things improved somewhat for the young composer and his mother. New lodgings were found for them which were altogether more congenial and contained a piano. Anna Maria was unwell for a time but her health improved. Wolfgang was offered the post of organist at Versailles, though Grimm advised against acceptance, realizing that composition was the young man's chief love.

On 18 June the Concert Spirituel opened with a magnificent symphony by Mozart known to us as the 'Paris', K297. He was bitterly disappointed with the playing at rehearsal and almost decided to stay away from the concert itself. However, at last he made up his mind to go, 'determined that if my symphony went as badly as at the rehearsal I would make my way into the orchestra, snatch the fiddle out of the hands of Lahoussaye and conduct myself.' In the event, all was well and the Parisians liked the piece ... 'particularly the last Allegro, because having observed that all *last* as well as *first* Allegros begin here with all the instruments playing in unison, I began mine with two violins only, piano for the first eight bars followed instantly by a forte. The audience, as I had expected, said "hush" at the beginning and when they heard the forte at once began to clap their hands. I was so happy that as soon as the symphony was over I went off to the Palais Royal where I had a large ice and said the rosary as I had vowed to do.'

Mozart gave his father this cheering news in a letter written at a moment of tragedy. On the day after the success of his symphony, Anna Maria had taken to her bed with a chill. Poorly nourished on cheap food and short of proper medical attention she rapidly got worse and on 3 July she died. Sitting by her bedside, Wolfgang could not bring himself to tell Leopold the bitter truth, saying only that his mother was very ill and that he had resigned himself wholly to the will of God. By the same post he begged a Salzburg friend, the Abbé Bullinger, to break the news to his father 'very gently. May God give him strength and courage.'

Wolfgang soon learned that Leopold and Nannerl were heartbroken and was reminded by his father, as if his own awareness were not sufficient, of the sacrifices his mother had made for him. At home the court organist, Anton Adlgasser, had died and there was reason to think Wolfgang could have the post if he returned forthwith to Salzburg. There were grounds for hope that permission for worthwhile travel abroad would not be withheld.

Mozart resisted. 'If I were to undertake the work, I should have to have complete freedom of action. The Chief Steward should have nothing to say to me in musical matters, or on any point relating to music. For a courtier can't do the work of a Kapellmeister, but a Kapellmeister can well be a courtier.' To Bullinger he wrote of 'the injustices which my dear father and I have endured at Salzburg which in themselves would be enough to make me wish to forget the place and blot it out of our memory forever.'

So Wolfgang remained in Paris for three further months, staying with Baron Grimm and Madame d'Épinay. A hoped-for commission from the Opéra did not materialise. As 'an act of friendship' he composed some music (*Les Petits Riens*) for the ballet master Noverre, which was used in a

totally forgotten piece by Gluck's rival Piccinni, and he
waited with impatience for the proofs of six violin sonatas
from a publisher.

Meanwhile Grimm, who had lent Mozart money,
aroused the young man's resentment by reminding him of

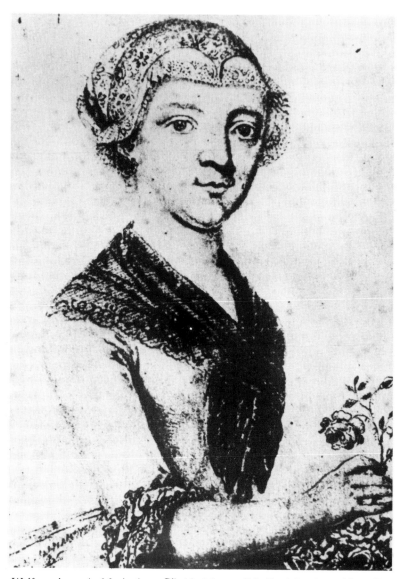

*Wolfgang's cousin Maria Anna Thekla Mozart ('the Bäsle'), pictured here. It
seems she shared Wolfgang's exuberant and sometimes scandalous sense of fun.*

his obligations and wrote pessimistically to Leopold about prospects in France for one who was 'too generous, not pushful, too easily deceived' and altogether lacking in the 'craft, enterprise and boldness' required for worldly success. On 26 September he was packed off for home on a coach which 'crawled at a snail's pace'.

Mozart himself was still in no hurry. After giving poorly attended concerts in Strasbourg, he returned to Mannheim, where he stayed for a month in the hope of a theatre commission. Then he went to Munich where Karl Theodor had now transferred his court, his orchestra and his opera, which meant that the Weber family were installed in the Bavarian capital.

There, Aloysia was enjoying some success as a singer and spurned the renewed advances of Wolfgang, whose future at that stage seemed to hold little promise, though this blow was softened to some extent by the presence in Munich of the cheerful 'Bäsle', who eventually accompanied Mozart back home. After presenting Karl Theodor's wife, the Electress Maria Elisabeth, with the violin sonatas which had been engraved in Paris, Wolfgang and his cousin left Bavaria and reached Salzburg on 15 January 1779.

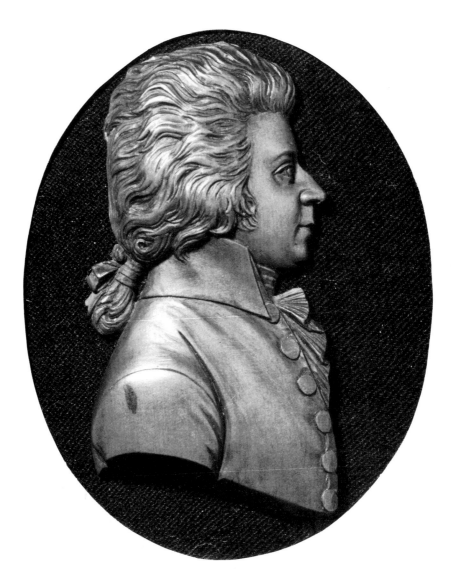

CHAPTER FOUR

THE FINAL BREAK
1779–81

*O*n his return to Salzburg, Mozart was appointed Court Organist and he remained at home for the best part of two years, carrying out the duties required of him by the Prince-Archbishop.

It was probably for a ceremony in the Spring of 1779, during which a crown was placed on a statue of the Virgin at the Church of Maria Plein on the outskirts of Salzburg, that Mozart wrote the Coronation Mass in C major, K317. For the cathedral he composed two settings of the service of Vespers and added to an earlier series of 'epistle sonatas' for organ and strings: they were so named because they were performed between the readings of the epistle and Gospel. Three symphonies date from this period – K318 in G, a short but spirited work, K319 in B flat for small orchestra and K338 in C, which has an andante movement of exceptional beauty. Perhaps the most splendid of all the Salzburg works is the Sinfonia Concertante for violin, viola and orchestra, K364, which heralds a new profundity from the young composer, still only in his early twenties.

Apart from composing and performing, Mozart was required as Court Organist to give keyboard lessons, so he was very fully employed during these two years spent at home with his father and sister. Meanwhile his reputation in the world outside Salzburg continued to grow, if slowly. The *Mercure de France* praised Mozart's symphonic style for its richness in ideas, adding, however, that it appealed more strongly to the mind than the heart. In the Spring of 1780, *La finta giardiniera* was given in German at Augsburg – probably the first time that an opera of Mozart's was given on a stage other than the one for which it was written. But in the same year any lingering hopes Mozart may have entertained about Aloysia Weber were finally extinguished when she married the court actor Joseph Lange in Vienna, and the routine of life at Salzburg became increasingly irksome to him, as we learn from the letters he wrote after leaving the city in November 1780 to complete an opera commissioned by the Elector Karl Theodor for the forthcoming Carnival season in Munich.

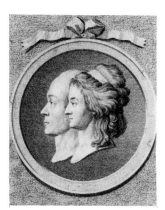

Aloysia Weber and Joseph Lange, married in 1779.

Mozart had begun work on what was to be the first of his great operas well before he left Salzburg, for the Court Chaplain there, Gianbattista Varesco, had been commissioned to provide the libretto. Once established in Munich, Mozart found it necessary to make many alterations to suit the talents of his singers and he was also at pains to simplify the text and make it more dramatically effective. Leopold Mozart acted as intermediary in a lengthy and acrimonious correspondence with Varesco, who eventually became very angry and demanded a higher fee. Since he had been asked to produce no less than four versions of the text and a good many additional alterations, he perhaps deserved better than to be dismissed by Leopold as 'a greedy, money-grubbing fool'. However, while keeping Varesco up to the mark, Leopold also treated his son to a torrent of advice. 'You must note all the [textual alterations] in your copy immediately, so that when you are composing the music, none of them may be overlooked,' Wolfgang was told; he was also warned, when composing, 'to consider not only the musical but the unmusical public. You must remember that to every ten real connoisseurs there are a hundred ignoramuses. So do not neglect the so-called popular style which tickles long ears.' There was also guidance about how to treat the orchestra in Munich: flattery was recommended as a specific for getting through long rehearsals, when the humblest viola player was as much in need of a pat on the back as anyone else.

It was left to Leopold to explain matters to the Archbishop when the six-week leave he had granted to Wolfgang ran out in mid-December, before rehearsals for the opera had even begun. There seems to have been no great pressure on him to return, but that did not prevent Wolfgang abusing his master in coded sentences, of which the following gives some idea: 'If only the Ass who smashes a *r*ing and by so doing *c*uts himself a *h*iatus in his *b*ehind so that *I* hear him *s*hit like a castrato with *h*orns and with his long ear *o*ffers to caress the fox's *p*osterior, were not so ... why, we could all live together.'

Mozart's sister Nannerl occupied part of her time sitting for a joint portrait with Wolfgang, who had himself been painted for the picture during the previous summer, and in mid-January she set out with their father for Munich, where they arrived in time for the dress rehearsal of *Idomeneo* on Mozart's birthday, 27 January. On the 29th, after two postponements, the first performance took place, to immense acclaim.

Idomeneo belongs to that well-defined genre of eighteenth-century theatrical entertainment, the *opera seria*. That is to say, it tells a story of classical antiquity in a manner akin to that of classical tragedy, which admits no light relief. Such pieces had often been loaded with irrelevant divertissements before the time of Gluck, who introduced a simpler, more dignified presentation in which every musical number was necessary to the unfolding story. Mozart, in his arguments with Varesco, was trying to achieve a similar effect.

The work which resulted is both powerful and passionate. It is the story of a King of Crete at the time of the Trojan wars. Praying to the sea-god for delivery from a storm at sea, he promises to sacrifice the first living thing he meets on shore. Alas, he is greeted by his son Idamante. A

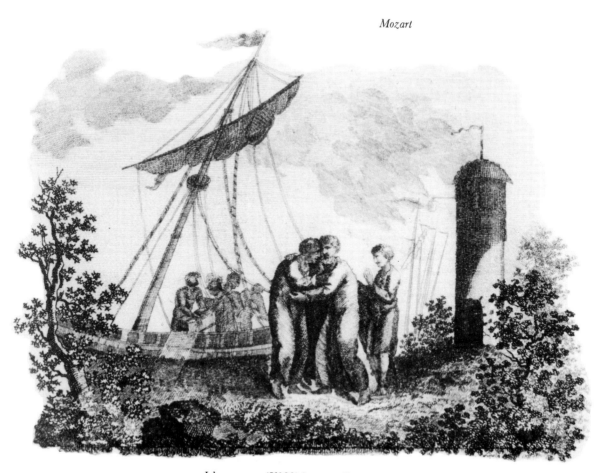

Idomeneo *(K366) is generally regarded as Mozart's first operatic masterpiece. First seen in Munich in January 1781, it tells of a king who unwittingly offers to sacrifice his son in gratitude to the sea-god for saving him from shipwreck. This vignette appeared in a vocal score of 1796.*

monster, which ravages the island when Idomeneo evades his vow, is killed by Idamante who, when he learns of his father's promise, offers himself as a sacrifice. At the last moment the voice of the sea-god is heard, sparing Idamante on condition that Idomeneo abdicates. Idamante becomes king, with Ilia, the woman he loves, as his consort. Among many splendid arias is Idomeneo's 'Fuor del mar' ('Out of the sea'), designed as a display piece of coloratura brilliance for Anton Raaff, the sixty-six-year-old tenor who created the part at Munich. In it, the king expresses his emotional suffering: although he has escaped the fury of the sea, an even worse storm rages in his breast.

After he had seen his opera successfully staged, Mozart was still in no hurry at all to return to Salzburg. He stayed on to make the most of the carnival season in Munich and paid a family visit to Augsburg with Nannerl and Leopold. Only after an absence of four months did Mozart pay heed, in mid-March, to the Archbishop's orders to join his household forthwith in Vienna. Colloredo had gone there to wait on Emperor Joseph II, who, following the death in November 1780 of Maria Theresa, now ruled alone, and to be near his ailing father, the Imperial Vice-Chancellor.

Required to perform on demand as a clavier player, Mozart was given 'a charming room' in Colloredo's house, but the domestic arrangements were not to his liking. 'The two valets sit at the top of the table,' he wrote home, 'but at least I have the honour of being placed above the cooks. I almost believe myself back in Salzburg!' Clearly Mozart had learned something from his father's tactics with fellow servants, for he added 'A good deal of silly, coarse joking goes on at the table, but no one cracks jokes with me, for I never say a word, or, if I have to speak, I always do so with the utmost gravity and as soon as I have finished my lunch, I get up and go off.' After his big success in Munich, it is easy to understand how deeply Mozart must have resented his return to servitude, underlined by the fact that others, like the orchestra leader Brunetti and the singer Ceccarelli, were allowed the freedom of choosing their own lodgings.

When the Archbishop's musicians gave a concert at the house of Prince Galitzin in March 1781, Mozart snubbed his colleagues by going there alone, and when he arrived, he walked straight up to the Prince and engaged him in conversation, leaving Ceccarelli and Brunetti to hover uncertainly behind the orchestra, 'not daring to come forward a single step'. According to his own account, all the nobility of Vienna had taken Mozart's part against the Archbishop when permission was refused for Mozart to appear at a charity concert for the Wiener Tonkünstler-societät; however, at Prince Galitzin's soirée, Colloredo changed his mind. The result was a big triumph for Mozart

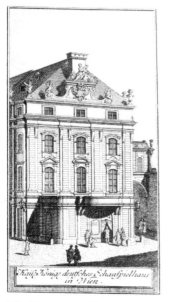

The Kärntnertor Theatre.

at the Kärntnertor Theatre in April. But causes of resentment continued to multiply. On the very night when he might have been playing before the Emperor for a big fee at Countess Thun's, Mozart was required for a concert at the house of Colloredo's father, and worse still, the Archbishop refused permission for Mozart to give a public concert which he believed would be very profitable. He wrote to his father: 'When I think that I must leave Vienna without bringing home at least a thousand gulden, my heart is sore indeed. For the sake of a malevolent Prince who plagues me every day and only pays me a lousy salary of four hundred gulden, am I to kick away a thousand? For I should certainly make that sum if I were to give a concert.'

At this stage, although toying with the possibility of an independent career, Mozart still intended to return to Salzburg when the Archbishop's visit to Vienna was over and improvised variations on a theme proposed by Colloredo at a farewell concert in Vienna at the end of April. However, when the Archbishop tried yet again to put Mozart down by ordering him to take back a parcel to Salzburg forthwith, the patience he was endeavouring to show for the sake of his father finally cracked. Wolfgang refused the commission, saying he needed to remain in Vienna for a few days to collect money owing to him. Bidden to leave Colloredo's house at once, he took refuge with the Webers. On 9 May, he had an open row with the Archbishop. 'Well young fellow,' Colloredo began, 'when are you going off?' Mozart said he could not go that day, making the transparent excuse that the coach was full. The Archbishop told him he had better go that day or he would have his salary stopped; Mozart was 'the most dissolute fellow he knew, no one served him so badly'; he was 'a scoundrel, a rascal, a vagabond'. Pleading for his father's understanding, Mozart's letter home continued: 'Then my blood began to boil, I could no longer contain myself and I said: "So your Grace is not satisfied with me?" "What, you dare to threaten me? ... There is the door! Look out, for I will have nothing more to do with such a miserable wretch."

At last I said "Nor I with you!" "Well, be off!" When leaving the room I said "This is final. You shall have it tomorrow in writing!"'

The following day Wolfgang tried to return to Count Arco the money he had been given for the journey and to hand in a petition for dismissal, but the diplomatic Arco told Mozart he should not take such a step without consulting his father. A week later another similar interview followed. Sensibly, Arco told Mozart that if he remained alone in Vienna he could not expect the fickle Viennese to support him for long, that he should stop giving the Archbishop the impression that he was 'insufferably insolent' and swallow his pride. But that was not Mozart's way. 'I treat people as they treat me,' was his reply. 'When I see that someone despises me and treats me with contempt, I can be as proud as a peacock.'

The final break came early in June. Once again Arco refused to accept Mozart's petition and, no doubt exasperated by the pressure put on him by the Archbishop, by Leopold and by the young man himself, shoved him out of the door with a kick. 'So that's the way to win people over, to soften them up!' wrote Mozart. 'Throwing them out of doors with a kick on the behind. That's the style!'

Now aged sixty-one, Leopold feared not only for his son's future but his own, since Wolfgang was threatening revenge on Arco, summing up his courageous if foolhardy attitude with the words: 'Although I am not a count, I have more honour in my heart than has many a count. Lackey or count, whoever insults me is treated by me as a rascal.' Feeling that he had finally thrown off his fetters, Mozart now abandoned the use of cypher in letters home, though there is evidence that from time to time they were still read by Colloredo. To such a man, Mozart must have seemed intolerably arrogant: 'I am more respected in Vienna than the Archbishop,' claimed Wolfgang. 'He is only known as a presumptuous, conceited ecclesiastic who despises everyone here, whereas I am considered a very amiable person.'

As Mozart set out to make a life for himself in Vienna, he

begged his father not to worry about his prospects. 'I have here,' he wrote, 'the finest and most useful acquaintances in the world. I am liked and respected by the greatest families.' Then, as now, good contacts were vital to the success of a freelance musician, and the more aristocratic they were in Imperial Vienna the better. The Emperor Joseph II has been described as the most thorough of the enlightened despots of the eighteenth century. A declared enemy of superstition and outmoded tradition, he sought to create a strong centralised state out of the disparate territories and nationalities over which he ruled. He promoted religious toleration, relaxed censorship and encouraged education, and although the total effect of his reign was to leave the Hapsburg Empire in greater turmoil than before, Vienna in the early 1780s was a stimulating place for a rising young artist.

Believing in the stage as an instrument of propaganda, Joseph decreed that the Burgtheater should become a national theatre with the object of bringing unity through

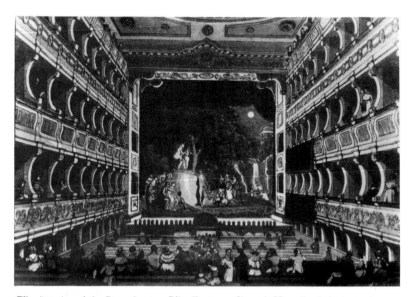

The interior of the Burgtheater. The Emperor Joseph II realised the importance of drama as a means of bringing unity to his widespread, polyglot domains, and made the Burgtheater into a national institution.

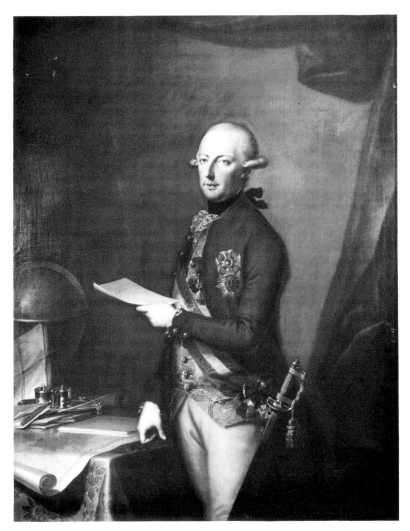

The Emperor Joseph II, pictured here in military uniform, was initially an enlightened ruler, encouraging education and religious tolerance.

culture to his diverse subjects. Though now banished to the suburbs, the popular theatre, stimulated by the spirit of rivalry, flourished as never before under the leadership of such men as Karl Marinelli, who built a new theatre at Leopoldstadt, and Emanuel Schikaneder, the future librettist of Mozart's *The Magic Flute* and already the most popular and accomplished theatrical figure of his time in Austria.

In 1780 Vienna was a city of 175,000 people which had doubled its population in forty years, a prosperous and cosmopolitan centre which flourished despite a series of wars in which Austria was often defeated. Though the majority of people were fervent Catholics, freemasonry was spreading rapidly and the absence of censorship allowed a stream of outspoken pamphlets to appear with such titles as *Is the Emperor Right?* and *The Degradation of the Lay Clergy.* On a more popular level there was the anti-clerical *Mamma wants to send me to a convent!*

Self-denial was out of fashion in a city denounced by some visitors for its excessive love of pleasure, a taste which matched in extravagance the decorative exuberance of Viennese Baroque architecture. Approaching Vienna from the river in the course of his Musical Tours, Dr Charles Burney was impressed by the 'forty or fifty towers and spires' which rose above the city, and although he found that the streets were 'rendered doubly dark and dirty by

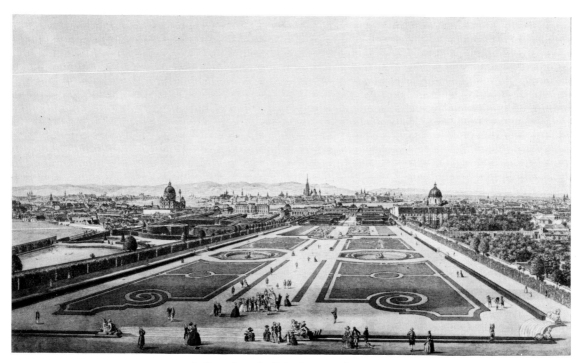

A view above the Belvedere over the terraced gardens in Vienna.

their narrowness and by the extreme height of the houses,' he thought the houses themselves were 'grand and magnificent in appearance' thanks to their 'elegant style of architecture in which the Italian taste prevails, as in music'.

It was a city where music abounded at all hours of the day and night. A band of 'French horns, clarinets, hautboys and bassoons', though 'miserably out of tune', serenaded Burney during meals and in the evening at his inn, *The Gold Ox*; one Sunday morning he was stopped in the street by a procession 'three miles long, singing a hymn to the Virgin in three parts', and he was surprised to hear even the soldiers on guard singing together in harmony. Innumerable festivals gave rise to dancing in the public pleasure gardens which, in any case, according to a visitor from Berlin in 1781, were always full of working-class people after five in the afternoon. As for their 'betters', they were not slow to subscribe to a forthcoming series of concerts provided the musician concerned was able to catch the popular fancy.

Mozart was right in thinking that if any city in the Europe of his time could give him a living, it was Vienna.

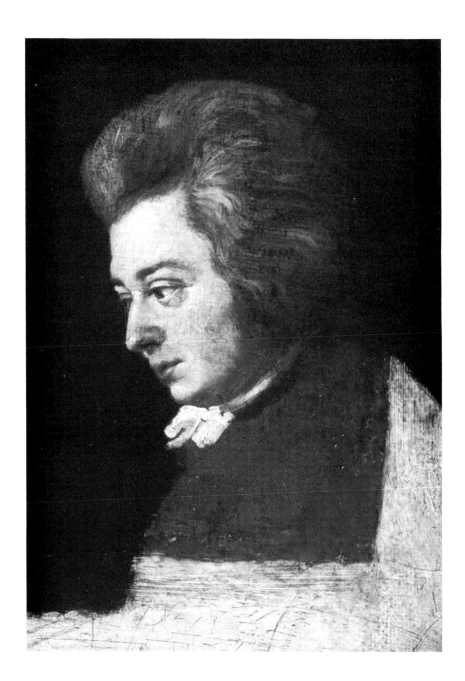

CHAPTER FIVE

SUCCESS IN VIENNA
1781–86

*M*ozart's life as a freelance musician began modestly enough. In 1781 he apologised to his father for sending him only thirty ducats because so far he had only one pupil and could 'only just make both ends meet'. But before the end of the month he was engaged to teach the daughter of an Economic Counsellor, Josepha von Auernhammer, a lady of influence as well as musical talent; the only difficulty here was that she was ugly ('as fat as a farm wench', said Mozart) and that she fell in love with her teacher.

The unattached Wolfgang attracted any number of rumours about his amorous activities, many of them circulated by dedicated enemies such as the Czech player Leopold Kozeluch, who was no doubt jealous of Mozart's talent and who preserved his own reputation by playing in public as little as possible. One Herr von Moll expressed the hope that Mozart would soon return to Salzburg as he was 'only in Vienna for the sake of the women', and further scandal was caused by his continued residence at the Webers', where it was supposed he was too intimately involved with Aloysia's sister Constanze. Wolfgang felt it necessary to deny all these allegations firmly in letters home to his father, asserting in July 1781 that he was only just beginning to live and that God had not given him his talent 'that I might attach it to a wife and waste my youth in idleness'. Mozart left the Webers, lodging briefly with the Auernhammers – a move hardly likely to improve his reputation in view of Josepha's known feelings – before taking a room on his own in the inner city.

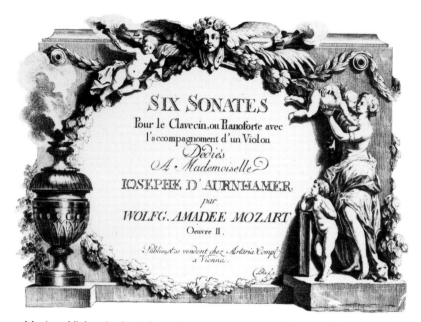

Music publishers in the eighteenth century constructed elaborate titlepages, as the frontispiece of Mozart's violin sonatas (K296, 376–380) shows. The sonatas were dedicated to Josepha von Auerhammer, an influential but alas unappealing pupil.

The year 1781 brought the publication of six sonatas for clavier and violin, and in July Mozart received the libretto for a play with music in the German tradition (Singspiel), from Gottlieb Stephanie, dramatist at the Burgtheater. This was *The Abduction from the Seraglio* (*Die Entführung aus dem Serail*), an entertainment strongly laced with the fashionable Turkish flavour, intended for a forthcoming state visit, though in the event production was delayed until the following year. Meanwhile personal problems continued to worry the young musician.

In December, despite his former resistance to the notion

of 'settling down', he broached to his father the idea of marriage. He had never been one, he said, to seduce innocent girls, but 'the voice of nature speaks as loud in me as in many a big lout of a fellow'; moreover, he had never been accustomed to look after his own belongings – 'linen, clothes and so forth' – and was convinced he could 'manage better with a wife' even on his existing income.

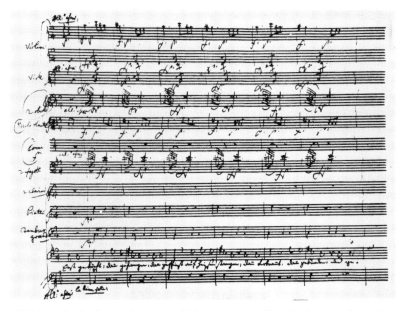

1782 brought the first performance of Mozart's opera The Abduction from the Seraglio *(K384). This piece from the manuscript of one of Osmin's arias shows the assurance of Mozart's scoring. When the Emperor remarked that the opera had too many notes, Mozart told him there were just the right number.*

Mozart was doing his best to rationalise a situation he could not avoid, for such was the gossip involving his name with that of Constanze Weber that the Webers' family guardian extracted a promise from him to marry Constanze within three years, in default of which he would have to make her a handsome annual allowance.

At the end of 1781, while these problems were still unresolved, Mozart took part in a keyboard competition before the Emperor at the Hofburg. His opponent, the acclaimed virtuoso and composer Muzio Clementi (1752–

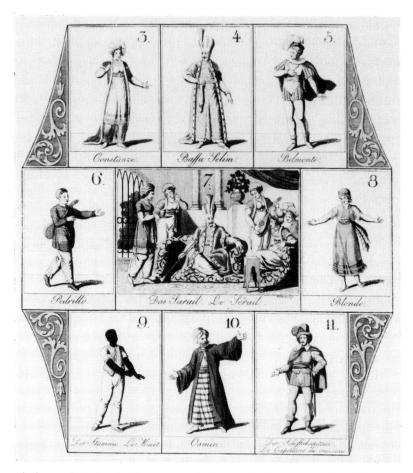

A picture-sheet showing the stage set (centre) and main characters from The Abduction from the Seraglio, c. *1800.*

1832), spoke of Mozart, who was regarded as the winner, in generous terms, but Wolfgang was less charitable. He dismissed Clementi as 'a charlatan, like all Italians ... His greatest strength lies in his passages in thirds. Apart from this he has not a kreuzer's worth of taste or feeling – in short he is simply a mechanicus.'

Mozart's constant hopes for an appointment at court were in no way advanced by the competition, though he was well paid for taking part in it. During the early part of 1782, however, he gave an important concert at the Burgtheater and helped to inaugurate a subscription series in the Augarten. July brought the first performance at the

Burgtheater of *The Seraglio*. It is said that the Emperor, who was present, remarked that the opera had 'very many notes', to which Mozart replied 'exactly the right number, your Majesty'. Although both the first and second performances provoked a certain amount of hissing from cabals organized by Mozart's enemies, the work was a success from the start. Gluck, the most respected operatic composer in Vienna at the time, requested an extra performance, and in the world outside Vienna *The Seraglio* was to become the most successful of all Mozart's stage works in his lifetime.

It tells the story of a lover, Belmonte, who rescues his loved one, Constanze, together with her English maid and Belmonte's servant from the harem of a Turkish Pasha. The Pasha, though in love with Constanze, magnanimously forgives them in the end. There is much superb music for the principal characters, including Constanze's great aria 'Martern aller Arten' in which she declares that whatever torture she has to endure, she will remain faithful to Belmonte. The piece owes a great measure of its popularity to the Pasha's comic servant Osmin, a character who obviously appealed to Mozart, for he requested his librettist to enlarge the part.

No sooner was *The Seraglio* launched than Mozart implored his father to give consent to his marriage with the real-life Constanze: 'My heart is restless and my head is confused; in such a condition how can one think and work to any good purpose?' On 3 August the marriage contract was signed and the day after the couple were married in St Stephen's Cathedral. The Baroness von Waldstädten gave a 'princely' supper for them, Gluck invited the young couple to dinner and Leopold's consent arrived, a little late but nonetheless received with great relief by Wolfgang: 'I kiss your hands and thank you with all the tenderness which a son has ever felt for a father, for your kind consent and fatherly blessing.'

That Leopold was still far from happy about his son's welfare is made clear in a letter to the Baroness, begging her to keep an eye on Wolfgang. 'Two opposing elements rule

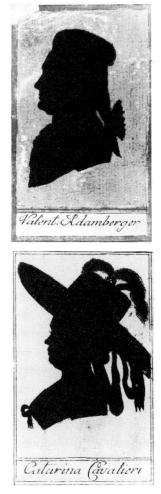

Two of the principal singers in the first performance of The Abduction from the Seraglio, *Valenti Adambergen and Catarina Cavalieri.*

Above and opposite:
On 3 August 1782, Mozart signed the contract binding him in marriage to Constanze Weber. Only five people attended the wedding including Constanze's mother and her guardian. Leopold's consent to the union arrived by post the following day.

his nature', said Leopold. 'There is either too much or too little, never the golden mean. If he is not actually in want, then he becomes indolent and lazy. If he has to bestir himself, then he realises his worth and *wants to make his fortune at once.* Nothing must stand in his way; yet it is unfortunately the most capable people and those who possess outstanding genius who have the greatest obstacles to face.'

Im Nahmen der allerheiligsten Dreyfaltigkeit, Gott des Vaters, Sohns und heil. Geistes. Amen.

It also appears from this letter that the elder Mozart was being victimised in Salzburg for his son's behaviour towards the Archbishop, though Leopold did his best to come to terms with his situation: 'I live quietly with my daughter and have a few friends who come to see me. Reading, music and an occasional walk are our recreation and in bad weather a very humble game ... of chess.'

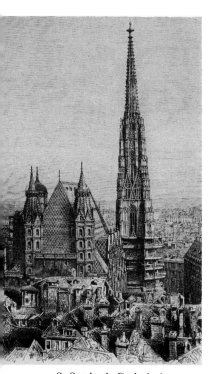

St Stephen's Cathedral was the setting for Mozart's marriage in 1782 and for his funeral service nine years later.

The pressure surrounding his marriage in no way blinded Wolfgang to Constanze's good qualities – her common sense and kind heart outweighing an absence of wit and a tendency to extravagance – and he was eager to take his new wife to Salzburg to meet his father and sister. Mozart started work on the grandest of all his settings of the Mass – in C minor, K427 – with the intention of having it performed during this projected Salzburg visit. No one knows exactly why the work was never completed but perhaps it was because the start of a new season in Vienna held out the promise of more pupils and concert opportunities, and for the time being the visit was postponed. There was, besides, the possibility of a permanent appointment as music master to the Princess of Württemberg: Mozart had been recommended by the Archduke Maximilian and had to mask his disappointment when the post went to Georg Summer, clavier instructor to the Imperial Court. He was able to convince himself that his income from pupils already matched the salary he might have expected from the Princess.

However, the need to make money by teaching became increasingly irksome to Mozart, for it took time which might have been devoted to his 'beloved composition'. He had to complete three piano concertos, apart from writing a good deal of small-scale instrumental music and dance music, and these marked the beginning of one of his finest achievements as a composer: the series of great dialogues for piano and orchestra which virtually created the piano concerto as we know it. The concertos in F, A and C (K413, 414 and 415) were described by Mozart as 'a happy medium between what is too easy and too difficult; they are very brilliant, pleasing to the ear and natural, without being vapid. There are passages here and there from which connoisseurs alone can derive satisfaction; but these passages are written in such a way that the less learned cannot fail to be pleased, though without knowing why'. The three concertos were published in the winter of 1782, at a time when his reputation stood high as 'one of the greatest virtuosi in Europe'. 'At his incomparable pianoforte,' wrote a member of the audience at an Augarten concert of this period, 'he several times caused us to feel sweet enchantment and the admiration due to him for his brilliant performance.' Nor was Wolfgang's fame confined to Vienna; in March 1783, a Hamburg music magazine indicated his standing when it predicted that the thirteen-year-old Beethoven was 'sure to become a second Wolfgang Amadeus Mozart if he progresses as he has already begun'.

The newly-married couple were able to move into progressively better lodgings, eventually attaining the coveted status of a first-floor apartment in April 1783. During the Carnival season that year, they had given an all-night ball in a house in the Wipplingerstrasse where they were staying at the time, though when writing to Leopold for the loan of his Harlequin costume, Wolfgang took care to inform his father that he had made the gallants pay for the privilege of attending his party. However, whether that was the case or not, it seems the Mozarts were already living beyond their means, for in the spring of 1783 Mozart asked the Baroness von Waldstädten for a loan to settle a debt.

To all appearances, Mozart was doing well. In March 1783 he took part in a concert arranged by his sister-in-law, Aloysia Lange, at the Burgtheater; it was attended by Gluck, who warmly praised Mozart's Symphony K297 (the one he had written in Paris) and invited the Mozarts and Langes to his home. A fortnight later Wolfgang was gratified by the presence of the Emperor at a concert of his own in the same theatre. It was a resounding success; the Emperor was delighted, and Mozart believed he might have been even more generously rewarded if the Imperial gift of money had been made after the concert, instead of being deposited at the box office beforehand, as the custom was.

In May, the question of a visit to Salzburg was again discussed, but as Mozart had never been officially dismissed by the Archbishop he thought he might be arrested when he got there. His situation in Vienna was altogether different; when the Mozart's first child was born in June, Baron Wetzlar offered to stand godfather, though this caused a passing difficulty with Mozart senior. Wolfgang had fully intended to name the boy Leopold, but just before the christening Wetzlar kissed the child and said 'so now you have a little Raimund' (the name of the Baron's eldest son). Mozart felt he could not offend his patron, so Raimund Leopold it had to be.

Leopold had dismissed as 'mere humbug' Wolfgang's fears about returning to Salzburg, and the young couple had set off in July for their long-promised visit to Mozart's native city. Parts of the incomplete C minor Mass were performed during the visit to St Peter's Church, with Constanze as soprano soloist, but the three-month family reunion was only a qualified success and on 27 October the young Mozarts left to return to Vienna via Linz, where they spent three weeks as guests of Count Thun. Mozart was asked to give a concert in the theatre, for which a major work was required, but this placed him in a difficulty. 'As I have not a single symphony with me,' he told Leopold, 'I am writing a new one at breakneck speed.' This was the Symphony in C, K425, now known as the 'Linz'.

Back in Vienna, where baby Raimund had died in his absence (from intestinal cramp), Wolfgang entered on the most flourishing period of his life. In the year 1784 he was in constant demand for concerts, giving no fewer than nineteen in the month of March alone. He was also composing at a feverish rate, so the Mozarts' domestic regime was severe; they were never in bed before midnight, and up at five or half past five most mornings; no wonder the maid they had brought with them from Salzburg complained of lack of sleep. The first report of Mozart's poor health dates from this period of excessive activity: in the summer he suffered what was probably a kidney infection, with violent bouts of vomiting.

During that year Mozart produced six of his finest piano concertos, one of which, K449 in E flat, he sent to his father in February, asking him not to show it to a single soul. Wolfgang had composed it for the daughter of a court coun-

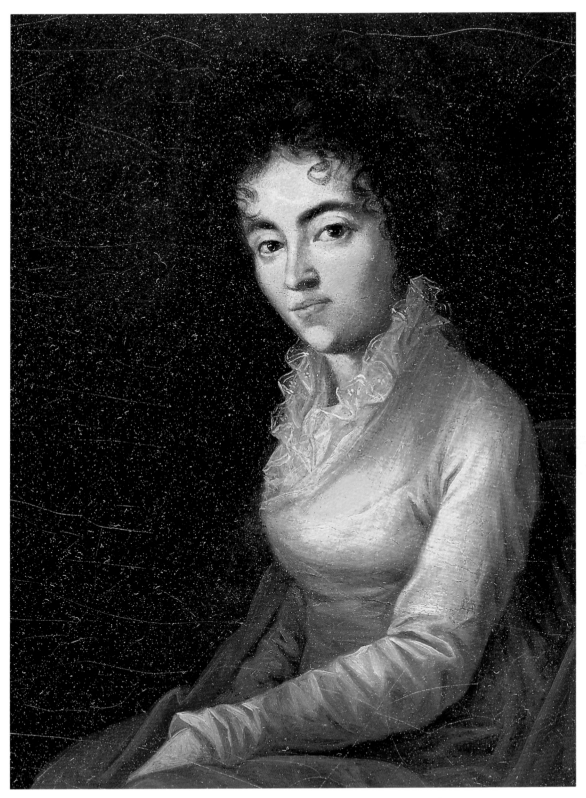

Constanze Mozart, painted shortly after her marriage to Wolfgang, by her brother-in-law Joseph Lange.

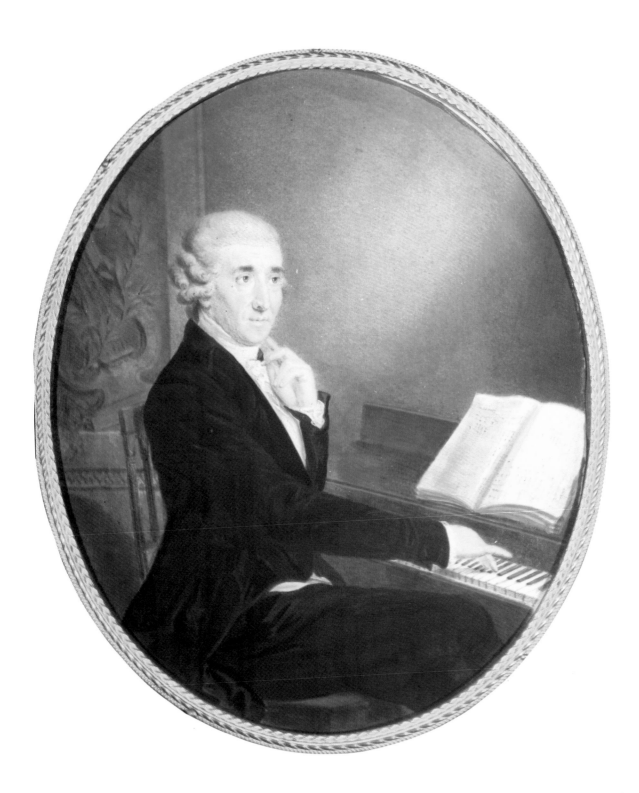

Joseph Haydn (1732–1809). Mozart was an admirer of this challenging and influential composer and was equally admired in return.

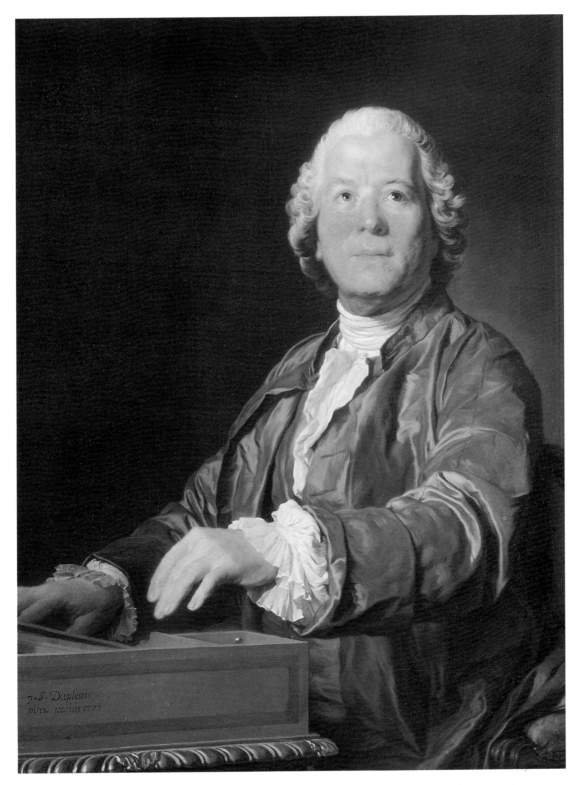

Christoph Willibald Gluck (1714–87). The influential German composer, portrayed here at the spinet, who pioneered musical simplicity in opera with Alceste *and* Orpheus and Eurydice. *During his retirement in Vienna, Gluck became friendly with both Mozart and Salieri.*

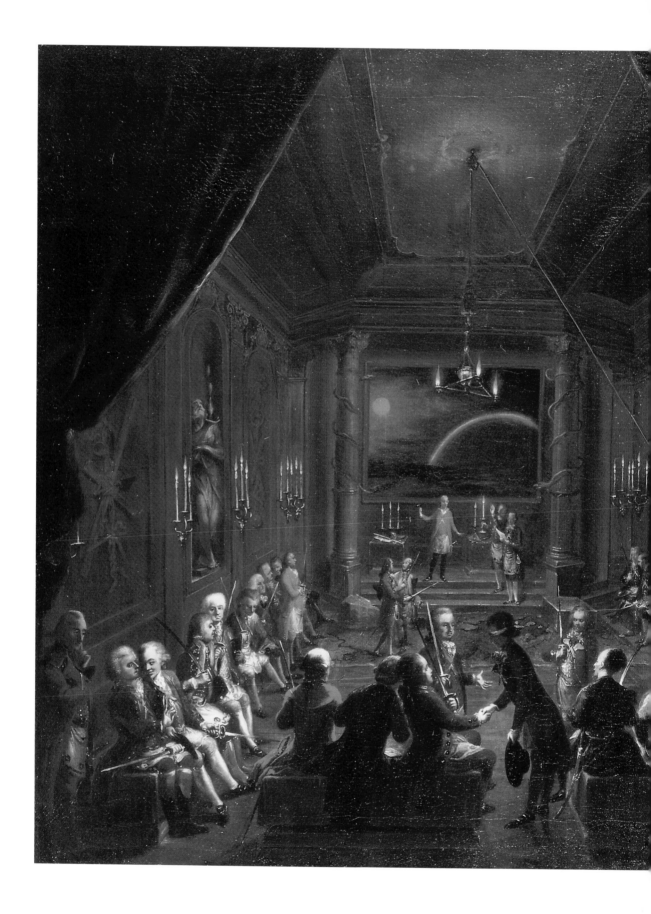

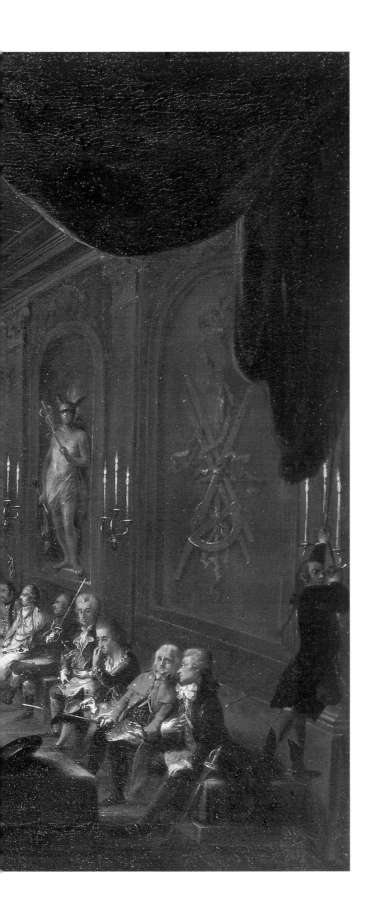

The egalitarian principles of Freemasonry strongly appealed to Mozart, who was elected apprentice at the Viennese lodge 'Beneficence' when he was twenty-nine. This anonymous painting shows a meeting of the Masonic lodge 'Crowned Hope' in Vienna. The figure on the extreme right is probably Mozart.

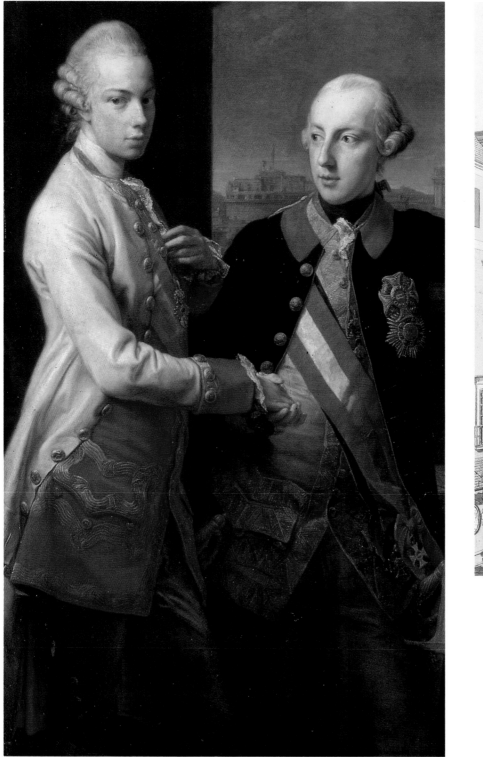

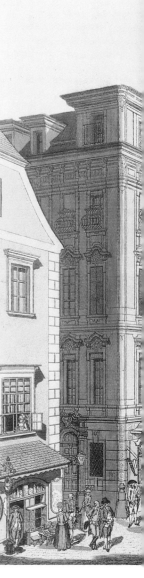

The Emperor Joseph II (right) with his brother Leopold, who succeeded Joseph to the Imperial throne in 1790.

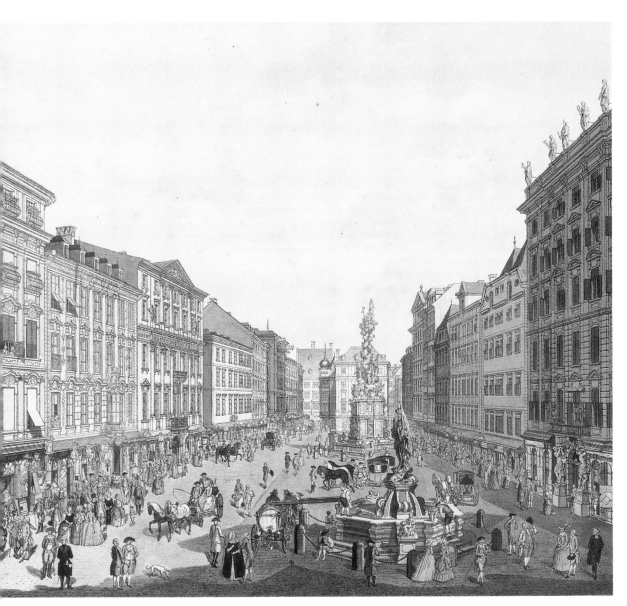

The Graben, shown here in an engraving of 1781, was, and still is, one of Vienna's most fashionable streets. Here, in the heart of the city, Mozart lived from 1781–2 and again in 1784. At that time his prospects both as composer and keyboard virtuoso looked bright.

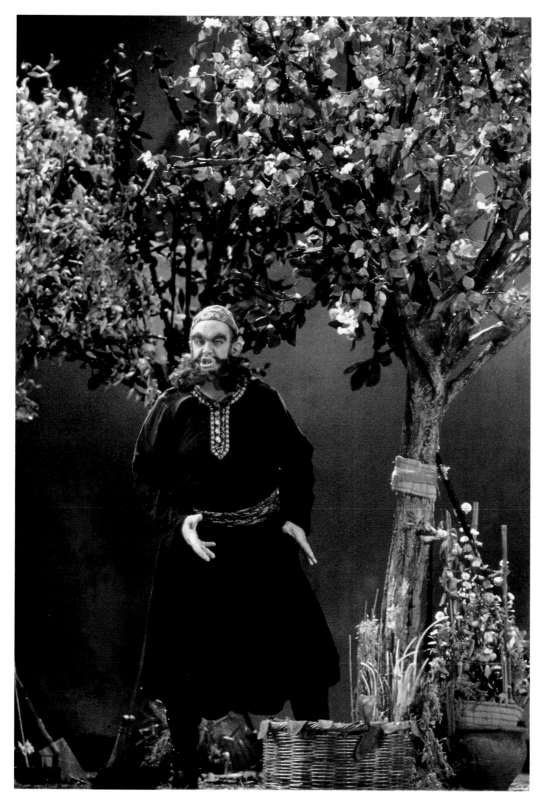

The Pasha's servant Osmin, played by Kurt Möll, in this 1989 performance of The Abduction
from the Seraglio *(K384), staged in the Royal Opera House.*

This is an autograph sketch for one of the piano concertos (K467a) which Mozart composed in the 1780s. Financial worries clearly loomed large since calculations are scribbled all over the music on this page.

cillor and been well paid – a much better arrangement, in Mozart's view, than giving his work to an engraver who would then swindle him by 'printing off as many copies as he likes'. He formed the intention of publishing in the future only by collecting subscribers in advance; the large number of people who were willing to subscribe for his concerts seemed a promising augury.

Apart from concertos, Mozart was producing music of several other kinds at this time, including works for one and two pianos, three superb wind serenades and a number of other chamber works including the six string quartets he dedicated to Haydn, which were published in 1785. These works were written under the influence of Haydn's own quartets, particularly those of op. 33, which are notable for their contrapuntal integration of four independent parts.

Mozart probably met Haydn in 1781 and a friendship grew up between them which was furthered by the quartet parties in which they both participated. The singer Michael

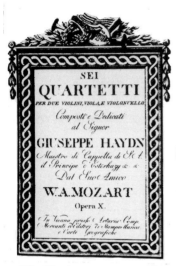

The Haydn quartets, a set of six string quartets which bear witness to Mozart's great admiration for Joseph Haydn.

Kelly referred to one such party at the house of the English composer Stephen Storace in 1784 when 'the players were tolerable; not one of them excelled on the instrument he played, but there was a little science among them, which I daresay will be acknowledged when I name them:

The First Violin .... **Haydn**
The Second Violin .... **Dittersdorf**
The Violoncello .... **Vanhall**
The Tenor [viola] .... **Mozart**.'

The 'Haydn quartets' were the result of 'long and laborious endeavour' on the part of Mozart, eager as he was to please the dedicatee. As for Haydn, his admiration for Mozart was unbounded, and it is pleasant to record that Wolfgang's father was able to experience this outstanding testimony to his son's success at first hand.

In August 1784, Wolfgang's sister Nannerl married a government official at St Gilgen, Johann von Berchtold zu Sonnenburg. Just before the event Wolfgang wrote to her, expressing the brotherly hope that the letter would reach her while she was still a Vestal Virgin – 'another few days and ... it is gone!' 'Our only regrets,' he added in the same letter, 'are for our dear father who will now be left so utterly alone.' One palliative, Mozart knew, would be to invite his father to Vienna, where he would be in his element helping to organise the incessant round of concerts.

Leopold reached Vienna on 11 February 1785, and the day after his arrival he joined Wolfgang and two other players in performing three of the 'Haydn quartets' in the presence of Haydn himself. It must surely have been gratifying when he heard from Haydn's own lips on this occasion the famous declaration: 'Before God and as an honest man, I tell you that your son is the greatest composer known to me either in person or by name. He has taste, and what is more, the most profound knowledge of composition.'

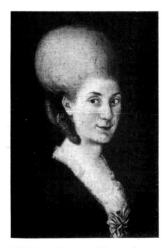

Wolfgang's sister Nannerl.

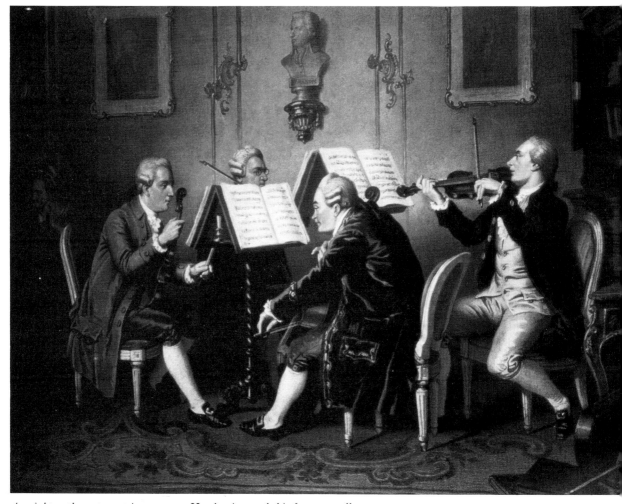

*An eighteenth-century string quartet. Haydn pioneered this form, usually
allowing the first violin to dominate over the other string instruments.*

So much for a great fellow-composer's seal of approval.
As for the popular view of Mozart at this time we can gain
some idea from Schink's rather gushing *Literary Fragments*
published in Graz: there Mozart is praised as 'great and
original in his compositions, and a master when seated at
the keyboard. His concerto on the Piano-forte, how excellent that was! And his improvisations, what a wealth of
ideas! What variety! What contrasts in passionate sounds!

One swims away with him unresistingly on the stream of his emotions.'

Predictably, Leopold was delighted by the acclaim which greeted his son wherever he went and by the money which appeared to be flowing in. A month after he arrived he told Nannerl in a letter that 'since my arrival your brother's forte-piano has been taken at least a dozen times to the theatre or some other house.' He rubbed his hands over the takings at a major concert in the Burgtheater on top of the proceeds from six subscription concerts, and offered the opinion that 'if my son has no debts to pay, I think he can now lodge two thousand gulden in the bank. Certainly the money is there, and so far as eating and drinking are concerned, the housekeeping is extremely economical.'

Just before his father arrived in Vienna, Wolfgang was elected to the Masonic lodge 'Beneficence' as an apprentice, but very soon advanced beyond this lowest of grades. In March 1785, Leopold was admitted to the same lodge and made even more rapid progress, being promoted from apprentice to master in little more than two weeks. This unusual haste was caused by Leopold's imminent departure from Vienna. For once following his son's example, he had overstayed the six weeks leave of absence granted him by the Archbishop, and under the threat of having his salary stopped if he stayed away any longer, he left for home on 25 April.

There now followed a period when Mozart's letters to Salzburg were fewer and further between. In November, Leopold complained to Nannerl that he had not heard from his son for a month; shortly afterwards he received a few lines giving the reason, or at any rate one reason: he was 'up to the eyes in work on *Le nozze di Figaro*', and Leopold was understanding enough to realize that 'there will be a lot of running about and discussions before [Wolfgang] gets the libretto so adjusted as to suit his purpose exactly, and no doubt according to his charming habit, he has kept on postponing matters and has let the time slip by.'

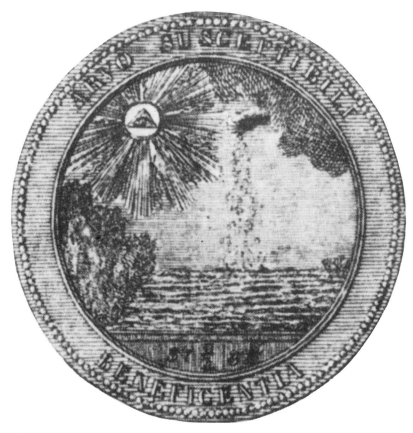

This is the seal of the Viennese Masonic lodge Zur Wohlthätigkeit *(Beneficence) to which Mozart belonged. In 1785 there were, in all, eight Masonic Lodges in Vienna, but in December of that year Emperor Joseph ordered that the number be reduced to not more than three.*

Mozart could not really afford to concentrate on composition at the expense of performing. Though we have Leopold's word for it that Constanze's housekeeping was not lavish, the couple did consider it indispensable to keep up appearances, and the struggle to make ends meet became ever more difficult. In November 1785, Mozart implored the composer and publisher Franz Anton Hoffmeister to help out with some money 'which I need very badly at the moment'. At about this time he drove himself to prepare three new piano concertos for the Lent concert season of 1786, while devoting most of his energy to his latest operatic venture, *The Marriage of Figaro.*

Exactly how Mozart came to decide on this subject is not clear. He had read through a large number of plays and had even begun to set one by Lorenzo da Ponte, the poet to the Imperial Theatres in Vienna; this subject, *Lo sposo deluso* (The Deceived Husband), was soon abandoned, probably on account of the weakness of the libretto. In January 1785, the Emperor instructed the censor to ban from the Viennese stage Beaumarchais's wittily subversive play *Le mariage de Figaro* 'since this piece contains much that is objectionable'. But the play, though not performed in Vienna, was printed, and from this Mozart and da Ponte fashioned a piece from which the politically offensive material was removed without making the characters into spineless puppets. Endowed with a ceaseless flow of Mozart's fine music, *Figaro* is one of the greatest and most human of all operatic comedies.

It is a story of intrigue in an aristocratic household. The Count is attracted by his wife's maid Susanna, who is betrothed to the valet Figaro, though Figaro in turn has to get out of an obligation to marry someone else. The page Cherubino is banished to the army by the Count for excessive flirting; the Countess is distraught because she thinks she has lost her husband's love. After many ingenious twists and turns, everyone's problems are resolved, thanks to the ready wit of the plebian Figaro rather than good sense on the part of his social superiors.

Mozart needed all the persistence he could command to get his new opera produced. The tenor Michael Kelly tells us that works by Gluck and Righini were awaiting production at much the same time and cabals were feverishly active in support of Mozart's rivals. Finally a decree from the Emperor himself settled the matter: *The Marriage of Figaro* was to be put into rehearsal forthwith. Perhaps Mozart had won a good measure of Imperial favour through the one-act opera *Der Schauspieldirektor* (The Impresario) he had composed for a private festivity at

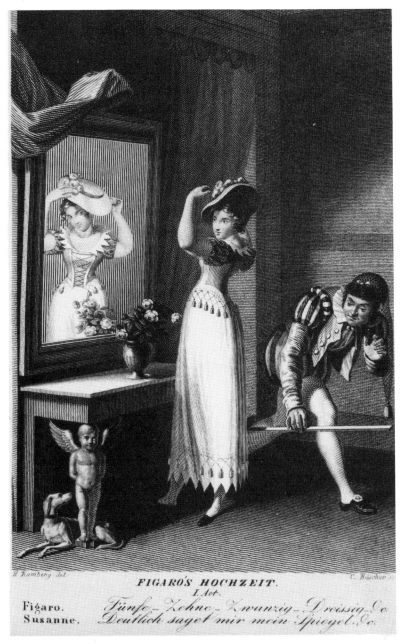

FIGARO'S HOCHZEIT.
I. Act.

Figaro. *Fünfe — Zehne — Zwanzig — Dreissig &c.*
Susanne. *Deutlich saget mir mein Spiegel &c.*

An engraving of 1827 showing the first scene of The Marriage of Figaro
*(K492). The maid Susanna is trying on her wedding hat. Her husband to be, the
valet Figaro, is measuring their married quarters in the house of their employer,
Count Almariva.*

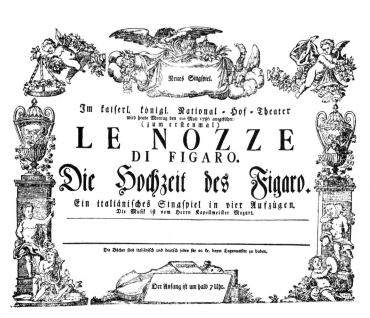

A playbill advertising the first performance of The Marriage of Figaro.

Schönbrunn in February 1786 – though he received only half as much money as his rival Salieri did for another piece given on the same occasion.

The first night of *The Marriage of Figaro* on 1 May 1786 at the Burgtheater must have been a real success, for practically every number was encored and the opera lasted nearly twice as long as intended. The effect of this was an Imperial ban on encores for ensemble pieces 'to prevent the excessive duration of operas', in its way a compliment to *Figaro*. There were technical problems on the first night and perhaps it took a little time for Vienna fully to take the measure of the new opera, as a Viennese newspaper report of July 1786 suggests: 'Herr Mozart's music was generally admired by connoisseurs already at the first performance, if we except only those whose self-love and conceit will not allow them to find merit in anything not written by themselves. The public, however (and this often happens to the public), did not really know on the first day where it stood. But now after several performances, one would be

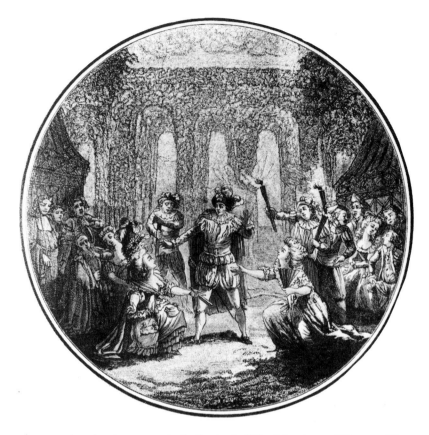

An engraving showing a scene in the final act of The Marriage of Figaro. *The count has made an assignation to meet the maid Susanna in the garden at night, but his wife takes her place and the count's unfaithful intentions are foiled.*

subscribing either to the cabal or to tastelessness if one were to maintain that Herr Mozart's music is anything but a masterpiece of art.'

If Mozart had been living today, he would have been well rewarded for his masterpiece with royalty payments and all kinds of other spin-offs. In the Vienna of those days he received a single payment of 450 gulden which was no more than he might have got from a successful concert, and did very little to delay the onset of chronic insolvency.

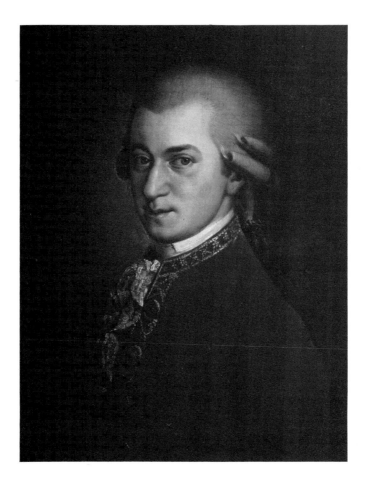

CHAPTER SIX

PUBLIC ACCLAIM, PRIVATE MISERY 1786–90

Although *Figaro* was given eight further performances in Vienna in 1786, none was for the composer's benefit, so Mozart began to think of further tours abroad as a source of income. Italy was considered, so was England – a project abandoned when Leopold flatly refused to look after his son's surviving children. For the rest of the year Mozart remained in Vienna, producing a series of fine chamber works, the great C major Piano Concerto K503 and the Symphony in D K504, which became known as the 'Prague'.

The music-loving public of the Bohemian capital had been strongly aware of Mozart's music since a production there of *The Seraglio*; soon after *Figaro* had been staged in Vienna, rehearsals began for a production of the opera in Prague, and by mid-December the city's newspapers were full of reports of its runaway success. 'No piece,' wrote one observer, 'has ever caused such a sensation'; after several performances the theatre was still full and a 'positive rain' of complimentary German poems was thrown down from the gallery.

When news of such a success was followed by an invitation to stay at Count Thun's palace in Prague, the Mozarts

97

hesitated no longer. They set off soon after Christmas and arrived on 11 January 1787 to a gratifying reception. On the very evening of their arrival, Mozart went to a ball given by a wealthy member of the aristocracy, Baron Bretfield, where the beauties of Prague, according to the composer, 'flew about in sheer delight to the music of my *Figaro* arranged for quadrilles and waltzes … Nothing is played, blown, sung or whistled but *Figaro*.' On 17 January, Wolfgang's presence at a performance of the opera was greeted by ecstatic applause as soon as the overture was finished; he directed the next performance himself from the

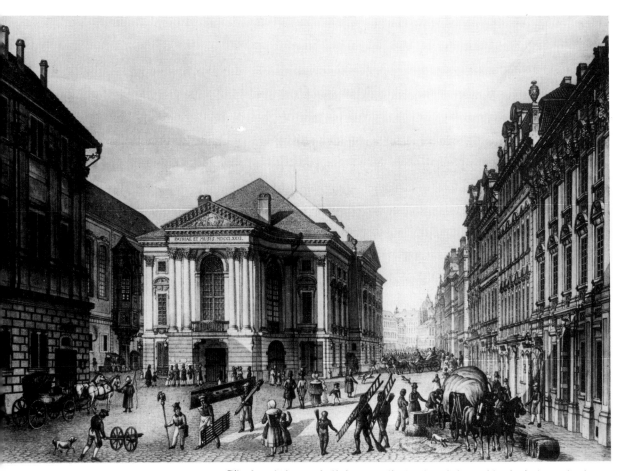

The Ständetheater, built between 1781–83 and situated in the fruit market in Prague. Mozart enjoyed a triumph with The Marriage of Figaro *and later with* Don Giovanni *(K527) at this theatre.*

keyboard, after a concert in the theatre the previous day which included the 'Prague' symphony and a full half-hour of improvisation from the maestro, including, by insistent popular request, variations on the hit tune of the day, Figaro's aria 'Non più andrai'. Mozart's triumph was complete. In the words of one newspaper, the *Prager Oberpostamtszeitung*, 'everything that was expected of this greatest artist was fulfilled to perfection'.

Before returning to Vienna in February 1787, Mozart had been commissioned by Bondini, the manager of the Prague theatre, to write a new opera for the following season, and

A half-yearly account of payments to the librettist Lorenzo da Ponte refers to the first Viennese performance of Don Giovanni *and da Ponte's work on a new opera for Salieri,* Il Pastor Fido.

he at once requested Lorenzo da Ponte to provide another Italian libretto.

The Venetian-born poet, at this time in his late thirties and destined to survive till he was nearly ninety, was in great demand. At almost the same moment he was asked for libretti by Mozart, Salieri and Vicente Martín y Soler, whose opera *Una cosa rara* had enjoyed a success rivalling that of *Figaro* the previous year. Da Ponte claimed to have assured a sceptical Emperor that he could cope with all three at once: 'I shall write at night for Mozart,' he said, 'and count that as reading Dante's *Inferno*. I shall write in the morning for Martín, the equivalent of studying Petrarch. The evening will be for Salieri, and that will be

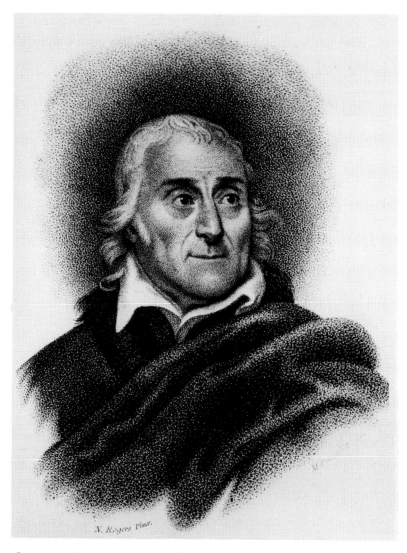

Lorenzo da Ponte, who wrote the libretti for three operatic masterpieces by Mozart – The Marriage of Figaro, Don Giovanni and Cosi fan tutte – was greatly in demand in Vienna. A bon viveur with a lively wit, he was driven by political enemies to leave the city and died in New York in 1838.

my Tasso.' If we are to believe da Ponte's memoirs, he settled down to work with a bottle of Tokay and 'a pretty sixteen-year-old girl (whom I had wished to love only as a daughter, but . . .). She came into my room at the sound of a hand-bell, which, to be truthful, rang a great deal: she fetched me now a biscuit, now a cup of coffee, now nothing but her own pretty face, perfectly fashioned to arouse poetic inspiration and the witty idea.'

For personal or other reasons, da Ponte was drawn to the Don Juan story and created a version of it for Mozart based on Goldoni's *Don Giovanni Tenorio* of 1736 and a more recent libretto by a Venetian rival called *Il convitato di pietra* (The Stone Guest). From this treatment of the story, da Ponte borrowed the appearance of the avenging statue of the Commendatore which brings about the final destruction of the libidinous Don Giovanni and provided Mozart with a magnificent dramatic opportunity. But he also allowed the composer's genius ample scope in other ways, for example with the contrasting characters of three of the Don's victims, Donna Anna, Donna Elvira, and the peasant girl Zerlina. There was light relief in the character of the servant Leporello, and material for the magnificent ensemble sequences which are among the glories of *Don Giovanni.*

The creation of the new opera was Mozart's chief preoccupation during 1787, though he also found time for other works, among them the string quintets in C major and G minor (K515 and 516) and the A major Violin Sonata (K526), as well as the famous *Eine kleine Nachtmusik* (K525). Symphonies by Mozart were performed at concerts in March, and in April the seventeen-year-old Beethoven came to Vienna with the intention of taking lessons from him, though the brilliant youth was recalled almost as soon as he arrived by news of his mother's illness. Mozart no longer gave big public concerts, partly no doubt because he had lost his novelty value for the Viennese, but also because he preferred to give his time to composition. In this role he was respected but often criticised because, as a Hamburg music critic put it, 'he aims too high in his artful and truly

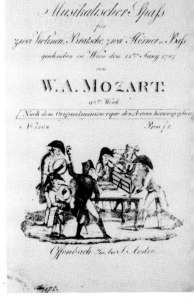

The title page of the first edition of Mozart's Musikalischer Spass *(Musical Joke) (K522), published in 1801. A satirical lithograph reflects the spirit of this amusing piece for strings and two horns, which provided the composer with some light relief in the midst of composing* Don Giovanni *in 1787.*

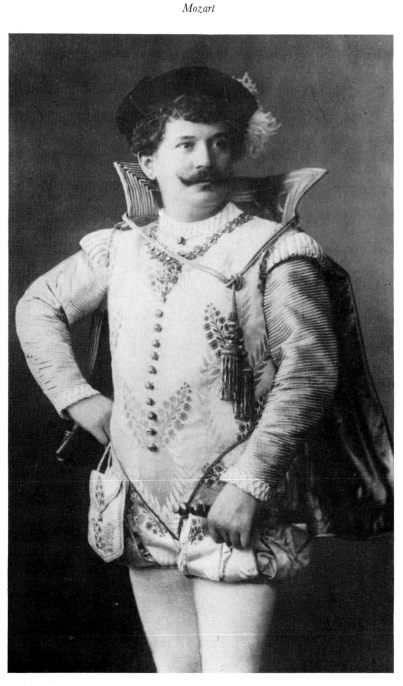

Leopold Demuth in the title role of Don Giovanni *in the Berlin opera production of 1908.*

beautiful compositions'. The same writer went on to make specific mention of the quartets dedicated to Haydn which he described as 'too highly seasoned'. Mozart's income

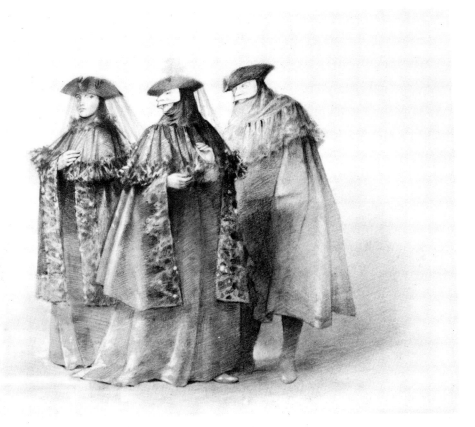

*Three masked figures wearing costumes designed by Mauro Pagano for a
production of* Don Giovanni *at the Salzburg Festival of 1987.*

declined as the time he spent composing increased, and
although he had made a good deal of money in Prague,
he decided to move at the end of April from central Vienna
to the then suburban Landstrasse where he had a
considerably lower rent to pay.

There was at this time the additional problem that
Mozart's health was poor, and he was further depressed by
news of his father's illness. Now sixty-eight years of age,
Leopold reported in a letter 'a great change in the condition
of my old body'. While expressing the fervent hope that his
father's condition would improve, Wolfgang replied with
self-revealing thoughts on the subject of death. 'I have for

many years,' he wrote, 'made myself so familiar with this best friend of man that his image not only holds no terrors for me but also brings me comfort and fortitude ... I never go to sleep without remembering, young as I am [he was thirty-one] that I may never see the following day. Yet nobody who knows me can call me melancholy or dejected in society.' This statement was borne out by acquaintances such as the singer Michael Kelly, who appeared in the original production of *Figaro*, and was a frequent guest of the composer. Mozart always received him kindly, and enjoyed beating him at billiards on 'the excellent billiard table in his house' – an amenity Mozart retained to the end. Kelly recalled in his reminiscences that Mozart was 'remarkably fond of punch, of which beverage I have seen him take copious draughts', but he also confirms that 'this remarkably small man, very thin and pale, with a profusion of fine fair hair of which he was rather vain' was essentially kind-hearted and 'always ready to oblige'.

At the end of May, Mozart had to endure the grief occasioned by news of his father's death. Fortunately there was an abundance of work to distract him, and on 1 October he left Vienna with Constanze for Prague to supervise the staging of *Don Giovanni*. The première had been planned for 14 October to celebrate the marriage of the Emperor's niece, the Archduchess Maria Theresa, but the opera was not ready and *Figaro* was revived instead under Mozart's direction. Rehearsals for the new piece proved difficult and various anecdotes about the final stages of preparation have survived, all more or less apocryphal. It is said that Caterina Bondini, as Zerlina, could not be persuaded to utter a sufficiently agonized shriek from offstage until Mozart crept up behind her and grabbed her so suddenly that she gave vent at once to the required cry; and Mozart is supposed to have written the overture during the dress rehearsal, though in fact it is more likely he wrote it out in the small hours a couple of days before the performance, kept awake with punch and gossip by Constanze.

The first performance when it came on 29 October was a

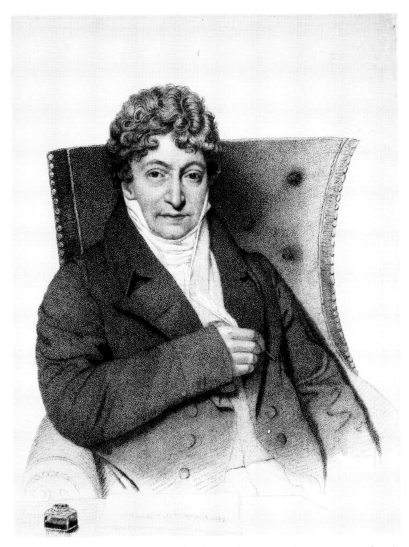

Michael Kelly (1762–1826), the Irish singer who created the roles of Don Curzio and Don Basilio in The Marriage of Figaro. *Mozart found him a genial companion, and his memoirs provide useful information about the staging of the opera.*

great triumph, in spite of Mozart's anxieties. 'When Herr Mozart entered the orchestra,' said a newspaper report, 'he was received with threefold cheers, which again happened when he left it. The opera is extremely difficult to perform but was given, in spite of this, after a short period of study. Everybody on the stage and in the orchestra strained every

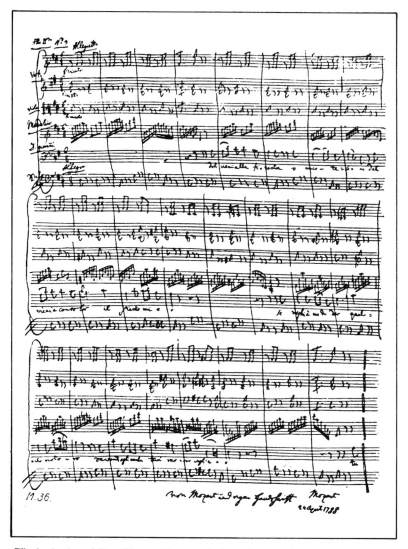

The beginning of Don Giovanni's serenade from the second act of the opera, with a prominent accompanying role for the mandolin. The date at the bottom, April 1788, suggests that this was Mozart's revised score for the first Viennese production of the opera in May of that year.

nerve to thank Mozart by rewarding him with a good performance.' Apart from receiving the usual fee of 50 ducats, the composer was also rewarded by the proceeds from the opera's fourth performance, given for his benefit.

Mozart arrived back in Vienna on 12 November, three days before the death at the age of seventy-three of Gluck, news which revived Mozart's hopes of a court appointment. As *Kammermusicus*, or Imperial and Royal Court composer, Gluck had been required to provide little more than a few dances for court balls in return for an annual salary of 2000 gulden, a sum described by the old man as 'too much for what I have done but too little for what I could do'.

Naturally Mozart hoped for the succession and this time he was not disappointed. Although he was only to receive 800 gulden annually, this was a sum a good deal larger than he received from the production of an opera, and should have provided him with a degree of financial security. The reason why it failed to do so has remained somewhat mysterious, since although Mozart insisted on keeping up appearances, maintained a servant, and was always well dressed, he and Constanze lived, as we have seen, with careful economy.

In May 1788, *Don Giovanni* was given for the first time in Vienna, and the Emperor attended one of the fifteen performances the opera received in the Austrian capital that year. It was not, however, an overwhelming success. The Emperor is said to have remarked to a courtier that it was 'too difficult for the singers', and told da Ponte that 'such music is not for the teeth of my Viennese'. When the comment was repeated to Mozart he is said to have replied: 'Give them time to chew on it!'

This was a difficult and depressing time for Mozart. He was by no means in the best of health and his income was not equal to the expense of living once again (as his way of life no doubt demanded he should) in the Inner City. He conducted a series of concerts organised by Baron van Swieten for which he updated Handel's *Messiah* in a style which no doubt appealed to contemporary taste but now seems inappropriate.

On an altogether different plane, perhaps for a projected season of concerts at the Casino, Mozart wrote over a period of six weeks that summer his three last symphonies, in E flat K543, G minor K550 and C major K551. He used clarinets instead of oboes in the Symphony No. 39 and the work reflects the warm emotion often associated by the composer with the key of E flat; No. 40 in the 'passionate' key of G minor has an urgent opening theme which sets the tone of an intense yet always graceful composition, and the majestic grandeur of the final symphony in C major, subsequently nicknamed the 'Jupiter', culminates in a brilliant fugal finale. Ironically, at the same time as he was producing these works of incomparable creative genius, Mozart was forced to postpone the publication of recent chamber music for lack of subscribers, and in June he wrote the first of a long series of begging letters to his fellow Mason, Michael Puchberg. Puchberg responded at first with relatively small loans and was then asked for a much larger sum to be repaid over a longer period. Early in 1789 Mozart asked for the loan of 100 gulden from the lawyer and magistrate Franz Hofdemel, then near the end of his Masonic novitiate, but was able to repay it as promised within four months – perhaps because of the assistance forthcoming from another member of Mozart's lodge, Prince Karl Lichnowsky.

In April 1789, the Prince invited the musician to join him on a business trip to Berlin, where there was much to be hoped for from the patronage of Friedrich Wilhelm II of Prussia, an able cellist and enlightened lover of music. There were stops on the way in Prague, where Mozart wrote home to tell Constanze how much he missed her, and in Dresden, where there were competitions on the organ and piano between Mozart and Dresden's leading keyboard player J. W. Hässler, whose abilities did not impress Wolfgang. In Leipzig, Mozart played on Bach's organ in St Thomas's Church to a large congregation, and gave a concert received with enthusiasm by a regrettably small audience.

The prices charged on this occasion may have been higher than was customary in Leipzig, but the fact is that Mozart, for all his reputation as a keyboard performer, was not universally recognised then as the genius we know him to be today. While *Figaro* was acclaimed in Hanover that

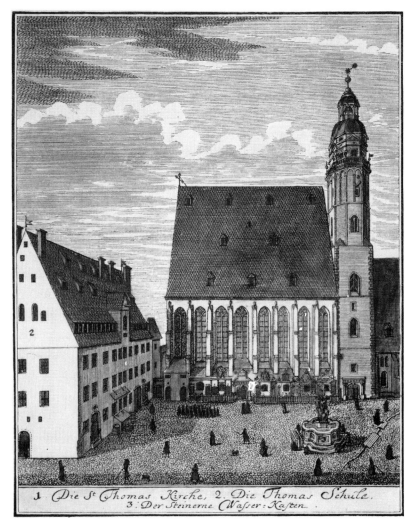

1. *Die St Thomas Kirche,* 2. *Die Thomas Schule.*
3. *Der Steinerne Wasser: Kasten .*

*St Thomas's Church in Leipzig where, in the spring of 1789, Mozart played on
the organ used by Johann Sebastian Bach.*

year as 'great and beautiful, full of art, fire and genius', a
critic in Frankfurt at much the same period declared that
the music of *Don Giovanni* was 'not popular enough to
arouse general interest'. A Copenhagen musical periodical
stated that for all his 'elevated ideas', Mozart did not find
ready acceptance because he had 'a decided leaning
towards the difficult and unusual'.

Among those who did appreciate Mozart's greatness was
Ludwig Tieck, whose memoirs were published in Leipzig

in 1855. He reported that in Mozart's lifetime the operas of Dittersdorf were more favourably received in Berlin that those of his rival, though *The Seraglio* was revived there as a gesture of welcome to Mozart when he arrived in the Prussian capital in the Spring of 1789. The story goes that, when Tieck entered the theatre well before the performance was due to start, he met 'a small unprepossessing figure in a grey overcoat' going from one music desk to another in the orchestra pit, looking carefully through the music. Tieck entered into conversation with the stranger about the theatre, opera and public taste and expressed his admiration of Mozart's operas above all. 'So you often hear Mozart's operas and are fond of them?' the stranger asked. 'That is very good of you, young man.' Soon the stranger was called away by someone on stage, and Tieck enquired the name of the person to whom he had been speaking. He was greatly moved when told it was Mozart himself.

Mozart performed before the King and Queen of Prussia in mid-May and was well rewarded, though he warned his wife not to expect him to bring any great profit back home. So indeed it proved, and although he returned to Vienna in June 1789 with the intention of writing six string quartets and six sonatas for the Prussian King, who had proved himself a prompt and generous client, Mozart was to complete only three of the quartets (with their cello parts designed to suit the talents of the King himself) and one of the sonatas. Very soon the appeals to Puchberg were renewed, for now Constanze, pregnant again, fell seriously ill with a foot complaint. Mozart, too, was unwell and unable to work. Anxiety no doubt inhibited his efforts at composition and there was no demand in Vienna any longer for his performing talents. 'Good God,' wrote Mozart to his friend in desperation, 'I am coming to you not with thanks but with fresh entreaties. Instead of paying my debts, I am asking for more money. If you really know me, you must sympathise with my anguish at having to do so.' When Puchberg did not immediately comply with the request for another 500 gulden, Mozart wrote again in mid-

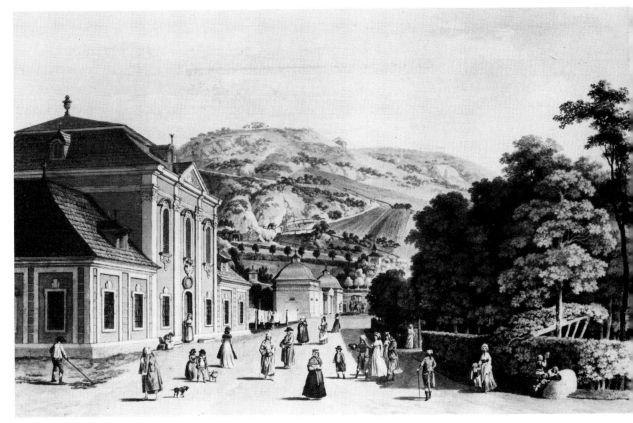

Baden, the fashionable spa near Vienna where Constanze sought a cure for persistent ill-health. Mozart wrote his well-known motet 'Ave Verum Corpus' for the Baden choirmaster.

July, reinforcing his plea with the news that Constanze would have to take a cure at Baden, a spa some 17 miles south of Vienna.

Constanze departed for the spa in August and Mozart visited her there: when he was not with his wife, he seems to have been in a permanent state of jealousy, and was always warning her in letters not to behave in a way likely to jeopardise their reputation. Not that there can have been any great justification for anxiety on this score; Constanze, apart from being ill, was well advanced in pregnancy, giving birth in November to a baby girl who died an hour later of cramp.

More encouraging for the composer was a highly

successful revival of *Figaro* in Vienna that summer and a commission from the Emperor for a new Italian opera, to be written once again in collaboration with Lorenzo da Ponte. *Cosi fan tutte* (All Women Behave Like That) was to occupy Mozart almost to the exclusion of all other compositions until the end of 1789. The one notable exception was the beautiful Clarinet Quintet he wrote for the clarinettist Anton Stadler, who gave the first performance of it at a concert in the Burgtheater that December.

Da Ponte borrowed some of the ideas for *Cosi fan tutte* (subtitled *The School for Lovers*) from *La grotta di Trofonio*, an opera produced in 1785 by Antonio Salieri, often regarded as Mozart's arch-rival; it was he and not Mozart who was appointed in 1788 as Kapellmeister, the chief musical officer in the Imperial household.

The story of the opera is beautifully constructed, an elegant and sometimes hilarious comedy which provided Mozart with a great range of expressive possibilities. Two young army officers, Ferrando and Guglielmo, take on a wager with the cynical Don Alfonso that their two girl-friends, Fiordiligi and Dorabella, will remain faithful in their absence. Off they go on active service, leaving their loved ones in tears. As a test of fidelity the young men return not long afterwards disguised as Albanians, and find that, after a while, the girls are ready to forget their promises to Ferrando and Guglielmo. At first shocked and angry, they eventually calm down under the influence of Don Alfonso, who instigated the whole affair, and all ends happily.

We know very little about the genesis of *Cosi*. Haydn and the long-suffering Puchberg attended a short rehearsal at Mozart's house on New Year's Eve and the opera was first performed with great success at the Burgtheater on 26 January 1790. It has remained among Mozart's best-loved operas ever since, although during the nineteenth century it was sometimes branded as immoral.

Less than a month after the première the Emperor Joseph II died, and with his departure the partnership of

Mozart and da Ponte came to an end. Joseph had champ-
ioned both poet and musician against the tales spread by
their enemies – Mozart claimed that Salieri never ceased to
intrigue against him – and after the Emperor's death, da
Ponte found it necessary to leave Vienna in a hurry. He fled
to Trieste and ultimately found his way to New York, where
he died in 1838 at the age of 89, his immortality guaranteed
by a trio of operatic masterpieces to which he had made an
indispensable contribution.

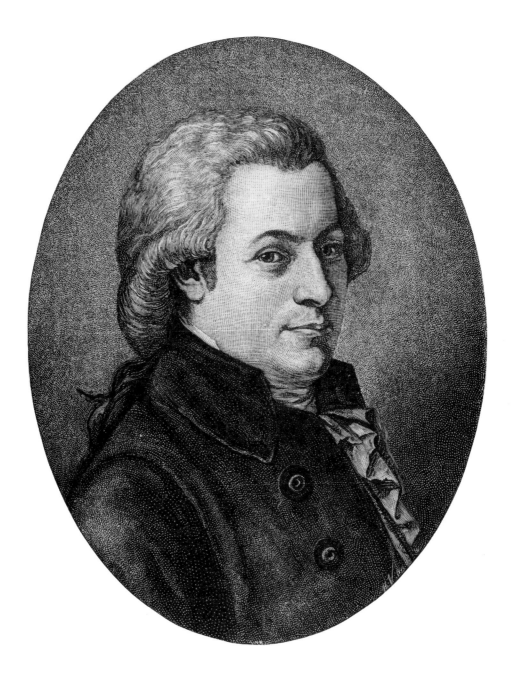

CHAPTER SEVEN

THE END AND THE BEGINNING

The new Emperor, Leopold II, soon made changes in his musical establishment, but any hopes Mozart might have had of succeeding Salieri as Kapellmeister were quickly dashed. He therefore applied for the post of second Kapellmeister, stressing his ability as a church composer, and continued to beg Puchberg for more money, this time on the grounds that if his poverty became known, it would damage his chances at court 'because unfortunately they do not judge by circumstances but solely by appearances'.

Nothing came of Mozart's attempts to secure a new court appointment, though he retained his position as court composer with a salary that came nowhere near keeping him and his family in the style he thought appropriate. Puchberg received a constant stream of begging letters in the summer of 1790, in which Mozart declared that financial worry was preventing him from finishing his quartets for the King of Prussia, reiterated the expense of his wife's persistent ill-health (which may have been caused by her constant pregnancies) and complained that he himself often felt too unwell to work, after nights rendered sleepless by pain. One medical theory suggests that Mozart may have

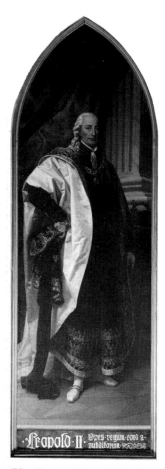

The Emperor Leopold II who succeeded his brother to the imperial throne in 1790.

been suffering from progressive kidney disease, whose symptoms include the 'pallid skin and bulging eyes' noticed in Mozart's appearance at this time.

Puchberg certainly gave assistance, for Constanze went to Baden again at midsummer, accompanied by her husband 'for economy's sake'; back in Vienna he had begun once again to take pupils as a way of making ends meet, including Franz Xaver Süssmayr, who was to gain a place for himself in musical history by completing Mozart's unfinished Requiem Mass. There was a bitter disappointment in September 1790 when the King and Queen of Naples visited Vienna for the double wedding of their daughters to the Archdukes Franz and Ferdinand; operas were commissioned from Salieri and Josef Weigl and a gala concert was organised, but Mozart was not invited to write anything or to perform.

In a state that must have been near desperation, he decided to follow the court to Frankfurt for the coronation there of the new Emperor on 9 October; he felt sure that the festivities would provide him with some opportunity. Pawning his silver to hire a carriage, he set off in a sudden revival of high spirits and told Constanze from Frankfurt that he was being invited everywhere, though every morning he stayed in his 'hole of a bedroom' to compose. A week after the coronation, Mozart gave a concert in the municipal playhouse which included the D major Concerto K537, consequently known as the 'Coronation'. One of those present, Count Ludwig von Bentheim-Steinfurt, remarked in his travel diary that 'there were not many people'.

Later in October there were visits to Mainz, where Mozart was paid rather more generously for a concert than he admitted to Constanze, and to Mannheim where the cast of the first production of *Figaro* in the city begged him to help with rehearsals. Finally on his way home to Vienna he paused in Munich, where the Elector invited him to play at a concert in honour of the King of Naples. Recalling his earlier humiliation, Mozart wrote bitterly to his wife: 'It is *greatly* to the credit of the Viennese court that the king has to hear me in a foreign country!'

An invitation awaited Wolfgang on his return home which must have been attractive. The London impresario Robert May O'Reilly had written offering Mozart £300 if he would come to England for six months and write two operas. At much the same time, Mozart was introduced in Vienna to Johann Peter Salomon, who also invited him to visit London. Haydn, as we know, accepted Salomon's invitation, though he was old enough to be Mozart's father, and Mozart considered he was unwise to travel so far when nearly sixty. The younger man was not willing to go to England, partly because he was already committed in Vienna and no doubt also because he was reluctant to leave his wife and friends yet again. Mozart is said to have waved farewell to the departing Haydn with tears in his eyes, and the prophetic words 'I fear we shall never see each other again.'

Da Ponte recalled in his memoirs how he too had tried to persuade Mozart to join him in London, and quoted a letter from the composer in which Mozart spoke of the imminent approach of death and of his imperative need to work while he was still able to do so. The letter may not be authentic, but there is no doubt of the extreme pressure under which he forced himself to labour during his last year. Sometime in 1790 he had received from the actor and impresario Emanuel Schikaneder, a fellow-Mason, the outline and part of the text of what was to become *The Magic Flute*; some parts of the score, including the humorous duet between Papageno and Papagena, were delivered by the spring of 1791. Schikaneder also wrote the words for a Masonic cantata Mozart had to complete for the opening of a new lodge in November that year. In March, Mozart performed his serene last piano concerto, K595 in B flat; he produced two great string quintets in D and E flat, K593 and K614; a commission arrived in July 1791 from the theatre in Prague for a new opera for the coronation in the Bohemian capital in September of the Emperor Leopold;

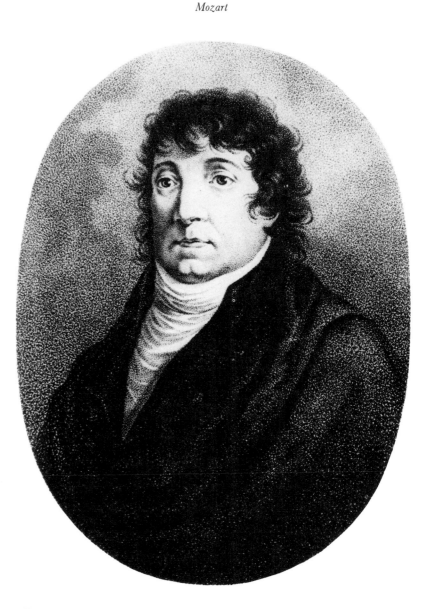

Emanuel Schikaneder (1751–1812) who commissioned The Magic Flute
(K620), also wrote the libretto and created the role of Papageno.

and during the summer, a mysterious stranger came to the
composer with a commission for a Requiem Mass, a
circumstance regarded by Mozart as a premonition of his
own death. In fact the mystery arose from a secret plan on
the part of Count Franz Walsegg-Stuppach, who wished to

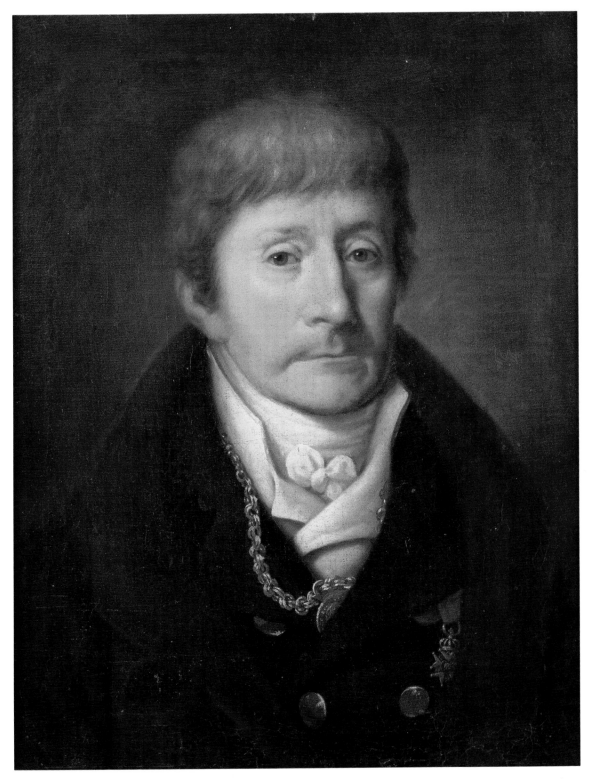

Antonio Salieri (1750–1825). To him came the worldly success Mozart craved. Although, as Peter Shaffer suggests in Amadeus, *he may have envied Mozart the spark of genius he lacked himself, there is no concrete evidence to suggest that he poisoned the great composer.*

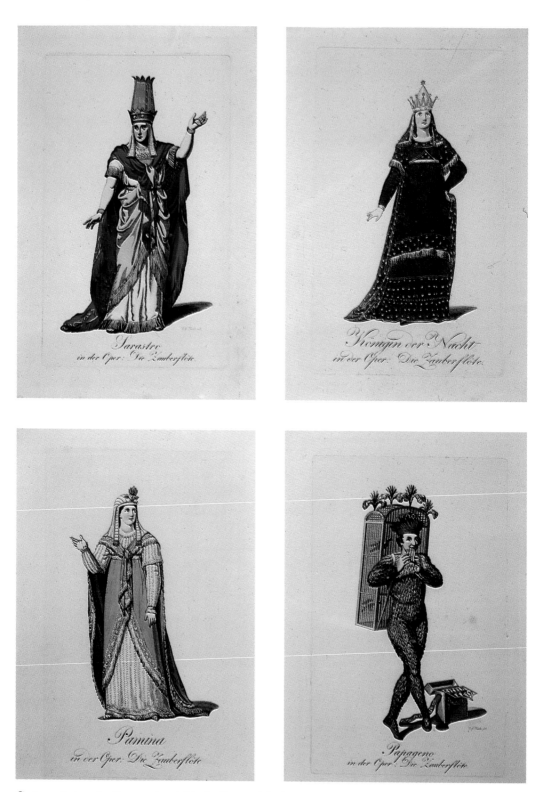

Costume designs for Sarastro (top left), the Queen of the Night (top right), Pamina (bottom left), and Papageno, by Heinrich Stürmer for a production of The Magic Flute *in Berlin in 1816.*

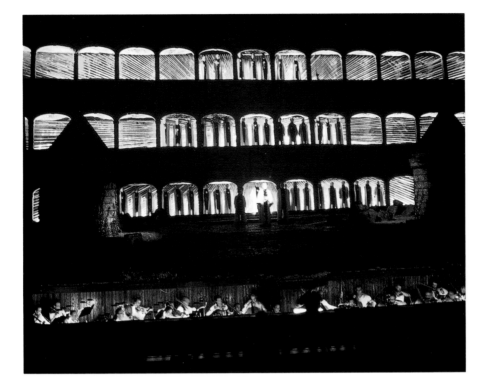

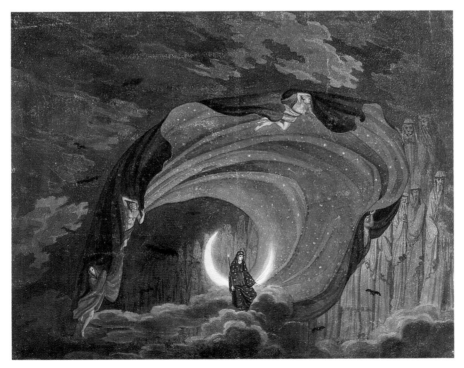

The Magic Flute. *Jean-Pierre Ponelle created this spectacular temple scene (above) for a production at the Salzburg Festival in 1978. The design by Simon Quaglio (below) provided a magnificent backdrop for the Queen of the Night in a Munich production.*

The beautiful city of Prague,
where Mozart enjoyed
spectacular triumphs with The
Marriage of Figaro *and* Don
Giovanni, *the latter specially*
commissioned for the Prague
theatre.

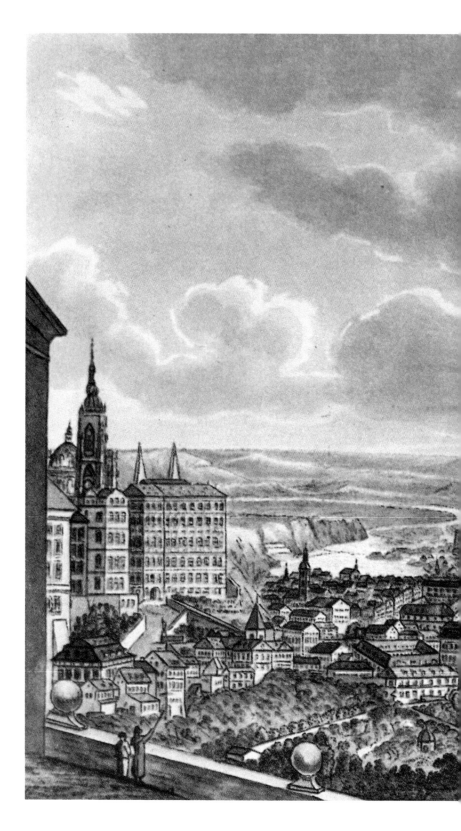

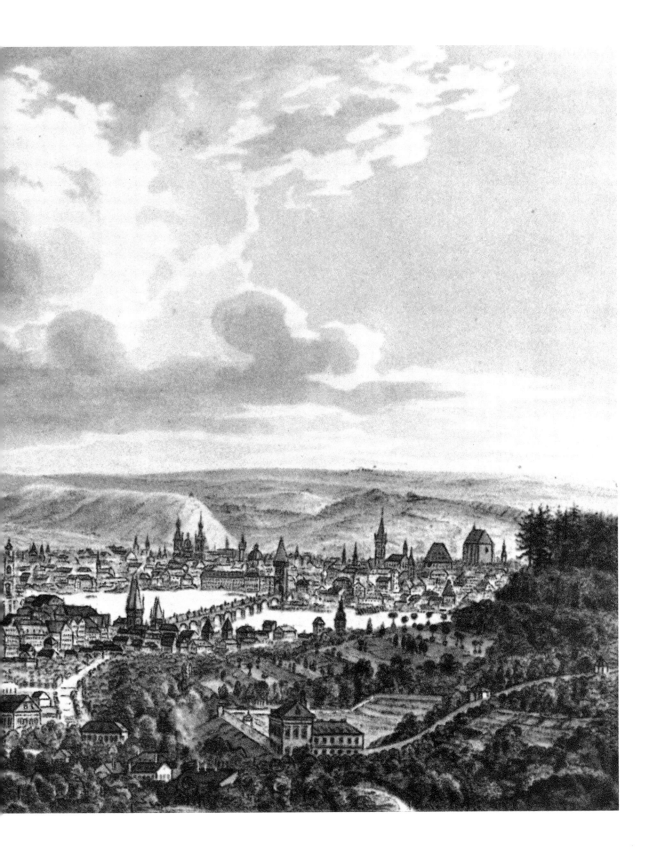

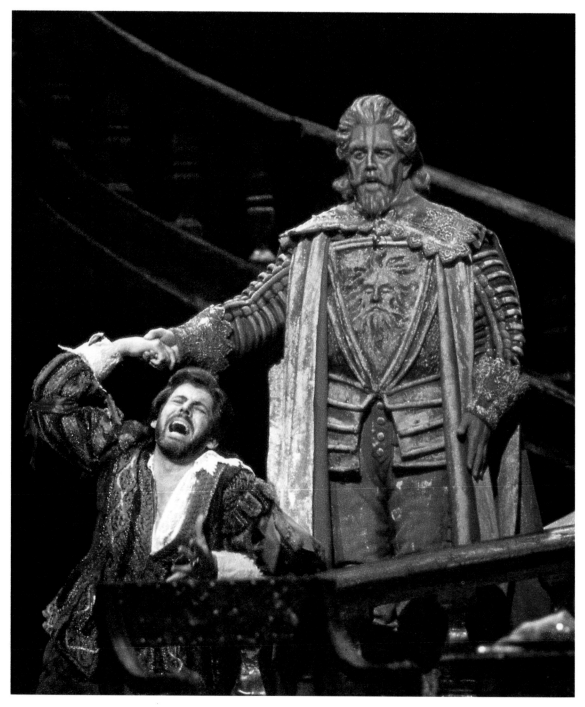

In this scene from Don Giovanni *the avenging statue of the murdered commendatore drags the corrupt protagonist down to Hell.*

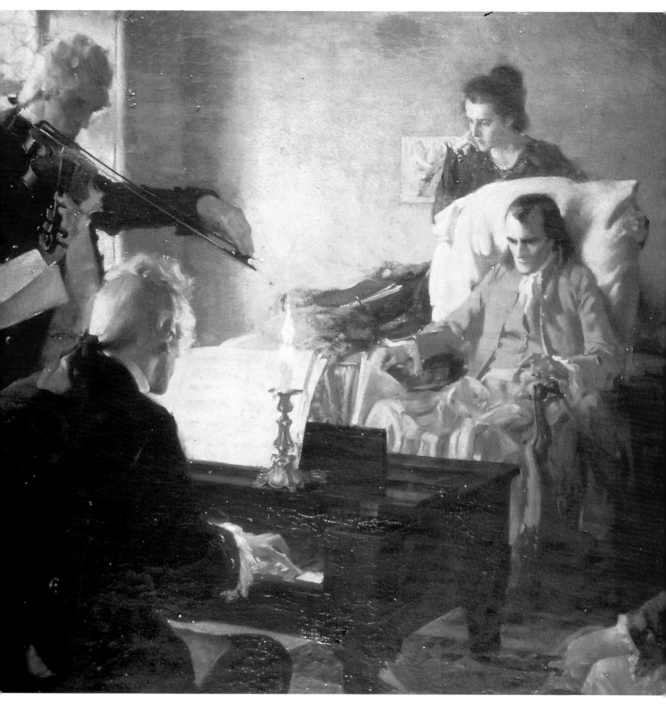

A fanciful recreation of Mozart's last hours. He is shown listening to a passage from his unfinished Requiem Mass (K626).

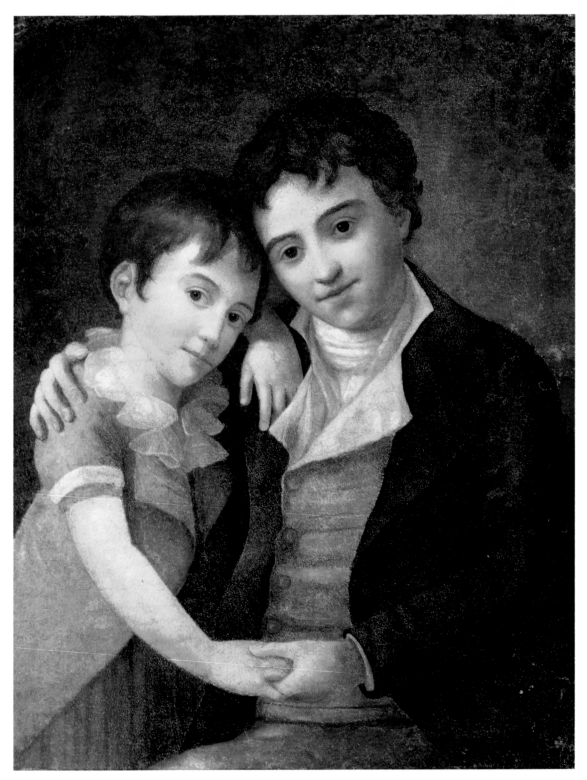

Only two of Wolfgang and Constanze Mozart's children survived infancy. They were Karl Thomas (right), born in 1784, and Franz Xaver, born in 1791. The elder boy gave up his musical studies to become a diplomat in Milan but the younger became a successful musician.

have the Requiem performed as a tribute of his own composition to the memory of his dead wife.

If Mozart's death was not actually hastened by overwork, as many believed, the pace of his activity in 1791 can have done nothing to improve his condition. We read of nights when he did not get to bed till 2 am and rose again to begin work for the day at four. Preparation of *The Magic Flute* brought him into contact with Schikaneder's theatrical company and he would often spend long social evenings with them, especially when his wife was absent, as she was again during the summer months of 1791, taking the waters at Baden. What hostile observers were quick to call loose living was explained by Mozart as part of his imperative need for congenial company. 'It is not at all good for me to be alone when I have something on my mind,' he explained to his wife in the course of describing how he spent one evening when she was away. 'I went to the Kasperle Theatre to see the new opera, then, when passing the coffee house, I looked in to see if Loibl was there, but there was not a sign of him. I again took a meal at the "Krone" simply in order not to be alone, and there at least I found someone to talk to. Then I went straight to bed...' Another letter is even more revealing of the composer's state of mind in the summer of 1791: 'I can't describe what I have been feeling, a kind of emptiness which hurts me dreadfully – a kind of longing which is never satisfied, which never ceases and which persists, nay rather increases daily ... if I go to the piano and sing something out of my new opera, I have to stop at once, for this stirs my emotions too deeply.' When Constanze returned to Vienna, bearing a sixth child on 26 July, one hopes that at least some of her husband's private misery was assuaged.

In the second half of August, the Mozarts set out for Prague for the production of *La clemenza di Tito*, the opera Mozart composed for the Emperor's coronation in that part of his dominions. The story, adapted from Metastasio, tells of the Roman Emperor Titus. It shows monarchy in a very favourable light, as might be expected on such an occasion.

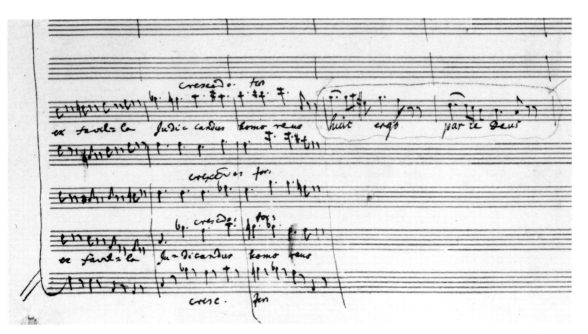

These are the last notes Mozart committed to paper, part of the Lacrimosa from the Requiem Mass. The work was subsequently completed by Mozart's pupil Franz Xaver Süssmayr.

In any case Mozart was doubtless still hoping to soften Leopold's hard-hearted indifference, and his Titus displays truly amazing clemency even to those who plot against his life and set fire to Rome itself.

The music, some of which was written in the carriage on the way to Prague with the assistance of Süssmayr, by now a devoted amanuensis, is generally not on the same level as the great works of Mozart's last period, but there is a splendid finale to the first act, and two of the arias have the added interest of obbligato parts for clarinet and basset horn which were performed by Anton Stadler. On his return to Vienna, Mozart found time to compose for Stadler a Clarinet Concerto whose autumnal beauties match those of the marvellous Clarinet Quintet.

Soon after his arrival in Prague, Mozart attended and may have conducted a festival performance of *Don Giovanni* and four days later, on 6 September, *La clemenza di Tito* was given before an audience which included the Emperor;

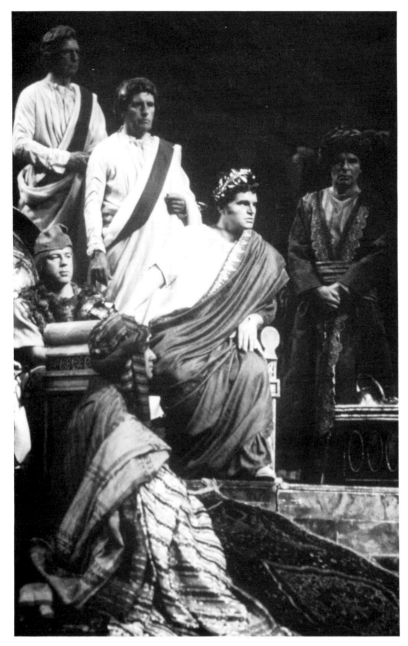

A scene from the Royal Opera House production of La Clemenza di Tito
(K621) in 1982.

after arriving an hour late, he accorded the piece a polite
reception. There was little of the glamorous socialising
which had attended the success of *Figaro*, and according to

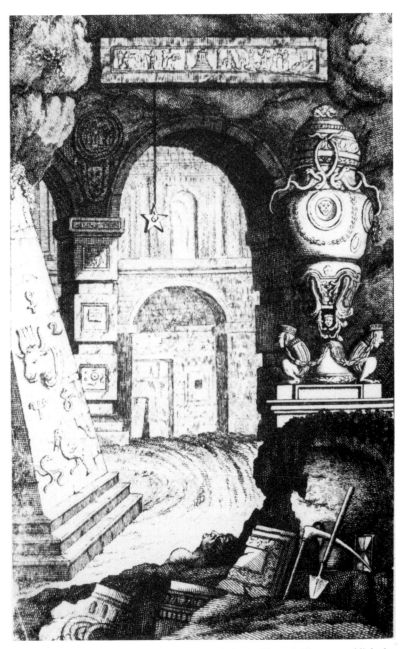

This engraving from the first edition of The Magic Flute *'s libretto, published in 1791, shows Egyptian motifs and Masonic symbols. Emanuel Schikaneder, the author, was also a mason, hence the masonic symbols.*

one account, by the time Mozart left Prague after this visit, he was obviously ill and taking medicine continually; though he was still capable of displaying a kind of 'gay seriousness'.

Back in Vienna, he was plunged into the final preparations for *The Magic Flute (Die Zauberflöte)*, which was first performed at the Theater auf der Wieden on 30 September, with Mozart directing from the keyboard. It was a success from the start: no less than twenty performances were given in October and Mozart had the gratification of seeing audiences grow in size as the run went on.

The Magic Flute is a strange mixture of solemn ceremony based on Masonic rituals and light-hearted comedy bordering on farce. The story arises from the eternal enmity between good and evil, personified in the characters of Sarastro the High Priest and the Queen of the Night. The Queen's daughter, Pamina, is held by Sarastro, and the young Tamino sets out to rescue her, believing, under the Queen's influence, that Sarastro is the evil one. Tamino is aided in his quest by a magic flute and by a bird-catcher, Papageno, who is equipped with a magic glockenspiel. Tamino soon discovers that he has been deceived about the nature of Sarastro and, having fallen in love with Pamina, is initiated into the priestly brotherhood. Both the lovers are subjected to ceremonial ordeals, and the Queen of the Night makes a final attempt to rescue Pamina, but the power of goodness triumphs and all ends happily.

The score is rich in great music throughout, but Sarastro's two bass arias and the coloratura displays of the Queen of the Night have become lasting favourites, together with Tamino's lovely tenor aria expressing his love for Pamina when he is shown her portrait, and Papageno's aria on his first entrance when he describes his profession as a bird-catcher.

Papageno was played in the first production by Emanuel Schikaneder himself, an accomplished and popular comedian, and Mozart enjoyed teasing him when the chance arose. Writing to Constanze, who again spent some time in

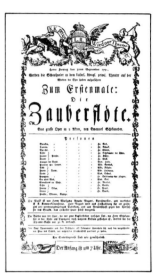

The playbill advertising the first performance of The Magic Flute *on 30 September, 1791. Mozart's name is less prominent than that of Emanuel Schikaneder.*

Baden during October, Mozart related how, on one occasion, he decided to take over the offstage glockenspiel which was sounded as Schikaneder mimed the action on stage. 'Just for fun,' wrote Mozart, 'at the point when Schikaneder has a pause, I played an arpeggio. He was startled, looked behind the wings and saw me. When he had his next pause, I played no arpeggio. This time he stopped and refused to go on. I guessed what he was thinking and played another chord. Then he struck the glockenspiel and told it to shut up! Everybody laughed because they realized for the first time that Schikaneder was not playing the glockenspiel himself.'

On 13 October, Mozart had the gratification of taking Salieri to a performance and witnessing his wholehearted approval of the work: 'he listened and watched most attentively, and from the overture to the last chorus there was not a single number that did not call forth from him a "bravo" or a "bello"!'

It is good to know that *The Magic Flute* brought a real measure of satisfaction to Mozart, though one report in a Berlin musical journal said that in spite of the cost of the production and the magnificence of the scenery, it 'failed to have the hoped-for success,' the writer adding that Vienna was still impatiently awaiting an operatic renaissance when Cimarosa arrived to replace Salieri as Imperial Kapellmeister. The same periodical, however, displayed greater perception in its critique of a Berlin production of *Don Giovanni* on 10 October 1791; it read: 'We must unite profound knowledge of the art with the happiest talent for inventing lovely melodies, and then link both with the greatest possible originality in order to obtain the most faithful picture of Mozart's musical genius.' Evidently there were some discerning individuals who valued Mozart at his true worth even during his short lifetime.

Constanze returned from Baden in mid-October, and while walking with her in the Prater one day, Mozart burst into tears, saying that he thought he had been poisoned and would not live long. Joseph Deiner, landlord of a

Viennese tavern, *The Silver Snake*, found him similarly depressed one day in November, 'looking unusually pale, his powdered fair hair in disarray and little pigtail carelessly tied'. Mozart had ordered wine instead of his customary beer, but left it untouched. 'You look quite ill and wretched, Maestro,' said Deiner. 'I heard you were in Prague and the Bohemian air had not done you any good. But you'll be alright!' 'No,' replied Mozart, 'I fear there won't be much more music making. I've got a chill coming on that I can't account for. You drink my wine. I'll have a fire lighted this very day.'

The composer recovered sufficiently to direct his new cantata (K623) at the dedication of a Masonic temple on 18 November, but two days later took to his bed with swelling

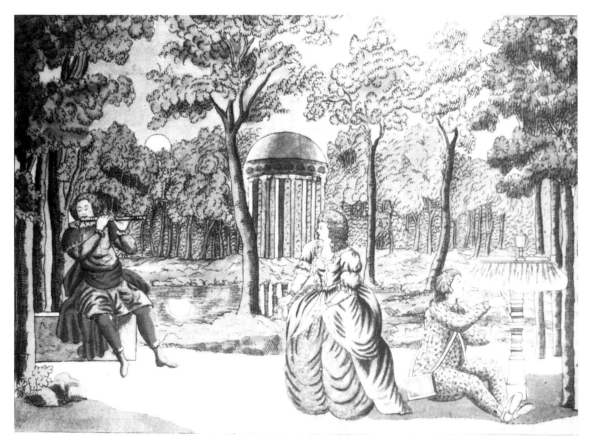

Tamino, Pamina, and Papageno, in the first performance of The Magic Flute.

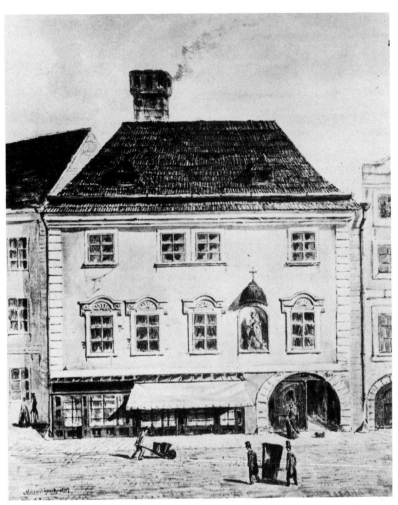

*No. 8 Rauchensteingasse, the house where Mozart died on the morning of 5
December 1791. He was thirty-five.*

of the hands and feet, a sort of paralysis and fits of vomiting.
During the next few days, between visits from his doctors,
Mozart continued to work feverishly on his Requiem,
explaining his ideas to Süssmayr and working out some
details on the pianoforte in his room; there were even short
rehearsals of parts of the work round his sick bed, including
one on 4 December in which he sang the alto part: during
the Lacrimosa he was unable to continue for weeping.
Someone sang the bird-catcher's song from *The Magic Flute*
to try and cheer him up, but Mozart knew that death was

not far off. Constanze's sister Sophie went for a priest, and Dr Closset was called that evening from the theatre, but he could do nothing. Mozart died at five minutes to one on the morning of 5 December 1791, at the age of 35. There has been much subsequent controversy as to the cause of his death. Some authorities believe that he died of a form of rheumatic fever; others who support the theory that Mozart was suffering from progressive kidney failure believe that he died following the onset of a uraemic coma.

In her husband's album, Constanze wrote soon after his death: 'Dearly beloved husband; Mozart – never to be forgotten by me or by the whole of Europe – now thou too art at peace – eternal peace! ! ... About one o'clock in the morning of the 5th of December in this year he left in his 36th year – alas! all too soon! – this good – but ungrateful world! – dear God! – For 8 years we were joined together by the most tender bond, never to be broken here below! – O! could I soon be joined with thee for ever. Thy grievously afflicted wife Constanze Mozart *née* Weber.

Constanze was to survive her husband by fifty years. She died in 1842 after marrying a man she first met in 1797, Georg Nikolaus Nissen. In the years immediately following Wolfgang's death she devoted herself to organising concerts of his works, touring widely in Germany and Bohemia without apparently showing any sign of the ill health which had pursued her during Mozart's last years.

Together with the tributes which appeared in the musical press, rumours began to spread regarding the manner of Mozart's death. Because his body swelled up after he died the idea gained ground that he had been poisoned, and Salieri's name was linked with the crime. This story became widely current again in the mid-1820s when Salieri, who had become mentally deranged, claimed in his ravings that he had done away with Mozart by poisoning him, and the suggestion has never been conclusively disproved. It does, however, seem extremely unlikely, and the Viennese physician Dr Eduard Guldener gains our sympathy with his public declaration of Salieri's innocence in 1824: 'I shall

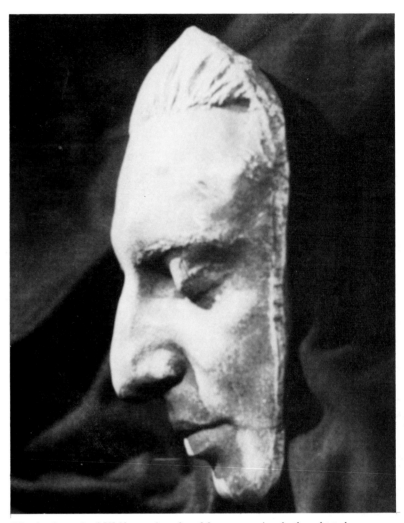

The death mask of Wolfgang Amadeus Mozart, previously thought to be spurious, is now accepted by some scholars as authentic.

Sperrs-RELATION.

Mozart's death certificate. The cause of his death has never been conclusively established, but here it is stated as 'severe miliary fever', later diagnosed as 'rheumatic inflammatory fever'.

have the greatest pleasure,' he wrote, 'if this can contribute to giving the lie to the horrible calumny on the excellent Salieri.'

Mozart's burial is another subject of controversy. It has often been said that he was given a pauper's funeral, but the evidence suggests that although it was very modest, it was not out of keeping with the fashion of the time. Very simple funeral arrangements were often made, in accordance with the express wishes of the late Emperor Joseph II. There was

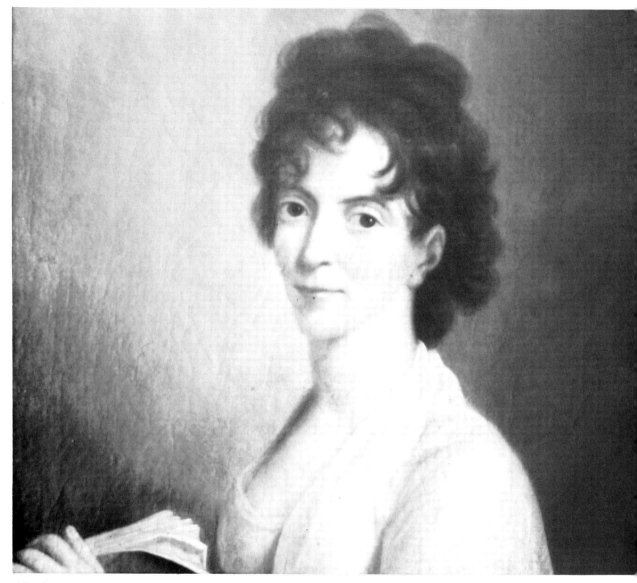

After his death, Mozart's wife Constanze expressed in her husband's album the wish to be reunited with him before long, but she eventually married again and outlived him by fifty years.

a short service in a side-chapel in St Stephen's Cathedral attended by a few fellow-Masons; others present included Baron van Swieten, who was quick to come to Constanze's aid, and Salieri. The fact that none of them followed the body to the cemetery of St Marx, where it was buried in a

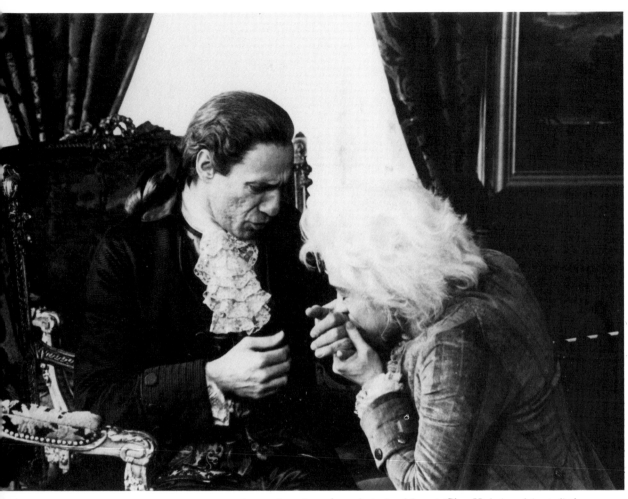

A scene from Amadeus *featuring Mozart (Tom Hulce) and (seated) the man who was rumoured to have killed him, Salieri (F. Murray Abraham).*

common grave, again seems to have been in accordance with the custom of the time among enlightened people.

A tablet now marks the spot in St Stephen's Cathedral where the funeral service was held, but Constanze had no memorial erected to her husband, feeling confident that posterity would see to that. She and her two surviving children, Karl and Franz Xaver, the last to be born, were soon receiving financial assistance from a number of sources. There were benefit concerts, Beethoven played a

Mozart concerto during a Vienna production of *La Clemenza di Tito*, Friedrich Wilhelm of Prussia paid a good price for some manuscripts and the Emperor Leopold provided a pension. Franz Xaver became a modestly successful musician, Karl a well-respected landowner in Italy, his estate purchased with receipts from performances of *Figaro* in Paris.

As for their father, two hundred years after his death we are still unable to do justice in words to the greatness of his genius. Amazing in all the many kinds of music he essayed, he was the creator of the piano concerto as we know it, superb in symphonic and chamber music, produced magnificent choral works for the church, and was arguably the greatest of all opera composers. For a time the true stature of Mozart as a composer was obscured, partly by the reputation for personal irresponsibility he left behind him. Two years after his death, an almanac of deaths for the year 1791 carried this unsympathetic paragraph about Mozart: 'In Vienna he married Constanze Weber and found her a good mother of two children of their union and a worthy wife, who moreover sought to restrain him from many foolishnesses and excesses. Despite a considerable income, he yet, in consequence of his exceptional sensuality and domestic disorder, left his family nothing beyond the glory of his name and the attention of a large public fixed upon them.' A diarist of the period noted the zest with which Mozart carried on his battle with Salieri and his other rivals, and alleged that he played billiards for high stakes all night long – 'he was very thoughtless, but his wife excused him'.

Karoline Pichler, writing her memoirs in the 1840s, recalled how she knew both Mozart and Haydn. 'They were men,' she wrote, 'in whose personal intercourse there was absolutely no sign of unusual power of intellect and almost no trace of intellectual culture, nor of any scholarly or other higher interests. A rather ordinary turn of mind, silly jokes and in the case of the former, an irresponsible way of life, were all that distinguished them in society.'

Looking back on Mozart's life, we can appreciate the perceptive insight of Mozart's sister Nannerl when she said quite simply that Mozart remained a child all his years. The practical matters which occupy and satisfy so many adults had no meaning for him. He was truly alive only when creating music in the solitude of his room, so his real existence remained hidden – as da Ponte put it, writing in New York in 1830 – 'like a precious stone buried in the bowels of the earth'.

Only when Mozart himself was buried did the world begin to learn what an abundance of life he had bequeathed to us.

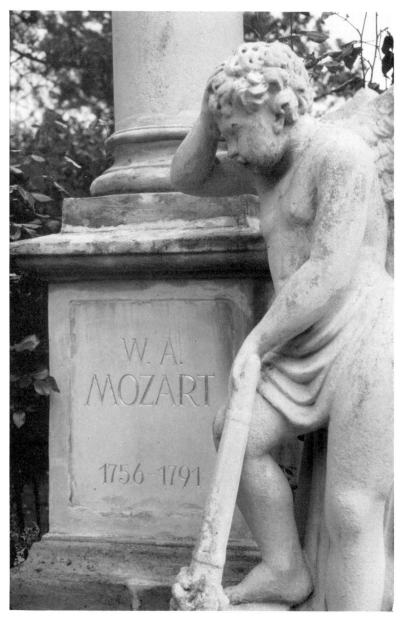

Mozart's memorial in the cemetery of St Marx in Vienna, where his remains were interred.

CHRONOLOGY

1756
Born at Salzburg, 27 January

1761
Composes his first pieces, an Andante and Allegro for solo keyboard

1762
Plays before the Elector of Bavaria. In September to Vienna, where Mozart and his sister Nannerl appear twice before the Empress Maria Theresa

1763
Beginning of the Grand Tour. Concerts in, among other places, Munich, Augsburg, Mainz, and Frankfurt, on the way to Paris, where they remain for five months. Mozart's first music appears in print: two pairs of keyboard sonatas

1764
Arrive in England and stay for fifteen months, meeting J.C. Bach

1765
Concerts in the Netherlands, where both children become seriously ill

1766
Back in Salzburg, Mozart arranges some concertos from sonatas by various composers and writes the Latin intermezzo *Apollo et Hyacinthus* for the university graduation ceremony

1767
To Vienna. Wolfgang and Nannerl both contract smallpox

1768

La finta semplice composed for Vienna but not in the event given there.
A one-act Singspiel, *Bastien und Bastienne*, commissioned by Dr Franz
Anton Mesmer, the inventor of 'magnetism therapy'

1769

Made third Konzertmeister to the Salzburg Court Chapel

1770

Leopold and Wolfgang in Italy; Count Firmian their chief patron in
Milan. Mozart writes his first string quartet. Meets the composer Padre
Martini and the famous castrato Farinelli. After hearing the Allegri
Miserere in the Sistine chapel, Mozart writes it out from memory. In
Rome he is made a Knight of the Golden Spur. *Mitridate* a great success
in Milan

1771

A second Italian visit sees the first performance of a serenata, *Ascanio in
Alba*

1772

Writes a dramatic serenata, *Il sogno di Scipione*, for the installation
ceremony of the new Prince-Archbishop, Count Colloredo, and begins
to receive an income of 150 florins as Konzertmeister, but Leopold and
Wolfgang are restless in Salzburg. Third Italian tour; *Lucio Silla*
performed in Milan

1773

Writes quartets K168–173 in Vienna. Several symphonies (the Salzburg
symphonies) this year and the following, notably K183 in G minor and
K201 in A major

1775

Premières of *La finta giardiniera* and *Il rè pastore*. Composition of five
violin concertos

1776

Several piano concertos. *Serenata notturna*. Haffner Serenade. Masses for
the Court Chapel

1777

Dissatisfaction with Colloredo erupts. Mozart leaves his service and
begins tour with his mother, visiting Mannheim, where he fails to
secure a court post but composes some flute quartets and concertos
and falls in love with a singer, Aloysia Weber

1778

Paris tour; his mother dies. 'Paris' Symphony. Leopold urges Wolfgang
to return to Salzburg; reluctantly he does. No major posts or
commissions offered

1779

Obtains expected post as Court Organist at Salzburg. Symphonies K318 and 319. Sinfonia Concertante for violin and viola K364. Coronation Mass

1780

Writes *Idomeneo* for Munich. Aloysia Weber marries the court actor Joseph Lange, who subsequently executes a famous (unfinished) portrait of Mozart

1781

Archbishop summons Mozart to Vienna for accession of Emperor Joseph II. Mozart finally leaves Colloredo's service and hopes for a better future in Vienna, where he also becomes increasingly intimate with Aloysia's sister Constanze. Competition with Clemenzi

1782

Die Entführung aus dem Serail (*The Abduction from the Seraglio*). Haffner Symphony. Marries Constanze

1783

Their first child, Raimund Leopold, born. After several delays, they travel to Salzburg for Leopold to meet Constanze; they stay about three months during which time the baby dies. Returning via Linz, Mozart composes K425, the 'Linz' Symphony, 'at breakneck speed'

1784

Begins catalogue of his works. Becomes a Freemason. Six piano concertos

1785

Reputation as a composer and pianist reaches its peak. Three new piano concertos. Publication of six string quartets dedicated to Haydn; receives accolade from Haydn

1786

Der Schauspieldirektor (*The Impresario*) performed in the Orangery in Schönbrunn Palace. Première of *Le Nozze di Figaro* (*The Marriage of Figaro*). Piano concertos in A (K488), C minor (K491) and C major (K503)

1787

'Prague' Symphony (K504) given on a visit there. After several months back in Vienna, returns to Prague for first production of *Don Giovanni*. String quintets in C major and G minor. Succeeds Gluck as court *Kammermusicus*

1788

Letters to Michael Puchberg, a fellow-Mason, pleading for loans. The last three symphonies

1789

Journeying via Prague, Dresden and Leipzig (where he improvises on Bach's organ) he visits Potsdam and Berlin, agreeing to write some quartets for King Friedrich Wilhelm II (K575, 589 and 590). Clarinet Quintet for Anton Stadler

1790

Première of *Cosi fan tutte*. Travels unofficially to Frankfurt to attend coronation festivities of new emperor, Leopold II

1791

Unsuccessful petition for post of Kapellmeister at St Stephen's Cathedral. Mysterious commission of Requiem Mass. *La clemenza di Tito* and *Die Zauberflöte* (*The Magic Flute*). Clarinet Concerto for Stadler. Death in Vienna, 5 December

FURTHER READING

Anderson, Emily (ed.) *Letters of Mozart and his Family,* London 1938; rev. edn ed. A. Hyatt King and M. Carolan, London and New York 1966

BBC Music Guides *Mozart Chamber Music* (A. Hyatt King), London 1968; *Mozart Piano Concertos* (Philip Radcliffe), London 1978; *Mozart Wind and String Concertos* (A. Hyatt King), London 1978

Blom, Eric *Mozart,* New York 1949; rev. edn London 1974

Brophy Brigid *Mozart the Dramatist,* London and New York 1964

Dent Edward J. *Mozart's Operas,* London and New York 1955 (3rd edn)

Deutsch, Otto Erich *Mozart: A Documentary Biography,* London 1965; Stanford, Calif. 1966

—— *Mozart and his World in Contemporary Pictures,* London and New York 1961

Hutchings, Arthur *A Companion to Mozart's Piano Concertos,* London and New York 1950 (2nd edn)

—— *Mozart: the Man, the Musician,* London and New York 1976

Keys, Ivor *Mozart: his Music and his Life,* London 1980

Landon, H.C. Robbins *Haydn: A Documentary Study,* London and New York 1981

—— and **Mitchell, Donald** (eds) *The Mozart Companion,* London 1965 (2nd edn); New York 1970

Levey, Michael *The Life and Death of Mozart,* London and New York 1971

Mann, William *The Operas of Mozart,* New York 1976; London 1977

Osborne, Charles *The Complete Operas of Mozart,* London and New York 1978

Ottaway, Hugh *Mozart,* London 1979; Detroit 1980

Raynor, Henry *Mozart,* London 1978

Sadie, Stanley *Mozart,* London 1966; New York 1970

Schenk, Eric *Mozart and his Times,* New York 1959; London 1960

LIST OF ILLUSTRATIONS

13 Mozart's birthplace, drawn from a photograph by Ludwig Hardtmuth. Copyright The Mansell Collection, Ltd, London.

14 Mozart and his two children, by Louis Carrogis Carmontelle. Copyright the British Library, London/The Bridgeman Art Library, London.

15 Maria Anna Mozart, aged ten. Copyright Mary Evans Picture Library, London.

16 Unsigned miniature on ivory of the young Mozart *c.* 1773. Copyright Mozart-Museum, Salzburg/Werner Forman Archive.

17 Tom Hulce as Mozart in *Amadeus* (1984), produced by Saul Zaentz, directed by Milos Forman, and based on the screenplay by Peter Shaffer. Copyright British Film Institute, Stills, Posters and Designs.

19 Map of Mozart's tours re-drawn by Samuel Denley.

20 Charles Burney. Copyright Österreichische Nationalbibliothek, Vienna.

21 Count Thun, surrounded by Masonic symbols. Engraving by Johan Georg Klinger, after a painting by A. Rähmel, 1787. Copyright Archiv für Kunst und Geschichte, Berlin.

22 'Feast to celebrate the wedding of Joseph II to Isabella von Parma' (10 October 1760). Copyright Schönbrunn Palace, Vienna/Archiv für Kunst und Geschichte, Berlin.

26 'Mozart's first visit to Paris', (November 1763 until April 1764). Lithograph, 1860, by Anton Ziegler. Copyright Archiv für Kunst und Geschichte, Berlin.

28 Titlepage of Mozart's sonatas for violin and piano (K6, 7). First edition. Copyright British Library, London.

29 J.C. Bach, by Thomas Gainsborough. Copyright the Mansell Collection Ltd, London.

31 Receipt acknowledging 'musical performances' from Wolfgang Mozart to the British Museum. Engraved, with details added 19 July 1765 by Mathew Maty, Secretary to the trustees. Copyright Mozart-Museum, Salzburg.

32 Pater Dominicus Hagenauer. Copyright Mozart-Museum, Salzburg.

33 This production of *Cosi fan tutte* (K527) first performed by the Royal Opera House in 1981. Copyright Dominic Photography, London.

35 View of Milan by Friedrich Bemhord Werner. Copyright Österreichische Nationalbibliothek, Vienna.

36 Engraving of Padre J.B. Martini. Copyright The Mansell Collection Ltd, London.

36 Thomas Linley the Younger, by Thomas Gainsborough. Copyright Dulwich Art Gallery, London/The Bridgeman Art Library, London.

37 Anonymous oil painting of Mozart as Knight of the Golden Spur, 1777. Copyright Mozart-Museum, Salzburg/Magnum Photos/Erich Lessing, Culture and Fine Arts Archives, 1986.

38 Pope Clement XIV. Copyright Österreichische Nationalbibliothek, Vienna.

38 *Mitridate, Re di Ponto* (K87), titlepage and dramatis personae of the first libretto, by Giovanni Montani, 1770, Milan. Copyright Archiv für Kunst und Geschichte, Berlin.

40 'A Portrait of the Young Mozart'. Copyright Sotheby's, London.

42 *God is our Refuge* (K20), autograph manuscript, 1765. Copyright British Library, London.

44 The titlepage from the first performance of *Lucio Silla* (K135), 1773. Copyright Archiv für Kunst und Geschichte, Berlin.

43 Scene from an Italian opera, by Gemälde von Giuseppe de Albertis, 1780. Copyright Museo Teatrale alla Scala, Milan/Archiv für Kunst und Geschichte, Berlin.

46 Letter from Leopold Mozart to his wife.

47 *La Finta Giardiniera* (K196), 1774. Titlepage of pianoforte arrangement. (Lithograph by Karl Ferdinand Heckel). Copyright Archiv für Kunst und Geschichte, Berlin.

49 Membership list of the Salzburg Court Orchestra, 1775.

51 Air-gun Shooting. Copyright Mozart-Museum, Salzburg.

52 Letter from Mozart about the 'Bäsle', Maria Anna Thekla Mozart, 10 May 1779. Copyright British Museum, London/Archiv für Kunst und Geschichte, Berlin.

54 View of Mannheim, the city and castle. Engraving by Hieronymus Wolff, after a painting by F.B. Werner, 1729. Copyright Archiv für Kunst und Geschichte, Berlin.

57 Aloysia Weber as Zemir in Gertry's *Zemir and Azor*. Engraving by Johann Esaias Nilson, 1784. Copyright Österreichische Nationalbibliothek, Vienna/Archiv für Kunst und Geschichte, Berlin.

58 The Isle du Palais and the Church of Notre Dame, Paris. Anonymous engraving. Copyright Österreichische Nationalbibliothek, Vienna.

62 Drawing of Maria Anna Thekla Mozart, *c.* 1777–78. Copyright Mozart-Museum, Salzburg/Archiv für Kunst und Geschichte, Berlin.

64 Boxwood medallion of Mozart, by Leonard Posch, 1789. Copyright Mozart-Museum, Salzburg.

66 Engraving of Joseph and Aloysia Lange, by Daniel Berger, 1785, after an original drawing by Joseph Lange. Copyright Mozart-Museum, Salzburg.

68 Vignette of Act II, Scene 6 from *Idomeneo*, engraving by C. Seipp, from a vocal score *c.* 1796. Copyright British Library, London.

70 The Kärntnertor Theater, Vienna, by J.E. Mansfeld, 1796. Copyright Österreichische Nationalbibliothek, Vienna.

72 Interior of the Burgtheater, St Michael's Square, Vienna. Copyright Österreichische Nationalbibliothek, Vienna.

73 Joseph II, portrait in Dragoon Uniform, by Joseph Hickel. Copyright Kunsthistorisches Museum, Vienna/Archiv für Kunst und Geschichte, Berlin.

74 View above the Belvedere over the Terrace Gardens of Vienna, by Karl von Schutz. Copyright The Bridgeman Art Library, London.

76 Mozart at the piano, unfinished oil painting by Joseph Lange, 1789. Copyright Mozart-Museum, Salzburg.

78 Titlepage of Mozart's violin sonatas (K296, 376–380). First edition 1781. Copyright the British Library, London.

79 *The Abduction from the Seraglio*, autograph manuscript 1782, from Osmin's Aria. Copyright Archiv für Kunst und Geschichte, Berlin.

80 A picture sheet with scenes and figures from *The Abduction from the Seraglio*, *c.* 1800, coloured engraving. Copyright Archiv für Kunst und Geschichte, Berlin.

81 Silhouettes of Valenti Adamberger, 1803, and Catarina Cavalieri, 1801. Copyright Österreichische Nationalbibliothek, Vienna.

82/83 Mozart's marriage contract, 3 August 1782. Copyright the British Library, London.

84 Engraving of St Stephen's Cathedral, Vienna. Copyright Mary Evans Picture Library, London.

87 Mozart's autograph sketches for Piano Concerto (K467a) *c.* 1785. Copyright Mozart-Museum, Salzburg.

88 Titlepage of the six string quartets (K387, 421/417b, 428/421b, 458, 464, 465), dedicated to Haydn, published by Artaria in Vienna, 1785. Copyright the British Library, London.

88 Painting of Mozart's sister, Nannerl. Copyright Mozart-Museum, Salzburg/The Bridgeman Art Library, London.

89 String Quartet, anonymous. Copyright Mozart-Museum, Prague/The Bridgeman Art Library.

91 The seal of the Viennese Lodge, Zur Wohlthatigkeit, 1783, from the Journal für Freimaurer, 1784.

93 Act I, Scene 1, from *The Marriage of Figaro* (K492). Engraving by Carl August Schwerdgeburth, from Orphea Taschenbuch, 1827. Copyright the British Library, London.

94 Playbill advertising a performance of *The Marriage of Figaro* at the Burgtheater, Vienna, 1 May 1786. Copyright Archiv für Kunst und Geschichte, Berlin.

95 Scene from *The Marriage of Figaro.* Engraving by Beguinet. Copyright The Mansell Collection, London.

96 Posthumous oil painting of Mozart, 1819, by Barbara Krafft. Copyright Gesellschaft der Musikfreunde, Vienna/Magnum Photos (Erich Lessing).

98 The Ständetheater, the fruit market, Prague, *c.* 1830 by Vincenz Marstadt. Copyright Archiv für Kunst und Geschichte, Berlin.

99 Half-yearly accounts for the Hoftheater, Vienna (1788–89), showing the payment to Lorenzo da Ponte for work done on Don Giovanni. Copyright Archiv für Kunst und Geschichte, Berlin.

100 Portrait of Lorenzo da Ponte *c.* 1820, by Michele Pekenino from a miniature by Nathaniel Rogers. Copyright Archiv für Kunst und Geschichte, Berlin.

101 Titlepage of Mozart's *Musikalischer Spass (Musical Joke)*, K522, first edition. Copyright British Library, London.

102 Leopold Demuth in the titlerole of *Don Giovanni* for the 1908 Berlin Opera. Copyright Österreichische Nationalbibliothek, Vienna.

103 Finale, Act I of *Don Giovanni* from a performance during the Salzburg Festival 1987, produced by Michael Hampe with costumes designed by Mauro Pagano. Copyright Pagano/Archiv für Kunst und Geschichte, Berlin.

105 Portrait of Michael Kelly engraved by H. Meyer from a drawing by A. Wivell. Copyright Victoria and Albert Museum, Theatre Library.

106 Autograph manuscript of *Don Giovanni.* Copyright Archiv für Kunst und Geschichte, Berlin.

109 St Thomas's Church, Leipzig, 1732, by Johann Gottfried Cruegner. Copyright Archiv für Kunst und Geschichte, Berlin.

111 Baden, from a drawing by Lorenz Jausdur. Copyright Albertina/Österreichische Nationalbibliothek, Vienna.

114 Portrait of Mozart, aged thirty-five. Copyright Mary Evans Picture Library, London.

116 Portrait of Leopold II, by Leopold Kupelweiser. Copyright Archiv für Kunst und Geschichte, Berlin.

118 Portrait of Emanuel Schikaneder, *c.* 1810, by Philipp Richter. Copyright Archiv für Kunst und Geschichte, Berlin.

120 Autograph manuscript of the Lacrimosa, from the *Requiem Mass*, the last music Mozart wrote. Copyright Österreichische Nationalbibliothek, Vienna.

121 Scene from the production of *La Clemenza di Tito* (K621) at the Royal Opera House, 1982. Copyright Clive Barda, London.

122 Engraving from the first edition of the libretto of *The Magic Flute*, 1791, showing an entrance to a temple, by Ignaz Alberti. Copyright the British Library, London

123 Playbill advertising the first performance of *The Magic Flute* at the Freihaus-Theater, Vienna, 30 September 1791. Copyright Archiv für Kunst und Geschichte, Berlin.

124 Coloured etching by Josef and Peter Schaffer of Act II, Scene 3, from *The Magic Flute*, from the first performance on 30 September, 1791, at the Freihaus-Theater in Vienna. Copyright Archiv für Kunst und Geschichte, Berlin.

126 Watercolour of Mozart's house in Vienna, painted by E. Hutter, now no. 8 Rauchensteingasse, Vienna. Copyright Archiv für Kunst und Geschichte, Berlin.

128 Mozart's death mask.

128 Mozart's death certificate.

129 Anonymous portrait of Constanze. Copyright Mozart-Museum, Salzburg/Werner Forman Archive.

130 Film still from *Amadeus*, 1984, directed by Milos Forman, written by Peter Shaffer, with F. Murray Abraham as Antonio Salieri and Tom Hulce as W.A. Mozart. Copyright British Film Institute Stills, Posters and Designs.

133 Endpiece. Statue with cherub. Copyright the Austrian Tourist Board, London.

COLOUR PLATES

1 Residenzplatz, Salzburg by F. Müller. Copyright Museum Carolino Augusteum, Salzburg.

2 The kitchen, Mozart's birthplace, Salzburg. Copyright Werner Forman Archive, London.

3 Mozart's House, Salzburg. Copyright Werner Forman Archive, London.

20 Joseph Haydn. Painting by Johann Zitterer, *c.* 1795. Copyright Historisches Museum der Stadt, Vienna/The Bridgeman Art Library, London.

21 Gluck at the Spinet. Painting by Joseph-Siffrede Duplessis. Copyright The Bridgeman Art Library, London.

22 Meeting of Masonic Lodge in Vienna. Anonymous painting, *c.* 1780. Copyright Historiches Museum der Stadt, Vienna/Archiv für Kunst und Geschichte, Berlin.

23 Joseph II with his brother, Leopold. Painting by Pompeo Batoni, 1769. Copyright Kunsthistoriches Museum, Vienna/Archiv für Kunst und Geschichte, Berlin.

24 Coloured engraving of the Graben in Vienna by Carl Schütz, 1781. Copyright British Library, London.

25 Kurt Moll as Osmin in the Royal Opera production of *The Abduction from the Seraglio*, 1989. Copyright Dominic Photography, London.

26 Anonymous portrait of Antonio Salieri. Copyright Gesellschaft f. Musikfreunde/Archiv für Kunst und Geschichte, Berlin.

27 Costume design for Berlin production of *The Magic Flute*, 1816. Stage design/set by K.F. Schinkel, costume by Heinrich Stürmer. Water colour by Karl Friedrich Thiele. Copyright Archiv für Kunst und Geschichte, Berlin.

28 Photograph of *The Magic Flute*, Act II, a performance from the Salzburg Festival, 1978. Set and costume by Jean-Pierre Ponelle. Copyright D. Anrather (1978)/Archiv für Kunst und Geschichte, Berlin.

29 Stage design for the Queen of the Night from *The Magic Flute*. Set by Simon Quaglio for performance of 27 November 1818 in Munich. Copyright Archiv für Kunst und Geschichte, Berlin.

30 View of Prague, *c.* 1790–93 after a drawing by Leopold Peucker. Copyright Archiv für Kunst und Geschichte, Berlin.

31 Scene from The Royal Opera House 1988 production of *Don Giovanni* featuring Thomas Allen as Don Giovanni and Gwynne Howell as the commendatore. Photo by Richard H. Smith. Copyright Dominic Photography, London.

32 A restrospective painting of Mozart on his death bed listening to his unfinished requiem, by Charles F. Chambers. Copyright The Bridgeman Art Library.

33 Oil painting of Franz Xaver (left) and Karl Thomas Mozart, by Hans Hansen, *c.* 1798. Copyright Mozart-Museum, Salzburg.

INDEX

Figures in italics refer to illustrations